DEATH IN THE FAMILY

DEATH
IN THE
FAMILY

JOHN CHIPMAN

DOUBLEDAY CANADA

Doubleday Canada and colophon are registered trademarks of
Penguin Random House Canada Limited

Library and Archives Canada Cataloguing in Publication

Chipman, John, author
Death in the family / John Chipman.

Issued in print and electronic formats.
ISBN 978-0-385-68084-4 (hardback).—ISBN 978-0-385-68085-1 (epub)

1. Smith, Charles (Charles Randal). 2. Coroners—Ontario.
3. Forensic pathology—Ontario. 4. Death—Causes. 5. Judicial error—
Ontario. 6. Justice, Administration of—Ontario. I. Title.

RA1063.4.C45 2016   614'.109713   C2016-902276-5
                                               C2016-902277-3

Jacket design: Five Seventeen
Jacket images: (x-ray film) Nick Veasey/Getty Images; (x-ray) Image from pp 55 of "Birth
fractures and epiphyseal dislocations" (1917) by Edward Delavan Truesdell/Internet Archive
Printed and bound in the USA

Published in Canada by Doubleday Canada,
a division of Penguin Random House Canada Limited

www.penguinrandomhouse.ca

10 9 8 7 6 5 4 3 2 1

Penguin
Random House
DOUBLEDAY CANADA

For Mom and Dad

CONTENTS

xi   PREFACE

PART 1: THE CHILDREN

3   Kenneth
91   Nicholas I
141   Jenna I
193   Nicholas II
233   Jenna II
277   Athena

PART 2: THE INQUIRY

343   Nicholas
349   Athena
373   Jenna
387   Kenneth

413   EPILOGUE
417   NOTES AND SOURCES
429   INDEX
437   ACKNOWLEDGEMENTS

Expert opinion is never a matter of right and wrong . . .
It just isn't that straightforward.

DR. JAMES YOUNG, FORMER CHIEF CORONER OF ONTARIO

IT WAS OCTOBER 2007, and I was driving home from work. CBC's *World at Six* was on the radio, and one of the top stories was about William Mullins-Johnson, who had spent more than eleven years in prison after being given a life sentence for molesting and murdering his four-year-old niece, Valin. Bill was one of the many victims of disgraced pediatric pathologist Charles Smith, and that cool autumn day he'd been back in court, where a panel of appeal judges had quashed his conviction and acquitted him of a crime that never occurred.

The story of Dr. Charles Smith's incompetence and negligence had been building for almost eight years by then, and while I knew the broad strokes, I had yet to connect with it in a meaningful way. Once the top pediatric forensic pathologist in Ontario and arguably the country, Dr. Smith had used his arrogance and guile in court to mask his incompetence on the job, and at least twenty people were wrongly accused or convicted because of his mistakes. It was a huge story, but the scope of the misery Smith had helped create didn't hit me until I heard that news report about Bill Mullins-Johnson.

Bill Mullins (the name he goes by now) had been living at his brother Paul's home in Sault Ste. Marie, Ontario, at the time of Valin's death. He and his brother were close. Bill was babysitting the three children of Paul and his partner, Kim Lariviere, the night Valin died.

The autopsy was done by a local pathologist, Bhubendra Rasaiah, who determined that Valin had been strangled to death. She had extensive bruising, including marks around her neck. Her anus was enlarged. A local

XII - JOHN CHIPMAN

pediatrician, Patricia Zehr, said the child had been sexually abused—the worst abuse she had ever seen. Dr. Smith consulted on the case from Toronto, co-authoring a supplementary report stating the child was being sodomized at the time of her death.

Initially, Paul didn't believe his brother was capable of something so horrific. He was a caring uncle, and the three children—six-year-old Jean, four-year-old Valin and two-year-old John—adored him. But as the police, Crown and medical experts laid out all their evidence at Bill's trial, Paul's faith started to waver. And when the jury said that word—guilty— Paul's younger brother was dead to him.

But Bill knew that he was not responsible for Valin's death. And he could think of only one other adult male who had been near Valin that night: his brother. Initially, Bill couldn't believe it either; he was sure there must have been some mistake. But as the Crown built its case at trial, as medical expert after medical expert took the stand, his faith also started to waver. And by the time he was convicted, Bill was convinced he'd be doing time for a crime his brother had committed.

A deep, visceral hatred took hold of the two brothers, and it consumed them. Paul sank into drug and alcohol abuse. His relationship with Kim collapsed. She left him, taking their two surviving children with her. Bill continued to maintain his innocence, and the penal system held it against him. His appeal was denied. He considered suicide.

And then, more than ten years into his sentence, Bill received a visit from David Bayliss, a lawyer with the Association in Defence of the Wrongly Convicted (now Innocence Canada). Bayliss told him he was re-investigating the case—he believed Bill was the victim of a miscarriage of justice. And he thought he might be able to prove it.

Convinced he already knew the answer, Bill asked Bayliss who he thought had killed Valin. Bayliss's response could not have been more shocking. He did not think anyone had murdered Bill's niece. He believed she had died of natural causes.

The bruising Dr. Rasaiah had seen during the autopsy was the result of blood pooling after the child's death. The signs of strangulation were caused during the autopsy itself. And indications of sexual abuse were part of the body's natural post-mortem process. The child's anus wasn't enlarged because she'd been sodomized; it enlarged as the muscles around it relaxed after death.

New medical experts found no evidence of foul play.

The Ontario Court of Appeal set aside Bill's first degree murder conviction, and entered an acquittal in its place.

"[The medical evidence] had my brother thinking that I killed his little girl. [And it] had me thinking that he killed his little girl because I knew I didn't kill her," Bill told the court at his appeal hearing in 2007.

The family would never know exactly why or how Valin had died.

The radio report included Bill's statement at his appeal, and it hit me like a bag of bricks. His story was almost biblical: two brothers turned against each other, each convinced the other had committed an unspeakable crime, only to realize years later that the crime had never happened.

Six weeks earlier, late in the summer of 2007, the courts had overturned another miscarriage of justice. It had taken a last-minute reprieve to save fourteen-year-old Steven Truscott from the gallows in 1959, when he was scheduled to hang for the murder of his classmate Lynne Harper. Truscott's death sentence was commuted to life in prison, and he spent a decade behind bars. His case became one of Canada's most famous wrongful convictions, but almost fifty years went by before the Court of Appeal for Ontario finally overturned his conviction. That was big news, but it was the story that followed that stuck with me: the one about Lynne Harper's family, who said they were still convinced Steven Truscott was guilty.

Who could blame them? They'd spent half a century believing one thing. It would be hard for them to concede that all their blame and hatred had been misplaced. But the Harper family could turn away from the truth; they could believe whatever they wanted, and it wouldn't matter. It wasn't like Steven Truscott was a part of their day-to-day lives.

Paul Johnson didn't have that option. Bill was his brother; there would be no turning away from the injustice he'd suffered. The two brothers would have to accept that their family was victimized twice, and it would be up to them to rebuild their shattered relationship.

I was working as a documentary maker with the CBC at the time, and I spent a lot of time with Bill and Paul and their families that fall, researching and reporting their story. The miscarriage of justice and Bill's lost years in prison were easy to appreciate, but the brothers' anguish went deeper. While Bill's wrongful conviction had rightly received most of the media attention, he was far from the only victim. Not only had Paul lost his daughter, but his faith and trust in his younger brother were stolen as well. That decade of hatred created an enormous chasm, but at least Paul had their shared history to help him rebuild their relationship. His children had nothing. Valin's older sister, Jean, grew up believing her uncle Billy was the monster who killed Valin. She could not remember him as anything else. Believing her uncle guilty was essential; it was her only way of making sense of Valin's death. It took her years to even consider another possibility.

Bill's ordeal had begun with his niece's sudden, unexplained death. But like all the cases involving Dr. Smith, that tragedy was only the beginning. Because of the accusations and investigations and trauma that quickly engulfed them, Bill and his family never had a chance to do the most important thing: to grieve Valin's death.

Of course, it took more than a single disgraced pathologist to cause this miscarriage of justice. For years Smith's reputation had shielded him from criticism. But when it finally began to crumble, attention was diverted from everyone else involved in Bill's case. No one other than Smith was ever reprimanded or disciplined. Dr. Rasaiah continued working at the same Sault Ste. Marie hospital. Dr. Zehr continued her practice as a pediatrician.

As I investigated Bill's case, I kept thinking: this is only one story. Dr. Charles Smith and the system that enabled him were responsible for so many more. Whose stories were those?

In June 2005, the Office of the Chief Coroner of Ontario ordered a review of all the criminally suspicious deaths and homicides that Smith helped investigate in the 1990s. In, 1992, he had assumed his position as the inaugural chief pathologist at the newly created Ontario Pediatric Forensic Pathology Unit, at Toronto's Hospital for Sick Children, a position he held until he was suspended a decade later. The review examined forty-five cases; it found problems with twenty. Thirteen of those had involved convictions. Shortly after those findings were announced in April 2007, the Ontario Government called a public inquiry to examine Smith's problematic cases and how systemic failures had contributed to the mistakes he made. (Smith worked as a pediatric pathologist for a decade before taking over the SickKids forensic unit. A subsequent review of that period of his career found another four problematic cases he'd worked on that ended with criminal convictions. Smith didn't respond to my request to speak with him directly for this book.) The Inquiry into Pediatric Forensic Pathology in Ontario is commonly called the Goudge Inquiry, after its chair, Mr. Justice Stephen Goudge.

Twenty cases are too many to examine properly in a single book. Most could carry a book on their own. But they break down into three distinct groups. The first are wrongful accusations: cases in which parents or caregivers were investigated but charges were withdrawn or never laid, or in which the accused was acquitted at trial—cases in which the justice system ostensibly worked. The second are wrongful plea deals, in which suspects—facing murder charges—felt their only option was to plead to a lesser charge even though they had done nothing wrong. And the third are wrongful convictions, like Bill Mullins-Johnson's, in which the accused maintain their innocence and are sentenced to life in prison. In this book I will examine one case from each of these three groups.

I will also investigate a fourth case. As I started researching this book, I wondered if anyone had got away with murder because Smith's involvement—as his career came to a crashing end—ultimately undermined a legitimate prosecution. Were any cases unduly tarnished because Smith had presented evidence? After all, he didn't get all his cases wrong. There *was* one such case, a case in which Smith's personal and professional failings led to the exact thing he was trying so fervently to prevent: the people responsible for a child's death getting away with it.

At least that's what it looked like initially. But after a year of investigating the case, I'm no longer sure. Dr. Smith, along with world-class lawyers and pathologists, may have got that case wrong too. And in a cruel twist, the two parents at the centre of it—parents I initially thought got away with murder—may be the biggest victims of all, forever living under a cloud of suspicion they have no way of legally escaping.

PART I

THE CHILDREN

KENNETH

....

ONE

who? why?

Two words. Two simple, three-letter questions. Yet finding their answers
had been anything but simple for Keith Hutton. Figuring out the truth had
consumed the seventeen-year-old for as long as he could remember.

Keith had always known he was adopted. His parents, Brian and Eileen
Hutton, were open with him and his brother, Eric, about that much. The
boys also knew they were biological brothers; they shared the same
mother. Keith was older by almost two years and more curious, at least
when it came to their adoption.

When he was eight, he'd written a full-page letter to Santa Claus asking
for his birth parents. Brian and Eileen found the letter in Keith's bedroom
before it made it onto the mantel with the milk and cookies. Keith remembers them being upset. Brian and Eileen may not have been the boys' birth
parents, they told him, but they were their parents. They'd raised them,
loved them, provided for them. And they were terrified that would be
forgotten if their birth parents re-entered the picture.

Keith never meant it to be like that. They would always be his parents.
He loved and respected them. He just wanted to know about his other set.

Brian and Eileen had always told Keith he could find out the truth
about his birth parents, but not until he was eighteen. Until then, he
wasn't legally allowed to seek them out. "You may think you're ready,
but you're not yet," his father used to say. "I know you want to know,

but we're following the rules for your own protection. You just have to be patient."

One Saturday in early December 2011, when Keith was eight months shy of his eighteenth birthday, Christmas came early. His father invited him to join him on some errands and perhaps grab some lunch along the way.

First stop was the bank. Keith assumed his father just needed to get some cash, but he walked past the ATM and headed over to the counter. Father and son followed the teller into the back, to a wall of safety deposit boxes. Brian pulled his long, narrow box out of the wall, and the pair was led into a small viewing room. The door clicked as the teller locked them inside.

Keith's father flipped open the box. It was crammed with documents. As Brian lifted a pile out, Keith noticed several coloured pages tucked away underneath. When he asked what they were, Brian said they were just some financial stuff, nothing of importance. But as Keith leaned in for a closer look, he saw stamped across the top page the words "Crown Ward."

While Brian was engrossed in some other documents, Keith slid the stack of papers his father was taking with him onto the smaller stack that included the coloured papers. He could barely contain himself when his father scooped up the entire pile and slipped it under his arm. His answers were coming home.

Keith remembers watching as his father took the papers upstairs and put them away in the desk in his office. After Brian went back downstairs, Keith slipped into the office, shuffled through the papers and pulled out the coloured ones. He hustled into his room, closed the door and hid them away.

Keith knew his father would be leaving soon for the hospital. Eileen had been dealing with some medical issues, and Brian spent as much time as he could with her.

"I'll be back in a couple hours," Brian called up before he stepped out into the frigid December night. Keith didn't answer. He was too over-whelmed with anticipation to speak. As soon as he heard the front door click shut, he pulled the documents out.[1]

As Keith scanned the pages his heart sank. There were no answers in them. They were just information sheets: tips on how to help your children cope with being adopted. He tossed the papers on the bed. He'd been so close. And then a thought hit him. He ran back to his father's desk and grabbed the rest of the paperwork.

Keith had found what he was looking for—his adoption papers.

His mother's name was Tammy Marquardt.

But as he read on, another name kept popping up: Kenneth. Then he saw something that dropped him down into his father's chair.

Brian's phone buzzed in his pocket. He was sitting beside Eileen's hospital bed. Keith's voice was loud enough that Eileen could hear it clearly too. He was demanding to know why he hadn't been told the truth. For a second Brian wasn't sure what his son was asking. Then Keith referred to the papers he had found. He now knew he had an older brother. And he knew his mother had killed him.

Brian and Eileen had been grappling for years with how they would tell the boys the truth about their birth mother. At least what they thought was the truth, what the social workers had told them at the time of the adoptions. But a couple of years earlier, the truth started to shift. And what was always going to be a complicated conversation became even more so.

Keith kept repeating that his mother was a murderer. Brian tried to calm him down, to explain that the situation was more complicated than those old papers revealed.

Tammy Wynne popped her first pill when she was four years old, and she's been struggling to stay clean ever since. She's not sure what that first one was exactly—something meant to calm her down, probably. Or calm down her mother, Margaret; that's whose pill it was, and that's who Tammy says gave it to her. Tammy doesn't remember herself as a particularly troublesome four-year-old, but like most children that age, there were squeals and screams, moments of rambunctiousness and temper tantrums.

"I was just excited to see my mom. I'd been at school all day and I just wanted to hang out and spend time with her," Tammy would recall later.

But some days the girl was too much for Margaret, and Tammy recalls that her mother would give Tammy one of her "nerve pills" and tell her to go play in her room while she went back to her soap operas.

Tammy liked the fuzzy feeling the pills gave her, and she quickly figured out where her mother stashed them. She would climb up onto the bathroom counter to get into the medicine cabinet, careful to line up the arrows on the bottle and lid just so, making sure to put the bottle back with the label positioned just as she had found it.

Margaret Wynne was an alcoholic. At least that's how Tammy remembers things and came to identify her. Booze flowed freely in the house. Young Tammy was happy to play bartender for her mother and her friends. She had her first drink at eleven, a shot of vodka followed by a shot of rye served up by her mother and her boyfriend. When she didn't cough on it, Margaret joked that it couldn't have been her first. There were plenty more shots to follow. She got falling-down drunk for the first time that same year, suffered her first alcohol-induced blackout, and was an alcoholic herself before she was a teenager.

And then there were the constant hospital stays. Tammy said her mother took her to hospital at least once a week for years. Tammy would later learn of a condition that she believes fit her mother's behaviour: Munchausen by proxy syndrome, in which a parent or caregiver fabricates, exaggerates or induces health problems in those under their care, usually to gain attention for themselves. Margaret was never diagnosed with the condition that Tammy knew, but it helped Tammy understand her childhood. Margaret was often convinced Tammy had a fever. Or pneumonia. Tammy rarely felt unwell, but that didn't matter. For years, Tammy pulled the ends of her bedsheets into precision hospital corners because that's where she'd learned to make a bed. "People sometimes like to call the hospital their second home. In my case, our house was my second home. The hospital was my real home."

In a later interview, Margaret Wynne strongly denied Tammy's characterization of her childhood and of Margaret's parenting. "Every word that comes out of that girl's mouth is nothing but B.S. Made-up lies."

Margaret said she was a social drinker, not an alcoholic. She said she never gave Tammy any of her own prescription medications. She said there were no prescription drugs in the house except for asthma medication, which both she and Tammy took. Margaret said she never gave Tammy alcohol. She did take Tammy fairly regularly to the hospital and her family doctor—two or three times a month—but only because Tammy was actually sick or pretending to be so for attention. Margaret said Tammy rarely stayed overnight in hospital.

Tammy's father had been out of the picture since she was small. Tammy got kicked out at sixteen and dropped out of high school the same year. She bounced between shelters and friends' couches, spending the odd night under an overpass as well. It was a tough situation, but no tougher than her life at home. And she'd met a guy.

Tammy's relationship with Rick Marquardt was tumultuous from the start. "Rick was a good guy, but he was a bit of a dog," Tammy explained. He was quick to hook up with someone else—anyone else—during their off-again phases. Tammy suspected he was doing it during their on-again times as well. But she was no angel either, seeing other guys in between her stints with Rick. Still, Rick was a welcome distraction from the dysfunction in the rest of Tammy's life. And then she got pregnant.

Today, Tammy says Rick was the father, but at the time, she told him the baby wasn't his. He was unemployed and drank too much. He already had a son, whom he didn't seem interested in raising. Robert Nelson was the other guy Tammy was seeing at the time. Robert was the better bet; he had a job and money. She told everyone, including Robert, that he was the father.

For the first time in her life, Tammy Wynne admitted she had a problem with alcohol and drugs. She was going to be a mother; she wanted to conquer her addictions. She joined Alcoholics Anonymous. She enrolled at an alternative high school that emphasized hands-on learning for students who struggled in traditional schools.

Kenneth Donald Wynne was born on May 18, 1991. He was a good baby, sleeping through his second night at home, but still Tammy found motherhood exhausting. The feedings, the diapers, the sleep deprivation; it was too much for the nineteen-year-old. By then Robert Nelson was no longer in the picture and she'd moved back in with her mother, but living at home just amplified her stress.

Through the pregnancy and aftercare program she had joined at her high school, Tammy and Kenneth were being monitored by Children's Aid. Tammy called a social worker one night when Kenneth was barely a month old. She could only get him to burp when he was sitting across her leg, his chin resting in the cradle of her hand as she gently patted him on the back. Tammy worried that if she dozed off during a feeding her hand might slip, and if she jerked back awake she might inadvertently choke him.

She needed a break. Children's Aid took him for the weekend.

However, a program worker at Rosalie Hall, a resource centre and home for young single mothers with which Tammy was involved, painted a more troubling picture. Cathy Sorichetti wrote: "On June 21st [1991], Tammy saw Maureen Edwards [from CAS] and asked that Kenneth be taken into care for the weekend. Tammy stated that she had been feeding Kenneth and he started to cry. No matter what she did he wouldn't stop. She said she put her hands around his neck and realized that she just had to squeeze for him to be quiet. Tammy was able to tell Maureen Edwards that she needed help because she did not want to hurt the baby."

Three weeks later, Tammy squeezed Kenneth's leg hard enough to leave a bruise. And Sorichetti wrote in her case notes that Tammy pulled her aside after a group support meeting, upset after a recent incident in which she had put her hand over Kenneth's mouth when he would not stop crying. The two women decided to contact Children's Aid, which made arrangements for Kenneth to be placed in a temporary foster home should Tammy need a break.

"Tammy felt good with this arrangement, as it allowed her a way out if it became necessary," Sorichetti wrote. "Although Tammy was stressed, this worker realizes that Tammy appears to be very aware of her limits and capabilities. Tammy is able to ask for help when needed."

In August a little luck fell Tammy's way. She landed a much-sought-after spot in the Massey Centre for Women, a residence in Toronto for vulnerable adolescent mothers that came with around-the-clock support.

Tammy needed it. Kenneth was a sick baby. He had asthma almost from birth. He was too young for a puffer, so Tammy had to use a special nebulizer mask that administered his medication as a mist. Keeping a mask sealed tightly over the face of a squirming, angry infant was no easy task. But the asthma wasn't the worst of his ailments. Kenneth was also prone to seizures. Tammy remembers the first one well. They had just moved to Massey Centre; Kenneth was barely six months old. He was sitting in his playpen when he suddenly slumped over. Tammy watched in horror as her baby's eyes rolled back in his head, the whites all that was visible through his narrowed slits. And then the convulsions started—full-out body-shaking tremors.

"It seemed to go on forever," Tammy said. "I remember thinking, 'Thank God he doesn't have teeth. He would have chewed his tongue off.'"

Tammy immediately took him to the Hospital for Sick Children, where doctors explained that he had suffered a febrile seizure ("febrile" meaning it was brought on by a high fever). Compared with epilepsy, febrile seizures are not dangerous, although in some cases they can evolve into epilepsy. The doctors told Tammy to monitor Kenneth, but said he should outgrow them.

But the seizures didn't stop, and Tammy repeatedly carted her son back to the hospital. Soon, doctors began to suspect that Kenneth was one of those cases in which febrile seizures make the jump to epilepsy. They prescribed phenobarbital, an anticonvulsant.

Tammy Wynne, a single mother with no family support, had an asthmatic newborn with epilepsy. Within months of Kenneth's birth, she was drinking again. Tammy says she managed to stay sober when she was looking after her baby, but anytime she could get a babysitter, it was back to Jack Daniel's.

Tammy's parenting progress reports, at least, were getting more upbeat. In May, after Tammy had moved to Massey Centre, a social worker named Jody McNamara wrote: "Tammy presents as really wanting to be a good parent, but I suspect she is frightened at times of parenting because of her own experiences with her own mother . . . I believe she is making every effort to meet her child's needs . . . I believe this young mother is coping with her new demands to the best of her ability/skills and appears to be meeting her son's basic baby care needs."

A Children's Aid report that month gave a similarly positive assessment: "There are no concerns in regards to Tammy's parenting of Kenneth. He is well taken care of, she attends to him and plays well with him. He is a very happy child and developing very well . . . given the opportunity, Tammy may likely make good choices for herself and Kenneth."

Her choices weren't all good, especially not when it came to men.

Aaron Wallace seemed like a nice guy. He sure worked hard to impress her, always had a nice car to drive—different nice cars, which probably should have been the first clue.

One night, he showed up at Massey Centre in a fancy sports car. They went out for dinner, Kenneth tucked into a car seat in the back. They were having fun, cruising around after dinner, when Tammy saw flashing lights reflected in the windshield. Aaron's eyes darted between the road and the rear-view mirror; his knuckles were paper white on the steering wheel. But instead of pulling over, he flattened the accelerator. When Tammy frantically asked what he was doing, Aaron admitted the car was stolen.

They weren't far from Massey Centre. Aaron raced into the parking lot and slammed on the brakes. He didn't stay long enough to say goodbye, and took off down the street, the police in hot pursuit.

They were both charged with motor vehicle theft, but the charges were dropped against Tammy after Aaron told police that she had no idea the car was stolen.

The second time it happened, Tammy should have known better. It was early 1992, and she was going stir-crazy cooped up in her apartment with Kenneth. Aaron suggested they rent a cottage for a weekend getaway. Tammy was excited until Aaron picked her up in a fire-engine-red Mustang he said his boss had lent him for the weekend. Tammy didn't voice her doubts too loudly. She wanted out of the city, and they weren't going anywhere without a car.

It was late when they finally set out, and Tammy soon fell asleep. But within minutes she was jolted awake when Aaron slammed on the brakes. Seconds later a police car crashed into the back of the Mustang, sending Tammy lurching forward toward the dash, then backward into her seat. As they raced through the darkened streets of one of Toronto's tonier neigh-bourhoods, two police cars close behind, Aaron confessed that he had stolen the car so they could go up north.

The night ended with Aaron smashing into a rock wall that surrounded a regal home. They hadn't even made it out of the city. Tammy remem-bers yelling obscenities at Aaron as he disappeared—again—into the dark-ness, police officers on his heels. Kenneth had a bump on his forehead; Tammy had sprained her ankle.

That's when she called Children's Aid the second time. She knew she wouldn't be able to look after Kenneth while she was on crutches. Aid workers took him for a week.

The second police chase ended things with Aaron. Rick Marquardt started coming around again. She told him that Kenneth was his baby, but then she got kicked out of Massey Centre after she let Rick sleep over. They moved into an apartment together, but broke up again and Tammy soon found herself without a place for her child to sleep.

They stayed at her mother's for a while but Tammy couldn't stomach living at home. She checked in to a shelter but didn't like the structure and rules. She stayed in a friend's basement apartment, but it was cold and musty; the bathroom sink fell off the wall and the place was constantly flooding. Winter was coming, and Tammy worried she would soon be sleeping on the street with an eighteen-month-old. Defeated, she called Children's Aid to tell them they needed to take Kenneth until she could find a place for them to live. Tammy said Children's Aid vacillated. Irate, she called the social worker back. She threatened to hurt Kenneth if Children's Aid didn't take him.

Desperate words born of desperate circumstances had the intended effect. Children's Aid seized Kenneth. The aid worker told Tammy she could have him back when she found a place to live. A week later she landed a spot in subsidized housing, yet it took more than three months to get Kenneth back. She visited him at his foster home almost every day. His health seemed to be improving, although the seizures hadn't completely stopped.

In the meantime, Rick wanted to make things permanent. One late-winter night, he popped the question. They were married on March 11, 1993, at city hall. It was her twenty-first birthday. The ceremony was a no-frills affair. Rick's friend Stewart Powell stood up for them with his girlfriend. They had no money for a honeymoon; all they could muster was a night of drinking at Stewart's girlfriend's apartment.

Kenneth was returned to her a month later, and the three of them settled into their new life together. Marriage vows did little to stabilize things with Rick, however. He was possessive but had a wandering eye. Tammy had a temper that often flared into fits of rage. Both were still drinking heavily. Tammy's apartment was in a sketchy part of town, on Shuter Street, but she was just happy to have a roof over her head. She put Kenneth in daycare and found work painting through a city-run job placement program. Rick was unemployed at the time and had a hard time believing Tammy had found a job so quickly. He accused her of running around on him. One night, she caught him cheating on her, and she attacked him.

Tammy needed some space, so she moved into her sister's place in Oshawa, a largely working-class city east of Toronto. But Rick came crawling back, and she let him in. They moved into a new apartment on Lloyd Street in downtown Oshawa.

Tammy kept telling him to knock it off. It was early September 1993 and Rick was messing around on their back deck. It had been raining and the wood was slick. He would take a couple of steps and slide across the deck, hands swinging, then a couple more steps and back the other way. Kenneth couldn't get enough of his dad's funny moves, and Rick was lapping up the youngster's giggles. Truth be told, Rick was good at becoming a father, not so good at acting like one. He'd shown little interest in Kenneth or his older son. And he had another child on the way, with a different woman. (He'd had a one-night stand eight months earlier, before he and Tammy were married.) Tammy felt it was important that Rick be a father to all his kids, even if they weren't hers. So she smiled at the unusual sight of her husband bonding with their son. And then the toddler started mimicking his father's slides across the porch.

Tammy tried to get Kenneth to stop. The deck was too slippery, and she was afraid he would hurt himself. The boy would stop for a moment, until Rick began sliding again. Rick said he was just about to tell Kenneth they should stop when the child's legs slipped out from under him.

Tammy scooped up her screaming son and squeezed him tight, trying to console him, but that only made him scream louder. When they'd finally settled him down, Tammy propped him up between her legs and tried to get him to walk. The youngster took one step and dropped like a stone. They rushed him to Oshawa General Hospital.

He had a spiral fracture along his femur, or thigh bone, and would spend the next month in traction, leg elevated, at the hospital. Tammy visited him every day but three. When he was discharged, on October 6, the doctor prescribed Children's Tylenol for his continuing pain, but Tammy was wary of giving it to him because of her own experience with drugs as a child. Kenneth was already taking epilepsy medication three times a day to curb his seizures. His doctor had started him on phenobarbital, but it had made him hyperactive, so now he was on Dilantin, which was more appropriate for young children. Still, the seizures had not stopped. Just after his first birthday, in May 1992, Kenneth had one at home; he fell and hit his head on a toolbox. Tammy was in another room when she heard a loud bang. She found her son unconscious, and although she was able to rouse him within a minute, she still called an ambulance. Kenneth was taken to the Hospital for Sick Children. He was examined and then allowed to go home with Tammy. The next day he had another seizure, and she took him back to SickKids.

In July 1993, she had taken him by ambulance to Oshawa General, where Kenneth had a full-body seizure that lasted eight minutes. A brain scan came back normal. The child had had a fever for the previous two days and had vomited earlier that day.

Kenneth also had several electroencephalogram, or EEG, tests done during these hospital visits. Although most forms of epilepsy will cause abnormalities in brain activity only during a seizure, a few kinds cause constant, unusual brain activity, even when the person isn't having a seizure. All of Kenneth's test results came back within the normal range for a child his age.

Marcellina Mian, a pediatrician at SickKids who was also the director of the Suspected Child Abuse and Neglect, or SCAN, program at the hospital, wrote to Kenneth's family physician, Shirley Caspin, in May 1993, detailing Kenneth's history of seizures. Mian said the toddler had suffered seven seizures during his two years of life. She said the first six were febrile seizures. But she wrote that the most recent seizure happened while Kenneth did not have a fever, which suggested it was a more serious grand mal seizure, caused by epilepsy.

In that same letter Mian noted that Tammy was concerned about Kenneth's speech development, feeling that it had started to deteriorate after Christmas. "He used to say bottle but now says 'ba' or 'babas,'" Mian wrote. "He says a few sentences but mostly uses single words."

Both grand mal and multiple febrile seizures have been reported to affect speech development.

Kenneth woke shortly before eight on Saturday morning, October 9, 1993. He'd been home from the hospital for two days. Tammy set him up in his highchair by the table with a bowl of Cheerios. The phone rang a little after eight thirty, and Rick answered. It was Jeanine, the woman now pregnant with Rick's third child. The big moment had arrived—Jeanine was in labour at Scarborough General. Rick soon left for the hospital.

Tammy and Kenneth wasted the rest of the morning in front of the TV until the cartoons gave way to pro wrestling. Tammy was not a fan, and didn't want to give Kenneth the chance to become one. She made him a peanut butter sandwich for lunch. He hadn't been eating well since his hospital stay, and she had to coax him into finishing it.

As usual, Kenneth resisted his nap. Getting him to go down—and stay down—had become a nightmare. He had his own room, but he would wake up three or four times a night, terrified of the shadows lurking on the walls. After a month at the hospital, everything looked foreign and frightening. So she had moved him into the spare bed in their room for the past couple nights, which seemed to help. Tammy offered to read him a book before his sleep.

She expected him to pick *Darkwing Duck* or one of the other Disney books he'd been stuck on recently, but he surprised her: he pointed at the Bible. Tammy was far from religious; a pair of Jehovah's Witnesses had offered her the Bible during a door-to-door visit. Taking a copy seemed like the only way to get them off her front step. Tammy had yet to crack its spine, and it had ended up among Kenneth's children's books, forgotten.

She tried to steer him toward a more conventional choice, but he would not be dissuaded. So Tammy plopped herself down on the couch. "'In the beginning God created the heavens and the earth,'" she began.

Kenneth cut her off. He took the book and started flipping through it. Tammy smiled at the sight of her two-year-old searching through the Bible as if he had any idea what he was looking for. He passed the book back to her, pointing to the page he wanted. He'd stopped at the book of Jeremiah, chapter 3.

Tammy read, "'People ask: "If a man sends his wife away and she leaves him and becomes another man's, should he return to her anymore?" Has that land not been utterly polluted? "You have committed prostitution with many companions, And should you now return to me?" declares Jehovah.'"

Hardly appropriate for a child, Tammy thought. But Kenneth was listening intently.

At one point the boy grabbed the book back. *Good*, Tammy thought, *he's had enough*. But Kenneth started flipping forward through the pages, landing now on Jeremiah, chapter 5. Again Tammy suggested they read one of his favourite children's books instead, but Kenneth was insistent. Tammy hoped this was only a passing fancy. Bible verses at bedtime would take some getting used to.

Tammy continued reading, and was glad when she noticed Kenneth's eyes getting heavy. As she was helping him lie down, he pointed to her stomach. "Brother there," he said.

Tammy had told him she and Rick were trying for another baby, and he was obsessed with becoming a big brother. She tried to explain that there wasn't a baby yet. But Kenneth wouldn't hear it, flashing his two-year-old stubbornness once again.

"Careful. Brother there."

She handed him his bottle. He was out in less than five minutes.

Tammy carried him to the spare bed. She pulled the sheet up over his legs to his waist and arranged his favourite teddy and blanket, the bottle nearby in case he woke up.

She wandered back out to the couch. It was almost one.

Tammy awoke with a start. She had only meant to lie down for a moment, but the clock said it was 4:15. On her way to the bathroom, she stood for a moment outside the bedroom door, listening; not a sound. He must have been tired; they'd slept the entire afternoon.

She slipped into the bathroom.

As she sat down on the toilet, she heard him calling for her. She called back to him that she'd be right there. He called for her again. This time his voice sounded muffled. He liked to play a game in which he held his teddy bear in front of his face, and pretended it could speak. That's what his voice sounded like.

She told him to stay in bed. He was back to crawling since he had broken his leg. The doctor had warned her that it could break again if he wasn't careful.

He kept calling for her, his voice still muffled, but now Tammy thought she heard panic as well.

She reassured him she was coming. Now she definitely heard panic and fear in his voice.

She had put Kenneth down at the top of the bed under a single sheet, but he had turned himself completely around, wiggling down to the bottom. All she could see were his thrashing legs; his upper body and face were buried in the sheet. One arm was twisted behind him, the other up above his head. He was an active sleeper, and sometimes his legs would get tangled up in the sheets. But she'd never seen him get himself turned around like this before. The sheet looked like someone was wringing it, and him, out in the wash.

Tammy yanked at the sheet, but it wouldn't come untangled. It was her damn hospital corners; they had cinched the sheet tight against the mattress and she couldn't get it loose with Kenneth flailing madly. Tammy pulled at the bunched sheet wrapped around his head, but that only made it worse. It was wrapped around his neck; if she pulled it the wrong way, she could end up choking him.

"Mommy!" He sounded scared and wheezy. She considered grabbing a pair of scissors but the sheet was bound so tightly around him that she didn't see how she could cut it loose without snipping him as well.

Tammy tried to get him to stop kicking. She had moved away from his head and was trying to work the sheet free from its open end near his chest and stomach.

And then he stopped kicking.

"Mom." His voice was quieter, with less force, and Tammy suddenly realized that his kicking might not have stopped voluntarily. Another minute, maybe two, passed as Tammy yanked at the sheet, and finally the ends were out from under the blanket. One, two, three; she kept unravelling the sheet until he was finally loose.

"Mommy's got you. It's okay," she said.

But it wasn't. His lips were purple. His face was a whitish grey.

"Wake up, Kenneth. Wake up!" she yelled, seizing him by the hips and shaking him as he lay unresponsive on the bed. When she picked him up, he was limp in her arms.

She sprinted out into the living room and lay him down carefully on the couch as she dialled 911.

"Police, fire, ambulance?"

"Ambulance," Tammy barked into the phone. "Come on, Kenneth. Come on."

"You have to calm down now," the operator said in the split second before the call transferred.

"He's not breathing!"

"Just calm down."

The ambulance dispatcher came on the line. Tammy gave her the address, explained how she'd found Kenneth.

"Okay, is he blue?" the operator asked.

"No, he's white. His lips are pale."

"His lips are pale. Are you sure he's not breathing?"

"I'm sure I don't feel anything! His stomach . . ."

"Okay, listen. Do you want to help him?"

"Yes!" Tammy replied. The dispatcher told her again that she needed to settle down, that the ambulance was on its way.

"Okay, have you ever done artificial respiration?"

"No." Tammy knew how to do CPR. She'd learned when she'd taken swimming lessons growing up, but she'd never had to use any of what she'd learned, not like this, with someone's life hanging in the balance. Her son's life.

"Can you lay him flat? Are you sure he's not breathing?"

"He's just pale."

"Did he have a seizure or anything like that?" the operator asked.

"No. He was just lying down for his nap," Tammy said. She had seen him have a seizure; had watched, horrified and helpless, as his eyes rolled back and his body convulsed. That's not what this looked like to her. He had been calling out, and his legs looked like they were thrashing, not shaking uncontrollably.

"Do you want to try to give him a few puffs of air?" the operator asked.

"How do I do that?" Tammy knew the answer, but it had left her.

"What you have to do is lay him on a flat surface, okay? Are you listening?"

"Yes."

"Okay, tilt his head back, all right, so his jaw is thrust forward." Tammy did as she was told.

"What I want you to do is put your mouth over his mouth."

"Okay."

"But don't breathe hard. You just give him a little bit."

"Okay."

"Just give him little puffs of air, okay?"

"Okay."

"All right, try it."

Tammy bent down over her son's body. She blew one breath, and then froze.

"How do I know what's too much?" she wailed into the phone, suddenly terrified that she'd made matters worse, that she'd blown up his lungs.

"Okay, they're there, the ambulance is there, okay," the operator said. "Just go and open the door and let them know where you are because they're just coming in the side door."

Two paramedics rushed in, firefighters right behind them. The firefighters pushed aside furniture to make room for the paramedics to work. They cut away Kenneth's grey sweatshirt and the T-shirt underneath. They searched for a pulse, but couldn't find one; listened for a heart beat, but couldn't hear one. A paramedic started mouth-to-mouth ventilations. Then he slipped a mask over the little boy's face as he scooped him up in his arms, performing CPR as they ran out to the ambulance. Tammy climbed into the front with the driver.

"Make him breathe!" she yelled over and over as they raced to Oshawa General Hospital.

TWO

RICK MARQUARDT GOT back to the apartment around 4:45 p.m. He hadn't felt welcome at the hospital. Jeanine's new boyfriend was there, and her mother was clearly not happy to see him. Pissed off, he left the hospital before the baby was born.

As he turned the corner onto Lloyd Street, all he could see were police cars: two parked out front, another unmarked vehicle in the driveway. He figured the police must be looking for him, and he wasn't keen to get arrested again. He snuck around the side of the building and knocked on the door of his friend's apartment. But after thirty minutes, the police showed no signs of leaving. He walked toward the front door.

A police officer quickly climbed out of his car to stop Rick from entering his apartment. Rick asked why, waiting for the handcuffs to come out. He was told his home was a crime scene.

The ambulance arrived at the hospital at 4:50. The paramedics were still administering CPR, though Kenneth had no vital signs. His pupils were non-reactive. The cardiac monitor was flat-lining.

Emergency room personnel immediately inserted an endotracheal tube down his throat and began ventilating him with pure oxygen. Doctors gave him multiple doses of adrenalin and atropine in an effort to restart his heart. At 5:01, doctors noted ventricular escape beats, an early sign of heart activity. At 5:03, a normal cardiac rhythm returned, along with a pulse.

Kenneth Wynne was alive, but just barely. He had not been breathing for at least twenty-five minutes.

Sheila Harding was the triage nurse that night. She spoke to Tammy shortly after Kenneth was admitted. She said Tammy was insistent that it took her twenty minutes to untangle Kenneth from the sheet. "She

said that each time she would untie one end, she would just find another
end," Harding said in her statement to police. "I repeatedly questioned
the 20 minutes it took her to untangle him, saying that it sometimes feels
like a long time in a situation like that, but she was positive that it was
20 minutes . . . She then said that she took the sheet off of his head and he
went limp like a newborn baby. He had stopped breathing, and she forgot
how to do CPR on a baby."

At the hospital, police interviewed Tammy four times. Each time, she
told them what had happened at the apartment; each time, her story was the
same. She was emotional at times, breaking down as one would expect
under the circumstances. But by the fourth time, she had had enough with
the constant questions. Tammy just wanted to see her son. She'd been at the
hospital for almost ninety minutes and still hadn't been allowed to see him.

At 6:21, Tammy walked into the resuscitation room with the hospital
chaplain. Kenneth looked tiny on the bed, his eyes closed, his body covered in tubes.

"Mommy's here," she said quietly, taking his tiny hand in hers. "You've
got to keep fighting, honey. Oh, Kenneth, I love you, please come back to
Mommy. You can do it. You're a fighter, Kenneth."

The chaplain listened quietly, along with Kathy Haley, an ER nurse.
Tammy's older sister, Carol, soon arrived at the hospital with her common-
law husband. The couple told the nurse about an incident when Kenneth
was a year old and someone had hit him hard enough to leave a handprint
and a ring impression on his face. Tammy claimed it was their mother
who'd hit him and had her charged for it. But Carol told Harding she was
never convinced their mother was responsible. At the time, she told one
of Kenneth's doctors that they were concerned his parents might be abusing him. They also accused Rick of being involved in three police chases
when Kenneth was in the car (getting both the driver and the number of
chases wrong).

Carol said Tammy had always had a quick temper and Rick's was violent. She told the nurse her sister had asked her to look after Kenneth
because she was scared Rick might go overboard with him if he was bad.

Harding said she would pass on their concerns to the doctor treating Kenneth.

After Kenneth stabilized, doctors told Tammy they were transferring him to the Hospital for Sick Children, in Toronto. She nodded. Her baby was alive. She asked if she could ride down in the ambulance.

Before the doctor could answer, a police officer who was hovering nearby said, "We can drive you down."

Tammy watched from the back of the cruiser as the ambulance pulled out in front of them. It looked so ordinary: No flashing lights. No blaring siren.

And then the cruiser made a sharp right into the parking lot of 17 Division of the Durham Regional Police.

"What are we doing?" Tammy asked. The ambulance continued south, lost in the rushing traffic.

"We've got some questions we'd like to ask you," one of the officers in the front said, without looking back.

Tammy's only thought was to get the interview over with. She needed to get to the hospital.

Staff Sgt. Sal Naccarato, one of the officers who'd driven her to the station, pointed to a chair on the other side of the table. The other officer, Det. Const. Rolf Kleum, hovered nearby.

Tammy again went over what had happened at the apartment earlier that day—putting Kenneth down for a nap, then falling asleep herself; hearing his first muffled calls from the bathroom, then finding him tangled up in the bedsheet. Tammy could feel herself getting more and more frustrated. She'd already answered the same questions four times at the hospital.

Rick was waiting in the hallway when the detectives finally let Tammy go. He was slumped forward in his chair, his hands nervously stroking the brim of his ever-present baseball cap. He had arrived a little earlier to give a statement himself.

He wrapped his arms around her as he asked what had happened. Tammy had been asked that question over and over again, but hearing it from him was too much. She could barely get the words out as her body convulsed with sobs. "Calling my name . . . all twisted up in the sheets . . . couldn't save him."

Rick nodded. "Don't worry. He'll be okay."

It was getting late, and Rick was worried there were no more buses to Toronto. They needed a ride down to SickKids. He asked an officer for a lift, and after some loud and forceful complaints, the officer agreed. Tammy continued to alternate between lucidity and hysteria during the ride to the city. Occasionally Rick would catch one of the officers eying them in the rear-view mirror and he'd gently nudge her to stop talking. If Tammy hadn't clued in to the police's suspicions yet, Rick had. She was barely coherent, but Rick was still worried that she might say something incriminating. He didn't believe she'd intentionally done anything to hurt Kenneth, but he didn't want to give the police any ammunition.

Kenneth looked peaceful, lying motionless, his eyes closed. The baseball game was on a nearby TV. Kenneth was a fan. He'd picked it up from Rick, a Blue Jays fanatic. Tammy liked watching the games as well. It was hard not to be a baseball fan in Toronto at the time; the Jays were the defending World Champions, selling out night after night. Sitting there in the ward, beside her comatose son, Tammy realized that many of her favourite memories involved the three of them watching games at home, yelling in agony or jubilation, depending on the score.

It was Game 4 of the American League Championship, the Jays at home against the Chicago White Sox. More than 51,000 people were crammed into the SkyDome only blocks away from the hospital. The Jays had taken a commanding lead in the series, winning the first two games on the road. But then they came home for Game 3 and got thumped 6–1.

It was after nine by the time Tammy pulled up a chair next to Kenneth's bed, and the Jays were down 5–3 heading into the bottom of the sixth inning. "Don't worry, Kenneth, we got this!" Tammy said excitedly to her comatose toddler. "We're coming around to the top of the order."

Pat Borders lined out to second base; one down. But lead-off man Rickey Henderson reached first on a walk, then went to second on a wild pitch. Devon White grounded out to the pitcher, but Henderson took third. Two down.

"Here we go, Kenneth, tying run is at the plate! Come on, Robbie!"

"You know he's in a coma. He can't hear you," the nurse said quietly. Tammy hadn't even noticed her come over.

"He can hear me," she said to the woman, staring at her until she looked away.

All-star Robbie Alomar worked the count to 2–2, then doubled into right field, scoring Henderson. "What did I tell you?" Tammy said. "You can always count on Robbie to come through in the clutch. Almost there, Kenneth. Here comes Joe Carter."

Carter took a ball, then fouled one off. Tammy gripped Kenneth's tiny hand in hers. Carter singled into the gap between third base and the shortstop. Alomar rounded third, heading for home. White Sox left fielder Tim Raines scooped up the ball. Alomar barrelled toward catcher Ron Karkovice as Raines's throw rocketed toward home.

"No!" Tammy cried as the umpire punched the air, calling out Alomar at home.

The White Sox scored two more runs, beating the Jays 7–4. Tammy looked over at Kenneth, his eyes still closed, his body motionless.

Det. Sgts. Paul Carroll and Sal Naccarato headed back to Oshawa General. They were curious about Kenneth's femur injury. They thought it could be indicative of abuse. The child had only been discharged from the hospital three days earlier.

Tammy hadn't informed Children's Aid about the injury. Kenneth's case worker only learned of it a week after the fact, when she showed up at the apartment for a visit. But the orthopedic surgeon who treated the toddler told Children's Aid that the injury was not necessarily the result of abuse; the injury could have happened under the circumstances Tammy described.

The detectives, however, heard divergent versions of those circumstances. They spoke with four nurses at Oshawa General, and each one remembered a different version of how the injury happened. Sheila Harding, the triage nurse, told the officers that Rick had said Kenneth was running and playing in the park at the time. "He said when Kenneth got to the crest of a hill, he slipped and fell. I remember thinking that was odd at the time because it had been raining. Why would a child that age be out playing in the rain?"

The other nurses' stories deviated only slightly. Ann Sanders, an ER nurse, said Tammy told her that Kenneth was running on a slippery floor or a hardwood floor and fell. According to Judy Brody, an admissions nurse, the child was playing outside when it happened, but she recalled Tammy telling her the accident occurred on the front porch, not the back deck. "She said he was sliding around on the wet floor when he did the splits. It was odd the way she described it. She said he was 'doing his James Brown act.'"

Dale Lewis, a pediatric nurse, relayed yet another version. "This was a couple days after the child was admitted," she told the officers. "I was in his room, and Tammy was sitting with him. He was such a beautiful-looking boy. He really was, and I remember I told her that. She smiled, said thanks. And then I asked how he broke his leg. She told me that she was washing the floor at the time and Kenneth was running around."

"Did she say how he fell?" Detective Carroll asked.

"I can't quite remember what she said, but I think it was that he just slipped, or maybe he tripped, like he stepped on a toy or something. But I do remember she went quiet after that. I asked her how he fell, like one leg went one way and the other went the other? And she looked at me, and just nodded yes."

A police synopsis lays out the nurses' stories, but it doesn't say whether the detectives had doubts about the explanations. Doctors at the Hospital for Sick Children, however, were suspicious about Kenneth's life-threatening injuries from the moment he was wheeled in. Dr. Sam Shemie, a physician in the intensive care unit, had primary responsibility for Kenneth's care.

"Unclear history," Shemie wrote in his progress notes. "[questions of previous investigation for child abuse, recent hospitalization for lower limb fracture, unsubstantiated allegations and blame from various family members.] General suspicion of non-accidental injury . . . will involve SCAN team . . . will need to decipher history from parents."

Shemie contacted Dr. Dirk Huyer, from the Suspected Child Abuse and Neglect team, along with Alex Nevin, an ophthalmologist, and William Logan, a neurologist, for help. Once briefed, Huyer agreed that there was reason to be concerned.

Nevin examined Kenneth's eyes for signs of abuse. His notes mirror his colleagues' suspicions, even though his findings came back clean. "Normal eyes," he wrote. "Does not R/O [rule out] suffocation or non-accidental injury."

Huyer met with Tammy to get a detailed medical history for Kenneth, and to hear firsthand what had happened. He also met separately with other family members and took careful notes.

Tammy's mother, Margaret, said she didn't trust Rick. She mentioned Kenneth's fractured femur, saying too many things were happening to the child in a short period of time. Her sister Carol said that wasn't the child's only injury; she recalled seeing a bruise on his face. The family laid out more concerns for Huyer: the child had been placed in foster care several times. Margaret said Tammy's apartment was rundown and disgusting; it was no place to raise a child. She added Rick once joked that Kenneth was going to go out as an abused child for Halloween. Carol said Rick pushed Tammy down a set of stairs. She came to live with Carol for a while after that.

"Rick is bad news," Carol said. "He'll stop at nothing to get her."

"If his stepfather did this to him, I don't know what I'll do," Margaret said. "There is something going on here. Too many things happen to the child; he shouldn't be this sick. It's probably his stepfather. He's a wife beater."

Tammy's family weren't the only people suspicious about Kenneth's parents. Silvana Maclellan, a child protection officer with Durham Children's Aid, noted that through the three days Kenneth was on life support at SickKids, Tammy appeared "upset, but in an inappropriate manner—is not reacting as staff would expect. She is saying she will kill herself if Kenneth dies."

Notes taken by hospital staff several times describe Tammy at Kenneth's bedside. Once, when she was with her sister, it was noted they were both emotional and crying. Another time, when Tammy was with Rick, they appeared to be "happy and talking."

The hours ticked by. Kenneth's condition was not improving. Doctors told Tammy his brain was swelling and there was little they could do to stop it.

Early on the morning of October 11, thirty-six hours after he was admitted, Kenneth's condition deteriorated dramatically as the brain swelling worsened. Later that day, Dr. Shemie told Tammy and Rick their son was clinically brain dead. It wasn't until Tammy heard the words that the truth finally hit home: her son wasn't going to wake up. Kenneth was gone. Child protection officer Silvana Maclellan noted that when Kenneth was removed from life support, Tammy showed "appropriate emotion for the first time in 3 days." Maclellan said authorities would "need evidence to prove this was dirty."

"I'm sorry, but I have to ask you this now," Shemie said. "Would you like to donate his organs? They could help save another child's life."

Tammy and Rick agreed to the organ donation.

She was sitting by his bed the next day, staring out the window at the whirring blades of a yellow emergency helicopter approaching the hospital. Was it coming to take Kenneth's organs away, she wondered, or bringing a child who needed them?

THREE

THE FUNERAL WAS held three days later in Scarborough. Tammy's mother made all the arrangements. Tammy pinned Kenneth's earring to his suit jacket. Rick dressed him in his favourite baseball cap and Air Jordan high-tops. Carol adjusted his cap at one point, revealing the sutures on his skull where he'd been sewn back up after the autopsy. Rick's ex-girlfriend Jeanine was there. Tammy congratulated her on her newborn.

Tammy was the only one who spoke at the funeral. She didn't prepare a speech, deciding to speak from the heart. She doesn't recall what she said, the words immediately lost in a haze of grief. Kenneth Wynne was buried at Pine Hills Cemetery. It was the first time Tammy had ridden in a limousine.

Mourners descended on the Scarborough Moose Lodge for refreshments afterwards.

"You're going to have to get over it," Tammy's aunt Kathy said to her over tea. "He's gone now. He's dead."

Tammy lost it, finally. She screamed every curse word she knew at her aunt, and then she ran from the hall.

Tammy opened her eyes. She was back in Pinehill Cemetery, standing over Kenneth's fresh grave.

Rick found her there hours later, still sobbing.

It was supposed to be a distraction, something to help them push off their grief. Game 4 of the World Series: the Blue Jays versus the Philadelphia Phillies. The Jays were up 2–1 in the series, looking to take a stranglehold.

Tammy and Rick had gone to a Scottish pub in Scarborough with Rick's friend Stewart and his girlfriend, Stacey Craig, to have fun and forget. But Tammy couldn't focus on the game. They'd buried Kenneth five days earlier. The cemetery was just around the corner.

Rick had been bugging Tammy all night to talk to the waitress; she'd lost a child of her own, and he hoped talking to someone who'd been through it might help. But Tammy was in no mood to talk. She just wanted to drink.

When Tammy went to the washroom, Rick waved over the waitress. "Could you go talk to her?" he asked.

The waitress found Tammy in an otherwise empty washroom. She asked Tammy how she was doing. Hesitantly, she told Tammy she knew what she was going through if she ever wanted to talk. Tammy's anger and grief erupted in a steady stream of vitriol and expletives. She rushed past the waitress, scared of what she might do to her if she stayed a moment longer.

What happened next is unclear. Rick remembers the waitress telling him Tammy had lost it and had taken off. They searched everywhere but couldn't find her, and then Rick thought to check the cemetery. It was less than a twenty-minute walk away. He says they found her in a parking lot across the street.

Tammy, though, remembers Rick finding her behind the bar, raving.

"I killed him!" she recalls screaming. "I killed my little baby!"

Stewart brought the car around, and they piled her inside. They drove to the cemetery where Kenneth was buried, parking across the street.

Tammy tried to bolt across the road. Stewart grabbed her, pulling her out of the rushing traffic. She turned to him, her eyes wild.

"It's my fault!" she screamed, pinning him against the car. "I killed my baby!"

Rick, fed up with her antics, disappeared. Stewart let Tammy go. Once free, she bolted through the traffic, screeching and sobbing. She made it across the road, but tripped on the sidewalk and fell to the ground in a heap.

She lay on her back, chastising herself for forgetting how to do CPR, screaming that she'd killed her child. Each time she accused herself, she slammed her head against the pavement. Blood started to colour the sidewalk.

Rick didn't hear the first knocks. It was late, and he was half-asleep.

Stewart was at the door. He told Rick that Tammy was in the psychiatric ward at Scarborough General. Police had picked her up on a "Form 1," which allowed her to be held involuntarily for up to seventy-two hours so doctors could complete a psychiatric assessment. Stewart drove him to the hospital, and Rick found her in the psych ward. Her room wasn't locked.

Rick took her by the arm, trying to get her to leave, but was stopped by a nurse.

Rick Marquardt is not a big man, but when he gets angry, that doesn't matter. He insisted that he was taking his wife home.

Doctors tried to dissuade him. They told him she was a danger to herself. They called security. None of it mattered. Rick was leaving with his wife. Security let them go, perhaps deciding to avoid a brawl in the hallway.

Whether it was from the stress and the grief or the medication they'd given her or all the booze she'd had the night before, as soon as she was back at the apartment, Tammy collapsed in bed.

She woke up to a loud, head-pounding argument. She stepped out into the living room to find two police officers standing in the doorway, with two paramedics behind them. Stewart Powell was there with Rick as well.

"Are you Tammy Marquardt?" one of the officers asked.

Rick yelled at her not to answer.

"Mrs. Marquardt, you have to come with us," the officer said as he and his partner moved toward her. Scarborough General had called police after Tammy had left.

"Like hell I do!" Tammy yelled.

Rick pushed the officer back out the door, where he lost his balance and fell down the stairs. Backup was called. Rick said he fought off four officers on his own until one of them knocked him out with a baton.

Tammy fell down the stairs herself as police officers dragged her out. Paramedics strapped her to a stretcher, stomach down. In the ambulance they gave her a shot of something, but if it was a sedative it didn't work, because she was still ranting when they arrived at Oshawa General Hospital. In the psychiatric ward, she was put in a straitjacket and strapped to the bed.

It was a small room with a large window at one end, two concrete walls, and another made of glass so hospital staff could keep the patients under twenty-four-hour surveillance. She was released after seventy-two hours. As she and Rick left the building, Tammy was surprised to find herself feeling good. She'd hit rock bottom, but she'd made it through. The toughest part was behind her, she thought. Better days were coming.

The knock at the door was firm and forceful. Tammy recognized two of the three officers, Carroll and Naccarato, from the night Kenneth died. Standing in her apartment now, they told her they wanted her to undergo a lie detector test. If she was telling them the truth, they said, she would have nothing to worry about. Tammy wasn't sure, but Rick told her to take the test. He said she had nothing to hide. They took her back to the station. The third officer, Det. Pat Sayer, administered the test.

Sayer connected electrodes to two of Tammy's fingers, then ran two thin straps around her chest and a blood-pressure cuff around her arm. The two other detectives left the room.

It wasn't until she was seated in that chair, strapped to a polygraph machine, that Tammy fully appreciated what was happening: police suspected foul play in Kenneth's death, and she was the only suspect. If that realization was terrifying, it was about to get worse.

After some baseline tests, Sayer began asking Tammy questions. Some were benign, banal even, but he kept circling back to the same question, the wording shifting slightly, but the meaning always the same. "Did you hurt Kenneth?" "Did you suffocate Kenneth?" "Did you do anything to cause his death?"

After the other detectives were led back in, Sayer announced that Tammy had failed the test. Based on the results, he couldn't say what had happened to Kenneth, whether Tammy had lost control or if Kenneth's death had been planned, but he could say that Tammy was deceptive in her answers.

The polygraph test was just the beginning; Detectives Carroll and Naccarato repeatedly showed up at the apartment over the next month. Sometimes they questioned Tammy there; sometimes they took her down to the station for a formal interview. The focus was always the same: tell us what happened. So Tammy told her story again and again.

The officers would listen intently, probing for inconsistencies, and then accuse her of killing Kenneth. Maybe it was an accident, one of them would say. You didn't mean it to happen. You were tired, he wouldn't sleep and before you knew it he wasn't breathing.

But no matter how hard they pushed, Tammy's story never changed: she had done nothing to hurt her child.

Dr. Dirk Huyer, of SickKids' Suspected Child Abuse and Neglect team, completed his report in November. He said he did not believe Tammy's story.

The clinical picture showed Kenneth had an ischemic/anoxic brain injury, caused by a lack of oxygenated blood reaching the brain. The child suffocated to death. The question was how. "The history that was provided by Tammy is inconsistent with Kenneth's serious clinical condition and ultimate death," Huyer wrote. "Sheets are porous and will allow air transfer through the material. It is very difficult to imagine a 2 year 4 month old baby becoming so trapped so seriously in a sheet independently such that 20 minutes were required to remove the sheet." The doctor also noted that Tammy never explained exactly how Kenneth's windpipe was blocked. "If the sheet was occluding the child's airway then he would have become unconscious and limp easily allowing quick removal of the sheet from his body." Tammy should have been able to get the sheet off the child quickly once he passed out, long before the oxygen depletion became life threatening. "At least 3–4 minutes usually pass before airway occlusion leads to loss of vital signs, ie., respiration and heart beat. This is a significant time period."

Huyer wrote that if the sheet had somehow choked Kenneth to death, there would have been marks on his neck, but there were no such signs on the body. The toxicology tests came back negative for anything unexpected. Huyer noted Kenneth's history of seizures but didn't think they were a factor in his death. He pointed to a laundry list of non-medical factors supporting an intentional injury: the child was under a continued supervision order maintained by Children's Aid; he had suffered previously unexplained facial bruising, along with a recent femur fracture; Tammy had a history of poor anger management; Kenneth was previously placed in foster care because of his mother's admitted inability to care for him, including her having involved him in a car chase; and multiple witnesses had thought Tammy's behaviour and apparent lack of grief during Kenneth's end stages in ICU at the Hospital for Sick Children didn't appear appropriate.

"Kenneth Wynne most likely suffered an asphyxia death which is without adequate explanation. Non-accidental asphyxiation is therefore a likely explanation," Huyer wrote. "Suffocation is one of the forms of non-accidental asphyxiation."

The doctor said the evidence suggested Tammy had suffocated her child to death, most likely with a pillow or piece of rolled-up clothing.

His report was addressed to a detective with the Durham Regional Police.

The knock came early. Tammy and Rick were still in bed. It was November 23, seven weeks after Kenneth's death. Tammy threw on a T-shirt and jeans and opened the door to Detective Sergeants Carroll and Naccarato.

They told her they were arresting her for second-degree murder. The detectives told her she had the right to legal advice.

Tammy didn't have a lawyer. She'd never thought to contact one. Rick said he would call his.

Naccarato signalled for her to turn around. He clicked on his handcuffs.

Tammy could no longer speak, she was crying so hard. The same thought kept running through her head: *I deserve this. I could have saved him. I knew CPR but I forgot how to do it. I'm getting what I deserve.*

The detectives took Tammy to Whitby Jail for processing. They ran her through a battery of tests—a full physical, blood test, urine test—then took her into an interview room. Carroll sat down across from her. Naccarato lingered behind his shoulder.

"We know you did it," Carroll told her, according to police notes. "The medical reports show that Ken didn't die because of being wrapped up in some bedsheets."

"Kenneth," Tammy said.

"Excuse me?"

"You said Ken. His name was Kenneth. He hated when people called him Ken."

"Okay. Kenneth. He didn't suffocate in some sheets. The medical experts know that, so you might as well tell us what really happened. I think you need some help. Would you like us to get your psychiatrist?"

Tammy didn't say anything.

"We've seen your [CAS] file," Carroll said. "We know about your anger issues, how you've lashed out at Kenneth in the past. Not necessarily physical abuse but verbal abuse. You know you've had a problem in the past."

"Yeah, and what did I do?"

"You asked for help. But this time you were too late. Kenneth was already dead when you called 911."

"Would you prefer to wait for your lawyer to get here?" Carroll asked.

"Yeah, I think I'd like to speak with a lawyer."

The two detectives got up to leave the room. They said they would wait until her lawyer arrived, but told her to knock on the door if she needed to go to the bathroom.

The detectives checked in on her over lunch.

"Your lawyer hasn't arrived yet," Carroll told her. "Do you still want to wait for him?"

"Do you have a gun?" Tammy asked him.

"Why do you want a gun?" he asked.

"Because if I had a gun I could kill myself. I want to die."

"I think you should come with us," Carroll said. They took her into another interview room, one that had a window onto the hall. The officers wanted to make sure she didn't try to hurt herself.

At the end of the day, Tammy was taken down to the segregation cells, two on the right, two on the left. Other inmates screeched at her as an officer led her into her cell. It was maybe eight feet by six feet, to Tammy's eyes. She could have reached from one wall to the other if she wasn't so tiny herself.

A thick slab of concrete protruded from one wall, a scrawny mattress on top. On another wall was a metal toilet attached to a metal sink. The door was solid metal, the only opening a small window with an even smaller flap underneath through which guards could slide her food. The door clanged loudly behind her as the guard slammed it shut, draining the light from the room.

Tammy didn't stay in Whitby for long. At her first bail hearing, the judge, in light of her past hospitalizations, ordered a psychiatric assessment. She was transferred to the Queen Street Mental Health Centre, in Toronto. It was much nicer than the Whitby jail. The women's wing was tucked away behind the nurses' station, but the common areas were co-ed. Tammy had her own room, and it actually felt like a room, with a desk, a chair and a proper bed. She was allowed to wear her own clothes.

But shortly after she arrived, two police officers came to her room to round her up. They told her they were taking her to St. Michael's Hospital. They shackled her hands and feet and drove her downtown. Tammy could feel people's eyes on her as the officer guided her out of the cruiser. With her legs shackled, she had to shuffle her feet as she was led inside. The officers took her into an office. A male nurse was waiting inside.

"Tammy Marquardt?"

Tammy nodded.

"Did you know you are pregnant?"

There must have been a mistake—Tammy had just had her period. But blood tests taken on her admittance to jail showed otherwise. Tammy's shackles were removed and she climbed up on the examination table, noticing the ultrasound machine for the first time. The nurse squirted a clear fluid onto the end of the wand.

A distinct thumpthumpthumpthump filled the room. Tammy recognized the sound. It was what Kenneth's heartbeat had sounded like at his first ultrasound.

"*Careful. Brother there.*" That's what Kenneth had said.

Tammy stayed on the inmate wing at Queen Street for almost three months. It was for the best. Booze and drugs were harder to come by on the inside (although not impossible) and, being pregnant, she had to look after herself.

Christmas came and went. As an accused child killer, Tammy was at the very bottom of the inmate hierarchy, even in the mental hospital. She did her best to avoid people and to stay out of trouble. She didn't get many visitors. Rick came to see her, regularly at first, but as the weeks turned to months his visits became more sporadic. She was finally released on bail on Valentine's Day, 1994. Her pre-trial psychiatric assessment found her fit for trial and stated that she was not certifiable on psychological grounds.

Forensic psychiatrist Mark Ben-Aron wrote in a letter to the court, "It is our opinion that if she is ultimately found by the court to be the perpetrator of the alleged offence, her mental state at that time was such that she would have been able to appreciate the nature, quality and consequences of her actions." From a psychiatric perspective, her assessors felt "the defence of not criminally responsible on account of mental disorder would not be available."

However, Dr. Ben-Aron did find that Tammy had severe "personality difficulties." He diagnosed her with paranoid personality disorder, with features of several other disorders, including borderline personality. Her mental health issues were not severe enough, however, to keep her institutionalized and not serious enough to account for her behaviour if she were found guilty of murdering her son.

After Tammy was freed on bail, she moved into Rosalie Hall, a resource centre and home for young single mothers. She had to report to the Toronto Bail Program three times a week and participate in drug and alcohol counselling. She would continue seeing Ben-Aron, her psychiatrist at Queen Street Mental Health Centre. When she arrived at Rosalie Hall, Tammy was more than four months pregnant and starting to show. The baby was due in August. It was a strange feeling: she'd barely processed Kenneth's death and now she was pregnant again. It was hard not to feel guilty about having another child so soon.

Another of her conditions was that she was not allowed to have any contact with Rick without permission. She'd never felt more alone in her life: mourning her son, separated from her husband, pregnant and awaiting her murder trial.

Tammy's case was crawling its way through the court system. She had two lawyers now. Steven Clark had represented Rick a couple of times on break-and-enter charges. This would be his first murder case, so he recruited a colleague, Edward Kelly, who had some experience with murder trials. They would pick Tammy up at Rosalie Hall and drive her out to Whitby for her court appearances. They walked her through the process, through the medical evidence and the Crown's case against her.

Tammy didn't understand most of what they told her. This was her first experience with the criminal justice system. She'd dealt with lawyers before, but only in Family Court. All she knew was she'd done nothing wrong. That's what she kept telling her lawyers, over and over: "I didn't do anything to hurt Kenneth. I didn't." They nodded, tried to reassure her. Tammy thought they were competent. Rick trusted Steven Clark, Steven Clark trusted Edward Kelly, so Tammy trusted them both.

Her uncle offered to retain a higher-profile lawyer. He said he could set up a meeting with Edward Greenspan, one of the best-known criminal defence lawyers in the country. Tammy told him not to worry.

"I'm in good hands."

On August 17, 1994, Keith Marquardt was born. Rick picked Zeus for a middle name; Tammy chose Vincent, a name she'd always liked. For the first hour, she was allowed to hold her new son and breastfeed him, and she did her best to bond with him as quickly as she could. Then he was moved into the nursery at the hospital. Tammy was allowed to visit him there only to breastfeed.

They stayed in the hospital for two or three days. Tammy was desperate for Keith to live with her at Rosalie Hall. The centre was just starting a pilot project to keep new mothers and their babies together for six months. But Children's Aid balked. Tammy was an accused child killer. They couldn't trust her with Keith, even with constant supervision.

Tammy was allowed to see Keith once a week, at the local Children's Aid office. She expressed her milk throughout the week and took it with her. She'd feed him right there in the office, her cooler of milk by the chair, the social worker hovering nearby.

—

Tammy's preliminary hearing was held over three days in late September 1994. Her lawyers told her not to invest too much in it. The purpose of a preliminary is to determine whether the Crown has sufficient evidence to warrant a trial. At this stage, the system is stacked in favour of the prosecution, but the prelim would be a good opportunity for Tammy's lawyers to hear the Crown's evidence against her.

Roughly eighty thousand people die in Ontario each year. Most are natural deaths. But any death that is sudden or unexpected, or may have involved violence, negligence or misconduct, is investigated by a coroner. Ontario coroners conduct about twenty thousand death investigations annually.

The purpose of the investigation is to answer several key questions: Who was the deceased? When, where and how did they die, and by what means? Deaths are divided into five categories, or manners of death: natural, accidental, suicide, homicide or undetermined. Homicides are the least common, making up about 1 per cent of cases. Pediatric homicides are even less common, well below 0.1 per cent of all deaths.

In the more complicated death investigations, coroners—who in Ontario are required to be doctors—rely on police and other professionals to help. Forensic pathologists conduct autopsies. And although coroners are doctors, they do not have the expertise to judge a pathologist's findings. Neither do police. Or Crown attorneys. Unless there is a compelling reason to seek a second opinion, a pathologist's findings are usually taken at face value.

Ten witnesses testified at Tammy's preliminary hearing. Chief among them was Dr. Charles Smith. Sitting in the courtroom in Oshawa, Tammy finally saw the man who had convinced police that she had killed her son.

Smith was the second witness to testify. He was thin and bookish and came across as reasoned and reasonable. The pathologist walked the court through his autopsy of Kenneth and his findings.

Smith conducted the autopsy on October 13, 1993, the day after Kenneth was removed from life support. The child's heart valves, kidneys and liver had already been removed for donation. Smith had not attended that procedure, but he had told the harvesting doctors that removing the organs would not affect his autopsy findings.

Detective Sergeants Carroll and Naccarato attended the autopsy, along with a police photographer. Smith prepared two reports after his autopsy— an autopsy report for internal use at the hospital and a post-mortem report that would be distributed more widely, to the coroner and the police investigating the child's death. Smith wrote "asphyxia" as the cause of death.

Asphyxia doesn't necessarily point to foul play; a number of natural processes can result in a body being deprived of oxygen and suffocating. In his autopsy reports, Smith did not say what he thought caused Kenneth to asphyxiate. Instead, he listed the findings that indicated asphyxia as the cause of death: petechial hemorrhages—or tiny reddish-purple blood spots resulting from burst vessels—he found on Kenneth's thymus gland, pulmonary pleura (the thin membrane around the lungs) and epicardium (part of the outer wall of the heart).

Smith also detailed the state of Kenneth's body after he was resuscitated, noting signs of hypoxic ischemic encephalopathy, a type of brain damage that occurs when a child's brain doesn't receive enough oxygen and blood. He noted signs of acute bronchopneumonia, or inflammation of the lungs. And he noted that the child had a healing fracture on his right femur.

But all these findings are non-specific: they could have natural or non-natural causes; they could occur by accident or by homicide. The cause of death should therefore have been listed as "undetermined."

In a "Short History" of the case in his internal hospital report, Smith included some troubling inferences that were hardly relevant to an autopsy, the details of which he mixed up and confused anyway. He wrote: "Social history indicates that the mother's husband (Robert Nelson) was not in the home at the time of the incident. Nelson (who married Kenneth's mother about three months ago) is not Kenneth's father. He was not present at the time because he was at a Scarborough hospital, attending to his girlfriend who was giving birth to his baby."

Smith told the court that Kenneth was in good health before he died. "He appeared to me, apart from the evidence of medical intervention, to have been a healthy boy who was appropriately nourished, appropriately developed, who had no evidence of congenital malformation and who showed no external evidence of injury apart from medical intervention."

In fact, Smith said one of the most significant findings of his external examination was the lack of injury. The same applied to his internal exam, although he noted that this was more challenging than normal. "One of the kind acts of Kenneth's parent or parents was to allow his organs to be used in other children, and so the findings in the internal examination were in part affected by the fact that such organ harvesting and transplantation had gone on." But he stressed that the harvesting had not compromised his ability to determine how the child had died.

Kenneth's respiratory system looked normal and healthy. So did his circulatory system. Ditto his gastrointestinal system and his genitourinary system. He noted the child had a healing fracture in his right femur. His head and scalp were free of injuries. The sutures, or joints between the bones of the skull, had come apart, which was typical when the brain swells. But Smith warned not to read too much into that.

"Swelling is a non-specific response to injury. If you twist your ankle, it will swell. If you stick your hand in boiling hot water, it will swell . . . So when we see a swollen brain in a situation like this, we know that there has been some injury to the brain, but whether that is a physical injury or an injury from lack of oxygen or lack of blood flow, it's not necessarily evident just looking at the brain."

He did find one thing of note: pinhead-size red blood spots—tiny hemorrhages called petechiae—on the surface of the child's lungs, heart and thymus. Smith said these showed the toddler died of asphyxia, caused by the body's failure to receive or utilize oxygen.

"The finding of those pinpoint haemorrhages, the pinhead haemorrhages, I should say, does not necessarily tell you how the asphyxia occurred. It doesn't tell you what the nature of the asphyxia is, and so it's necessary to look for other evidence of asphyxia or the manner of the mechanism of asphyxia."

Smith reported that the child's hyoid bone, found in the upper neck, was intact. In strangulation cases, the hyoid is often fractured, but Smith discounted that in Kenneth's case because of his age. "Because of the nature of the development of the hyoid in a child," he explained, "it is a much more pliable or flexible structure, and it is exceedingly uncommon for the hyoid to be fractured. It is examined as part of the autopsy, but it is not necessarily a meaningful observation in a very young person."

Smith said he also found petechiae on the brain, but he said these were indicative only of the swelling, and said little about what might have caused them.

In strangulation cases, he explained, petechiae are often found in the skin around the eyes or in the cells of the eyes themselves. But Kenneth's eyes were clear. "If [petechiae] had been present, that would increase my confidence in stating that Kenneth had suffered some form of neck compression," he testified. But he said that the absence of petechiae around and in the eyes was not definitive evidence that Kenneth had not been strangled. Petechiae can fade, Smith said, and he didn't do the autopsy until four days after Kenneth was brought to hospital.

Smith said that when he did his microscopic exam, however, he found a couple more clues. First, he could find no signs of a pre-existing disease. And second, there was evidence, albeit microscopic, of bleeding in the neck around the thyroid cartilage, or Adam's apple. But he said that finding wasn't definitive of anything on its own. "Apart from the microscopic focus of haemorrhage in the neck which may be a pointer to his mechanism of injury, and I say 'may' because I can't state with absolute certainty that it is. It may be a pointer to his mechanism of injury or it may not be, but the only positive findings we have are those."

Smith seemed to be saying that he was confident he knew how Kenneth died—asphyxia—but based on his post-mortem findings (or lack thereof) it was hard to say exactly what caused the asphyxia. Crown Sheila Cressman asked him if an epileptic seizure could have been the cause.

"The bottom line is that down the microscope or with my autopsy examination, I cannot assure you that he did not die from a seizure," Smith replied, adding that such a cause would be a "very, very unusual or uncommon event."

It should have been good news for Tammy. The pathologist said he didn't have enough evidence to be certain how Kenneth died, and he couldn't rule out a seizure as a factor. But he also said he didn't believe Tammy's explanation that Kenneth suffocated after getting tangled in his bedsheet.

"I do not believe that that is an accurate explanation for his death, no."

"Can you explain why not?" Cressman asked.

"The concept of asphyxia occurring in such a way that a person is able to phonate, that is to speak or to scream or to make any kind of vocalization," Smith explained, "is inconsistent with an asphyxia wherein there is obstruction to air passage. He said that although he had not examined the bedclothes, there was no way a plain cotton sheet could block airflow enough to cause suffocation.

Cressman asked him, "Is there anything else in that explanation which could trouble you in terms of its credibility?"

"Well, I have trouble with the length of time of the untangling," he responded, referring to the 20 minutes Tammy said it took to unknot Kenneth from the sheet. "I don't know what Ken was like and let me speak not as a pathologist perhaps, but as a parent. I mean, I don't know how many times I have untangled my own children from bedclothes and playing in bedclothes, and I can't believe for a moment that it's a 20 minute process.

"I find it perhaps surprising even if the story about being in the bathroom and hearing screaming or calling out for 10 minutes and did not generate a response, but there, I'm not making the statement as a forensic pathologist . . . I just, I find the story unbelievable in its various aspects, some of which are unbelievable based on my understanding of forensic pathology, and some are just my own experience as a parent."

The effect was devastating for the defence. Suddenly the lack of pathological evidence didn't make Kenneth's death look like a tragic, unexplained accident. It made Tammy look devious in trying so hard to hide all the signs of what she had done.

The Crown also called Stewart Powell and Stacey Craig, who had gone to the bar with Tammy and Rick in the weeks after Kenneth's death. In their testimony, Tammy's outbursts outside the bar and outside the grave-yard didn't sound like the grief of a distraught, broken mother. They sounded like guilt boiling over.

Stacey told the court that she tried to comfort Tammy after she got upset behind the bar. Tammy was screaming that she had killed Kenneth. At first, Stacey didn't believe her; she just thought Tammy was upset.

"How did you try and comfort her?" Crown Lisa Cameron asked. "You said you put your arm around her shoulders?"

"My hands [were] on her shoulders. [I] told her 'No,' that she hadn't killed him and she said, 'Yes I did. I killed my son.' And I said, 'Tammy, you didn't kill your son.' She looked me straight in the eye and said, 'Yes I did.'"

"And when she said that, how did it make you feel?"

"Uncomfortable. I believed what she was saying."

Stewart Powell said that after they had gone to the cemetery that night, they were sitting on the grass across the street. "We started talking about stuff, and about stuff that had gone on; how Kenneth was before, and all this. She got up and started running toward the street so I ran up, stood in front of her. She tried getting around me to get to the road. I pushed her back. She fell down. I went to give her a hand up, and that's when she got me around the collar of my shirt and looked me dead smack in the eyes and said that 'I killed Kenneth.'"

"And what did you do?" Cressman asked.

"I walked away."

"And why did you walk away?"

"Because I was at the point, when she did that, I felt like ripping her head off."

"Why did you feel that way?"

"Because the way she grabbed me and the way she told me, it was her admitting, I felt like it was her admitting, I felt like it was her admitting to me that she did kill Kenneth."

"And did you believe her?"

"Yes, I did."

Tammy's sister, Carol Wynne, also testified. She told the court that she let Tammy and Kenneth stay with her for a week in the summer of 1993, while Tammy was getting back on her feet.

"Did she ever say anything about herself and Kenneth that struck you as unusual?" another Crown, Lisa Cameron, asked.

"When she first came in, she asked me if I could watch over her because she has a very bad temper and she didn't want to take it out on Kenneth."

The preliminary hearing wrapped up. Tammy Marquardt was ordered to stand trial for second-degree murder.

With her trial moving forward and her time with Keith capped at a single weekly visit, Tammy needed to find something positive for herself. She settled on an unlikely source: school. Years earlier, she had dropped out of high school five credits short of what she needed to graduate. Now, she enrolled at Sir Robert L. Borden Secondary School in Scarborough, travelling there from Rosalie Hall each day. She kept to herself for the most part. Tammy was turning twenty-three and facing murder charges. She didn't have a lot in common with her classmates.

She worked hard, attending both day classes and night school; she was determined to make up her credits in one semester so she could graduate in June, before her trial started. And she reached her goal. Though her life was in turmoil, she attended her graduation ceremony, the first person in her family to have graduated from high school.

While she attended school, Tammy saw less and less of Rick, who had returned to his philandering ways. Another of his exes had given birth to a son, who was just three months younger than Keith. The woman insisted Rick was the baby's father. Divorce papers were delivered to Tammy, unannounced, in April 1995.

FOUR

TAMMY WAS ALONE and scared when the jury trial started on October 2, 1995, almost two years to the day after Kenneth died. Months earlier, the Crown had offered her a plea bargain: she could plead guilty to the lesser charge of manslaughter and get five years, likely serving significantly less than that. The offer was still on the table.

Tammy's lawyers were torn. Steven Clark liked her chances at trial. He didn't think the Crown had enough to prove the murder charge. But Edward Kelly was less sure. He encouraged Tammy to consider the plea. She was facing life in prison, with no shot at parole for at least ten years. If she was convicted, the judge would have the discretion to lock her up for even longer. But Tammy wasn't interested. It wasn't right.

Tammy had forgotten how to do infant CPR. That's why she blamed herself for Kenneth's death. She would have to live with that tragic failure for the rest of her life. But the Crown, the police, the medical experts, they were accusing her of hurting her son on purpose. Of killing the one good thing in her life.

She hadn't hurt him, and she wouldn't say that she had. Tammy told her lawyers there would be no plea deal.

Mr. Justice John McIsaac would preside at the trial. Edward Kelly was right to be worried: it was a one-sided affair from the get-go. Several rulings on pre-trial proceedings went against Tammy. All but two of the autopsy photos submitted by the Crown were allowed as evidence. Photos of dead children never help a defendant, but the judge said that their value in helping the jury understand Dr. Smith's testimony out-weighed any prejudice they might cause. Pictures of Rick and Tammy's apartment were also allowed. Justice McIsaac ruled that they would help the jury visualize the scene of Kenneth's death. But they also showed that Kenneth was being raised in a filthy apartment. Justice McIsaac said,

"They show Ms. Marquardt to be a messy housekeeper. I cannot see how they would have any tendency to create in the minds of the jurors a possibility that, for that reason, she is more likely to have committed the crime which the Crown alleged."

During the trial, the judge also allowed two expert medical witnesses—who hadn't yet given their testimony—to remain in the courtroom while other medical experts testified. Normally, witnesses are barred from hearing others' testimony during trial, as it might influence their own, but Justice McIsaac made an exception "because some of the expert witnesses would be in a better position to testify if they are able to hear the other experts."

As testimony was about to begin on the first day of trial, Justice McIsaac had a word of warning for both the Crown and the defence when it came to questioning Smith. "I'm going back to my former life and I had occasion to have Dr. Smith as a witness and he becomes incensed if the deceased child is ever referred to as 'it,'" the judge cautioned. "So don't ever do that because he's going to jump on you and it's going to have a potentially negative impact on the trial if he does that. We've got to. Both sides have got to be careful to not refer to the deceased child as 'it.'"

The Crown called twenty-nine witnesses, seven of them doctors. All the witnesses painted a grim picture of Tammy's parenting abilities. Maureen Edwards, the Children's Aid social worker, testified that Tammy told her that "sometimes when she was feeding the baby or burping him that she imagined that she was putting her arms around his neck. She would know enough at that time to put the baby down." The social worker did say the young mother told her she would separate herself from the child when his crying was overwhelming her. And Tammy admitted to her that she yelled at Kenneth a lot out of frustration.

The case continued to pile up against Tammy in that Whitby courtroom. Witness after witness took the stand to pick apart her explanation, her behaviour, her grief.

Carol Wynne said that she found Tammy's behaviour at Kenneth's funeral odd. "It seemed to me that that funeral was a party. The only time I see her cry was actually during the service."

"And why do you use the word 'party'?" asked Crown prosecutor Sheila Cressman.

"Because she was walking around [with] smiles on her face; both her and Rick. And for a funeral, that's not proper."

Other witnesses painted similarly damning pictures of Tammy's behaviour after Kenneth died. Stewart Powell, for instance, said he found her demeanour at the funeral troubling. "The one thing that sticks out in my mind the most is when we said we were sorry and she went, 'Shit happens,'" he testified.

"What was her demeanour at that time?" the Crown asked.

"Weird. She was joking. She had a sense of humour about the whole thing."

Stewart also recounted Tammy's outburst behind the bar they had gone to. He said Tammy was fighting with Rick because he felt she'd had too much to drink. She was hysterical. Stewart's girlfriend, Stacey, was holding and consoling her as the pair sat on the ground behind the bar. "She was trying to break the hold that Stacey had on her and she was screaming that she had killed Kenneth." Stewart testified that she yelled this over and over, at least ten times. She also screamed that she'd forgotten CPR, but only added that caveat once or twice. Stewart didn't take her admissions too seriously. "At that time, I thought it was just the alcohol talking," he said.

His feelings changed when they ended up at the cemetery later that night, after Tammy told him forcefully she had killed Kenneth. "By her reaction and the tone of her voice and the way she was acting, I felt that she meant what she was saying."

Tammy's defence lawyer Steven Clark began his cross-examination. He asked Stewart if he himself had been cheerful at times at the hospital, as he was alleging Tammy had been at Kenneth's funeral. "Do you remember laughing or sharing a laugh with Rick while you were viewing the child in the room, sir?"

"Yes, Rick and I did. We were thinking about how Kenneth was at times that I had been over there and it was not a laugh like it was funny. It was just remembering times when Kenneth was well."

"Because otherwise it might be pretty unusual if someone was laughing looking at a person who was perhaps dead at the time, wouldn't you agree?"

"Yes," Stewart responded.

"You say you did it because you were thinking of the good times."

"Yes."

"That was a way you could help yourself cope with a very difficult situation, isn't that correct?"

"Yes, sir."

"And do you think the same might apply to Tammy Marquardt, the child's mother?"

"It is possible."

Clark also asked him about his own behaviour when he believed Tammy confessed to him that she killed Kenneth. "Did you try to probe any further to ask her details?"

"No, I did not."

"Did you ask her, 'What do you mean by that?'"

"No."

"Did you ask her, 'Did you smother him?' 'Did you strangle him?' 'What do you mean you killed him?'

"I did not ask any questions because I just walked away," Stewart testified.

"And you walked away because you told us that you felt like killing her yourself."

"Yes."

"Meaning you were so upset by her change, or at least your perceived change in what she was saying, that you started to believe that she killed her son, isn't that right?"

"Yes."

But if that's how he felt at the time, Clark said, why didn't he immediately tell Rick? Stewart answered that Rick had gone into the cemetery, and he didn't want to go in there.

Clark also questioned why, if Stewart believed that Tammy had confessed, he didn't tell the police at the earliest opportunity. After all, Stewart was at Rick and Tammy's apartment when police showed up to admit her to hospital for a psychiatric evaluation. "Why didn't you tell the police?"

"Because I was too busy concerning myself with keeping Rick calmed down and trying to talk him—to allow the police to talk to him."

"Mr. Powell, the police were right there. You had an opportunity I'll bet within a half-hour of this whole incident of telling them what happened, didn't you?"

"Yes, I did."

Stewart said he gave a statement to police "about two days later."

Clark had him look at the date of his statement. "The event occurred on October 21st, sir, is that right?"

"Yes."

"And this is dated November 24th, more than one month later."

"Okay," Stewart answered.

"So why was it a month later, not two days later?"

"I really couldn't tell you. Maybe I was trying to forget the whole thing."

Rick Marquardt's testimony was barely more favourable. He testified that on the morning of October 9 he left the apartment to be with his ex-girlfriend who was having a baby. That fact aligned with the Crown's theory that Tammy was angry about Rick's infidelities and took it out on Kenneth. (Although Rick's testimony didn't support that theory. He said Tammy was fine with his going to see his ex at the hospital.) Rick also testified about Tammy's outburst behind the bar.

"When you were out the back, what do you remember happening out there?" Crown Lisa Cameron asked.

"Tammy screaming she killed him because she forgot her CPR. She said it numerous times."

But Rick didn't think it was a confession. He put it down to the booze and grief and guilt talking. And while he was careful to qualify his words—she killed him *because she forgot her CPR*—he also understood the implications of what he was saying: he was helping the Crown build its case against his former wife.

—

Some of Tammy's earlier statements to social and child protection workers were raised at trial. Social worker Maureen Edwards had assisted Tammy through a pregnancy and aftercare program at Rosalie Hall. She saw Tammy both before and after Kenneth was born, and told the court about a home visit she had made in June 1991, when Kenneth was just over a month old.

Tammy, she said, "initially reported that things were going quite well, but then started to talk that everybody was giving her lots of different advice and that was confusing for her. There were problems between herself and her mother. She talked about it being difficult to soothe Kenneth when he was crying. That she spoke at one point—said that sometimes she was feeding the baby and burping him and imagined that she put her arms around his neck. She knew enough to put him down at that point and we talked about different strategies when babies are crying, what she could do to ease her frustration." She added that she and Tammy discussed whether placing Kenneth in foster care for a few days would be a good way to give her some relief, a step Tammy decided to take.

During cross-examination from Steven Clark, Edwards clarified that Tammy said she *imagined* putting her arms around Kenneth's neck, not that she had *actually* done that. Edwards also clarified that the aftercare program was voluntary and that Tammy was under no obligation to participate.

But another social worker, Cathy Sorichetti, said Tammy told her a slightly different—even more troubling—version of that incident. Tammy attended a support meeting for new mothers at Rosalie Hall the next month, on July 18, 1991. Sorichetti was the social worker overseeing the gathering. "Tammy approached me after the meeting and said again that she was feeling stressed. She recalled a time to me, a previous time, where she had felt stressed out and Kenneth had gone into care and how at that time she had felt her hands going around his neck. This time Kenneth was crying and she felt her hand go over Kenneth's mouth and that she realized at that time that she could just cover his mouth for him to be quiet and that frightened her. She said so—as soon as she realized that she stopped, and she covered her ears and screamed."

Sorichetti said she asked Tammy if she felt Kenneth should be placed in foster care again. "She didn't want that to happen. She felt that he wasn't in immediate danger and that she was telling me this because she needed some support." Sorichetti said she didn't feel the child was in immediate danger either. Under cross-examination, she said the concerns Tammy raised were common among new mothers attending the support group.

Frances (Frankie) Holmes, a child protection worker with the Toronto Children's Aid Society, was assigned to supervise Kenneth's care in 1993. She told the court about two visits she had with Tammy in late January. Tammy was living in a basement apartment at the time. It was musty and cramped, so she was trying to find something better. "Tammy was feeling quite stressed in caring for Kenneth, looking for an apartment," Holmes told the court, "and she expressed some concern that she might hurt him." Tammy asked that Children's Aid place Kenneth in care until she got their living arrangements sorted out. Holmes said she agreed, but decided to give Tammy a day to see if she could sort it out herself. She visited her again on January 26. Tammy still felt that placing Kenneth in temporary care was the best option.

"Once that decision was made I was going back to my office and arranged a temporary placement. It wasn't likely to happen that day, just the process was set in motion," Holmes explained. "However, later I went back to my office then I got a telephone call from Tammy. And at this point she was expressing much more distress, she was crying and she was demanding that Kenneth be removed that day. So I immediately went back to her apartment, and from her apartment arranged a placement and Kenneth was put into a foster home that day."

A temporary placement was ordered for three months. Tammy wasn't happy it was going to be for that long. "I wasn't thrilled either," said Holmes, "but we also had this understanding that the child could be returned sooner if the other expectations were met." She said it was always her preference to return the child to the parent as soon as possible.

During his cross-examination, Steven Clark pointed out that it was Tammy herself who initiated the temporary placement. "This was her request that she wanted it done," he said to Holmes. She confirmed that it was.

Clark said, "This wouldn't have crossed your mind unless she raised it necessarily."

"No, I wouldn't have acted," Holmes replied. "From what I knew up to then I would not have removed him from her."

Marlene Wikaruk was working as a hostel supervisor at the YWCA in Oshawa in 1993 when Tammy and Kenneth moved in for a month in July. She told the court about a conversation she had with Tammy a week after she moved in. "She stated that she squeezed Kenneth's leg. She didn't realize how hard until she saw a bruise appear and I told her we would have to call the Children's Aid Society." Wikaruk said Tammy understood that and was fine with it.

"Did she appear calm or excited?" Crown Sheila Cressman asked.

"No, she didn't seem excited. She seemed calm; a rather fragile little person."

Under cross-examination, Wikaruk said it was an unusual conversation. "It does surprise me because she came to me unsolicited." Wikaruk reported the bruise to Children's Aid. She said Tammy and Kenneth stayed unsupervised at the YWCA for another three weeks.

Silvana Maclellan was the Children's Aid child protection worker who took over Kenneth's supervision when Tammy moved to Oshawa. She told the court that she got a call from Frances Holmes in early July asking her to monitor the case now that Tammy and Kenneth were living in her region. Holmes also told her that Tammy had told a worker at the YWCA where she was living that she was "losing it." Maclellan met with Tammy and Kenneth on July 12.

Steven Clark asked her, "I take it that the information that you had received from those other Children's Aid workers was to the effect that Tammy was losing it, is that fair to say?"

Maclellan replied that was correct.

"That didn't appear to be your impression . . . is that fair to say?"

"Yes."

"She was very calm and when she spoke to you about these various incidents, she was trying to speak maturely or responsibly about her position?"

"Yes," Maclellan agreed. She and Tammy discussed the bruise on Kenneth's leg, but Maclellan didn't document what it looked like. "The bruise was consistent with her explanation of how the bruise got on his leg and it wasn't significant," she explained.

"But if you're going out there to investigate the very bruise," Clark countered, "why wouldn't you have put what you just told us now?"

"I didn't see it as abuse at that time." Maclellan said that at the time she had no concerns about Tammy looking after Kenneth on her own.

Shirley Caspin, Tammy's and Kenneth's family doctor, testified that she saw Kenneth fifty-eight times in the twenty-eight months of his life. "Perhaps a little more often than usual" was how she characterized the frequency of visits. "It was a new child for mom. She had a lot of questions."

Caspin told the court that she was aware of three seizures the child had, but they weren't concerning because she believed they were associated each time with a fever. "The main thing you follow in children with seizures is their neurologic development and that's done very, very routinely," she testified. "There are routine milestones done every three months on children until they are two. He was absolutely at his milestones if not better. So there was absolutely no damage that could be appreciated as a result of these seizures."

However, Miroslav Ort, a pediatrician in Oshawa who had also treated Kenneth, testified that Tammy gave him different information. "She told me he had seven attacks of seizures, two with fever and five without any fever." He said Tammy told him the seizures lasted one to ten minutes, and that Kenneth was being treated with phenobarbital. "That's one of the basic first-line drugs for epilepsy in children," Dr. Ort explained, adding that Kenneth was eventually taken off the medication because it was making him hyperactive. Ort then prescribed Dilantin. He also ordered a brain scan and an electroencephalogram, or EEG. Both came back normal.

Defence lawyer Edward Kelly asked the pediatrician the significance of the EEG results. "Even if the test is normal, that in itself doesn't say for certain that the child doesn't have some significant abnormality."

Ort agreed.

"So it's not uncommon for doctors to take more than one test?"

"That's correct," Ort replied.

Ort said he saw Kenneth on July 6. He later learned the child was taken to Oshawa General twice the next day. "He was brought to the hospital at 18:26 to the emergency room and the chief complaint was nausea. That means he was just prone to vomiting. He was sent home and the diagnosis was possible viral infection. I would like to say that at that time the temperature was 35.6 [Celsius]. That means no fever. He was brought back at 9:36 p.m. and at that time he was brought back with a so-called seizure. Again, temperature was 36.2. No fever."

He said the second diagnosis was seizure disorder. "We also use the diagnosis . . . not to label the child as epilepsy. When you say seizure disorder, it doesn't look so bad as when you say he has epilepsy."

Paramedics, doctors and nurses were called to testify about the treatment Kenneth received at the hospital.

Dr. Caswell Rumball was one of the first to see Kenneth in the ER at Oshawa General that afternoon. He told the court that Kenneth wasn't choking on anything at that time.

Defence lawyer Steven Clark asked him, "Did you make any notes or have any recollection as to whether there were any obstructions at all in the mouth of the child?"

"I did not make any such note and I have no recollection of anything like that," Rumball replied.

"Would you have made any note or would you have any recollection as to whether there were any fibres or materials around the mouth of the child?"

"If there was a foreign body or something notable I would have noted that, but I did not."

Dr. Sunil Mehra, then head of pediatrics and neonatology at Oshawa General, took over Kenneth's care once Dr. Rumball and ER staff had re-established his heartbeat and stabilized him. But Mehra told the court the child was still completely unresponsive.

"What other observations did you make?" Crown Sheila Cressman asked.

"His pupils were very dilated and they were fixed. They were not responding to any light stimulus at all."

"And what does that observation indicate to you?"

"That means that the child has sustained a degree of hypoxia or lack of oxygen for a period of time," Mehra said.

"And are you able to determine for what length of time he would not have had oxygen?"

"No. It doesn't tell you for how long, but it tells you the gravity of the situation. If the pupils are fixed and not reacting, then we know the prognosis is very guarded in this case."

Cressman asked Mehra if Kenneth appeared to have a fever. Mehra said he did not.

"Was there any indication from what you saw about Kenneth that he was in a post-seizure state?" Cressman asked.

"No."

"What would you expect to see if he were in a post-seizure state?"

"In post-seizure state," Mehra explained, "the child could be flaccid, not responsive, but generally the vital signs are all maintained. They have a good heart rate and they still have a good breathing pattern. So, these are benign convulsions we call it which don't last more than a minute to two and the vital signs are maintained all the way through."

But under cross-examination, Mehra said the child did have some "twitchiness" while he was being treated, although the pediatrician said this was most likely caused by hypoxia, or lack of oxygen to the brain.

Clark asked him, "Would you agree that if a child had a seizure of some kind that there might not be physical signs that were noticeable?"

"There may not be any physical signs at that time."

"And if someone is in a post-seizure state would you usually try to correlate that with some history provided by someone who might have been there?"

"Yes."

"And would you agree it's not just one simple observation as to what an individual might look like in that condition?"

"In medicine, you have to always correlate the findings with the history available to you."

"It's pretty hard to do one without the other?"

"It's difficult, yes," Mehra replied.

Sheila Harding was the nurse who first greeted Tammy when she arrived at Oshawa General. Tammy had explained to her what happened at the apartment. Harding told the court she had a hard time believing it took Tammy twenty minutes to untangle the toddler from the bedsheet, but Tammy was adamant.

"How did she appear at the time she was telling the story?" Cressman asked her.

"Very calm," Harding replied. "Very calm for someone that knows that the child—like Kenneth had come in what we called VSA: vital signs absent. And for someone that knew that their child was in that condition, normally I would expect a much more anxious, upset mother, but she didn't present that way. She was quite calm and just answered my questions the way they were asked." She recalled that Tammy was not crying and did not ask to see Kenneth. "She kept saying to me, 'They just better make sure he doesn't die.' She kept saying that over and over and over."

"What was her tone when she would say that?" the Crown asked.

"Almost like a threatening type of tone. Like I felt it was unusual to say it in the way she had said it. 'They better not let him die. They better not let him die,' as though there was almost like something else coming behind it."

The nurse said Tammy was strangely emotionless when she took her to see Kenneth. "She said, 'Kenneth, my darling, please don't leave. Mommy is here. Mommy doesn't want you to leave.'"

"And what was her emotional, her apparent emotional state at that time in terms of did she appear upset?" Cressman asked.

"No, she did not. She did not cry."

Const. Scott Terry was one of the first officers at the hospital, and he had a different memory of Tammy during their interactions. "She would go into, I called hysterics or convulsions, where she could barely breathe and she was hyperventilating at times and really upset where through the interview I would stop and then I would let her go through her little, you know, her motions of being quite upset . . . to a point that I saw that she was calming down a bit, so then I would suggest could we get back to some more information or could we get back to what you were telling me."

Terry told the court that Tammy didn't know initially how long it had taken her to untangle Kenneth from what she described at the time as blankets. The police officer had to suggest times to her. "She hesitated and she was kind of hemming and hawing because she, I don't think, [could] come up with a figure and that's why I suggested was it 5, 10, 15, maybe even 20 minutes." Terry said she chose fifteen minutes, but it appeared that she was guessing.

Sam Shemie, Kenneth's main doctor at SickKids, said Tammy's explanation for what happened didn't make sense to him. When he called it "suspicious," the judge asked him not to use that word in front of the jury.

Dr. Shemie said that drug screening tests found Dilantin in Kenneth's system. The child was being given it to treat his seizures, but the levels were low, "below therapeutic." If Kenneth did have a seizure before or at the time of his injuries, Shemie believed he didn't have enough medication in his system to control it.

And a neurologist testified that taking a child off Dilantin could result in a seizure.

But no one believed Kenneth was having a seizure at the time Tammy found him, including Tammy herself. She believed he was conscious, that his thrashing was controlled. It was different from the seizures she'd seen him have before. The Crown's medical experts agreed that Kenneth wouldn't have been able to call out for help in the midst of a seizure.

And even if he was having one, the medical experts doubted that it could have been responsible for the brain damage the toddler had suffered. William Logan was a pediatric neurologist at the Hospital for Sick Children when Kenneth was transferred there. His assessment: Kenneth was in a coma, and brain dead. "The term that's generally used is cerebral death," Logan testified.

Crown counsel Lisa Cameron asked him, "Would a seizure of any kind cause a person to be in Kenneth's state?"

"No," Logan replied. "You can have brain damage from seizures but they're almost always very prolonged seizures . . . [and the damage is] not usually to the degree that Kenneth had. In other words, they will be in a coma, but they will still have some brain activity and still respond to some extent." He said he didn't think Kenneth had suffered a prolonged seizure. All the earlier ones he'd suffered had been relatively brief. "The ones that are more serious are ones that cause the patient to stop breathing and to turn blue. They go on for a long, long period of time. We're talking 30, 40, 50, 60 minutes, two hours, three hours. Very long."

So what did the doctor think had led to Kenneth's coma and brain death? He couldn't say for certain, but he didn't think Tammy's explanation could account for his condition. Her story, he felt, "was quite unusual," and he struggled to connect the events as she had described them with a two-year-old in cardiac arrest. Oxygen depletion to the brain would explain the coma, but what explained the oxygen depletion? Dr. Logan didn't see anything in Tammy's story that could.

During cross-examination, Edward Kelly asked Logan about other possibilities. "Doctor, there is an area of research of inquiry relating to epilepsy and it relates to the issue of sudden death due to epilepsy. Now, I'm not going to pretend that I know a lot about this field at all, and I presume you do or as much as anybody can know. Is it not the case, though, that this is an area of concern to neurologists?"

"It's a concern in the sense that we don't quite understand it," Logan answered, "but it's not a concern from the point of view of being very frequent."

"It's a very irregular activity or very uncommon?"

"Yeah."

"But it does involve, as I understand it, some type of discharge from the brain causing the heart to beat in an irregular way. Is that fair to say?"

"That's fair to say. That's one of the theories," the neurologist replied.

"One of the theories. And we're really at that stage with this inquiry, we're really at the preliminary stage of the inquiry."

Dr. Logan agreed that research into what is called sudden unexplained death in epilepsy, or SUDEP, was still in its early stages.

The defence lawyer then asked if previous neurological disorders such as seizures were always evident at autopsy.

Logan answered that no, seizure activity might not always show on an autopsy.

Kelly said emergency personnel didn't find anything blocking Kenneth's throat, but could the child have suffocated because his tongue rolled back during a seizure and blocked his airway?

No, Logan said, he was pretty certain that didn't happen.

"It's fair to say," Kelly told him, "that you're concerned about the history provided in this case given the child's clinical history, but is it also fair to say you can't provide us with a certain explanation for the cause of the child's death?"

"I think the cause of death was cardiorespiratory arrest. What I can't tell you is why he had that, if that's your question. I think that's a sufficient cause for the death, but why he had that, I can't tell you."

Kelly didn't ask the neurologist whether the diagnosis of SUDEP should have been considered in Kenneth's death. Crown Lisa Cameron did, though, on re-examination.

"The topic of sudden death due to epilepsy was raised. Do you feel that that applies in Kenneth Wynne's case?" she asked Dr. Logan.

"No."

"And if someone is having a seizure and choking, would they be speaking?"

"They wouldn't," Logan replied. "If they are choking, they wouldn't be able to speak, generally."

FIVE

DR. CHARLES SMITH began his testimony just before noon on Tuesday, October 17, the second-last day of trial. He was the twenty-eighth of the Crown's twenty-nine witnesses.

Justice McIsaac asked the Crown, "What is the area you're wishing permission that he be allowed to give evidence upon?"

"Pediatric forensic pathology," Cressman replied.

"Any difficulty with that, Mr. Clark?" the judge asked defence counsel.

"It's a fairly lengthy CV," Steven Clark answered, "but it only took me one or two pages to satisfy myself that this witness is qualified to give expert-opinion evidence in the area of forensic pediatric pathology. Please proceed."

Charles Smith took the stand. The pathologist wore glasses and had neatly trimmed hair.

Crown prosecutor Sheila Cressman asked him, "Are you able to tell us approximately how many pediatric autopsies you would have performed over the course of your career?"

"No, I can't," Smith said. "More than a thousand, but I don't know how many."

He told the court he was the director of the Ontario Pediatric Forensic Pathology Unit, "the only pediatric forensic pathology unit of its kind in existence as far as we know," he said.

"In Canada, or where?" Cressman asked.

"My understanding from the chief coroner is anywhere."

"In the world?"

"That's my understanding."

The unit was established in 1991 by Toronto's Hospital for Sick Children and the Ontario Ministry of the Solicitor General. It was the first regional unit of its kind, Dr. Smith testified, although similar units would be established in the next few years. The unit's work focused on

completing autopsies of children and infants in Toronto and the surrounding area. It would also handle pediatric death cases from across the
province as needed.

Smith had been appointed the unit's inaugural director in 1992, even
though he had no training in forensic pathology at that time (or anytime
afterward). He may have conducted more than a thousand autopsies by that
point in his career, but only ten to fifteen of them had involved criminally
suspicious cases. Pediatric forensic pathology is a challenging field.
Pathologists spend their days dissecting dead children, and the spectre of
child abuse hangs over many criminally suspicious cases. Smith was already
the staff pathologist at SickKids in charge of autopsies, recognized for his
devotion and dedication to coroner's cases. He didn't have any specific
training or expertise, but he was willing to take on a job no one else wanted.

In acting as a forensic pathologist, Smith's job was to determine a child's
cause of death, mechanism of death and, when possible, manner of death.
They are three related concepts. Sometimes the cause and mechanism of
death are the same. Sometimes they are different. An example: a victim
has a gunshot wound. The gunshot was the cause of death. But blood loss,
not the gunshot itself, was the mechanism.

The manner is the type of death. Going back to the gunshot wound, it
could be a homicide, a suicide or an accident. It may not be possible for the
pathologist to determine which from the autopsy alone. It's left to the coroner
(or medical examiners who serve a similar role in other provinces) to figure it
out, and the coroner enlists the police to help in the investigation.

Forensic pathologists are asked to pinpoint time of death and injuries,
although both are exceedingly difficult. In pediatric cases, timing is often a
key issue, because it helps to determine who could have caused the fatal
injuries. (Timing wasn't an issue in Kenneth's case, as Tammy was the only
person with access to him at the time he was found struggling in his bedsheets. Timing would, however, play a crucial role in several other cases in
which Smith was involved.)

Smith testified that the cause of Kenneth's death was asphyxia. A
person will lose consciousness about fifteen seconds after oxygen is cut off

from the brain, he told the court. Death occurs after two to five minutes of oxygen deprivation.

Smith testified that he found microscopic evidence of hemorrhages, or bleeding, "adjacent or alongside some of the small skeletal muscles . . . in the neck." The finding pointed to possible strangulation, accidentally by the bedsheet or intentionally by a person. But either way it was likely mild and not fatal. That's because neck compression also leaves petechiae in the tissues around the eyes, Smith explained, and Kenneth didn't have any there.

Smith said he did find petechiae scattered across the surfaces of Kenneth's lungs, heart and thymus, which are non-specific. (He said he couldn't rule out the transplant surgery having caused the petechial bleeding. Kenneth's liver, kidneys and heart valves were removed for donation after he died.)

Smith said Kenneth's brain was "markedly swollen," another by-product of asphyxia, but one that he said pointed more toward suffocation. (Asphyxia can also be chemical or metabolic. The chemical hydrogen cyanide, for example, can disrupt breathing at the cellular level, causing death.) The swelling was so severe it was pushing apart the individual plates that make up the skull.

Could a severe asthmatic attack or seizure have been responsible? Could it have been strangulation or suffocation? Could a tangled sheet around Kenneth's neck tighten enough to cut off the flow of oxygen? Could he have suffocated under it? Or did Tammy intentionally strangle or suffocate Kenneth?

Cressman asked him, "Was there any finding on Kenneth's body to help you explain how the asphyxia occurred?"

"It's probably easier for me to tell you how it did not happen . . . and that will answer your question, if I can do that," he replied. He said he had found no evidence of a natural disease process in the lungs that could explain asphyxia. Although an acute asthmatic attack could cause fatal asphyxia, Smith said he had found no evidence that Kenneth had suffered one.

He said Kenneth's death was consistent with "impaired supply of oxygen that can occur as a result of abnormalities in the environment"—such as a child being locked inside a sealed refrigerator, he explained, or drowning. "Airway obstruction will do it, and that can be things like putting; if a child puts a plastic bag over their face or their head region, that is a diagnosis of asphyxia caused by airway obstruction, lack of oxygen."

Hanging or neck compression would have the same result, he explained, but one would also see marks on the neck, bleeding in the soft tissues of the neck and petechial bleeding in the area around the eyes and across the scalp, none of which were present in Kenneth's case. Smith said he didn't think the sheet was tight enough around his neck to be a factor, and he saw no signs that it was. Choking on an inhaled object like a marble or a piece of hotdog could also cause airway obstruction, but he said that didn't appear to be a factor in Kenneth's asphyxia.

"So, what I'm left with in Kenneth is this: He has evidence of asphyxia. I have no natural disease that explains the asphyxia. I have some microscopic evidence of hemorrhage in his neck that would be consistent with neck injury, but I can't say whether that neck injury was accidental or non-accidental. It would appear to be not a severe or prolonged neck injury if it was real, such that we see the petechial changes in or around his eyes or in the region of his face. So, what I'm saying is that he died of asphyxia. The asphyxia could be environmental, could be an environmental lack of oxygen, could be something like a plastic bag or a gentle suffocation."

Cressman asked him if Kenneth's death could have been caused by a seizure. "I can't accept the explanation," he replied, "unless you have other evidence to support it. I don't have evidence of that at all." Epileptic deaths, he said, are typically seen in teenagers or adults, and he saw no evidence to suggest it was a factor. "Epilepsy is . . . often associated with changes that can be seen in the brain down the microscope and I don't have evidence of that."

Cressman said, "If I'm able to tell you, Dr. Smith, that during much of the time Kenneth was wrapped in the bedsheet his mother reports that he was calling out to her, 'Mommy, Mommy,' up until at least fairly close to the time he was actually unwrapped, does that assist you in dealing with the seizure hypothesis?"

"If that's true," Smith answered, "then the seizure hypothesis is not at all a tenable explanation. Now, you need to understand something here. Seizures are very common in the dying process in children. So I cannot say that Kenneth did not have a seizure, but if what you tell me is true, the seizure did not cause death."

Later in his testimony, Smith said that although he was unconvinced, he couldn't rule out the possibility that Kenneth may have died from a seizure.

The pathologist often qualified his opinions with statements like "unless you have other evidence to support it" or "in the absence of another credible explanation." These qualifiers put the onus on the defendant to come up with an explanation for the injuries. But it's the pathologist's job to consider all potential causes and mechanisms of death. When medical evidence is not definitive, the manner of death should be listed as unascertained, or undetermined, as opposed to a natural or accidental death, or a homicide or suicide.

In the end, Dr. Smith testified that his findings from the autopsy were consistent with suffocation with a soft object or having the head placed in a plastic bag. The pathologist also said someone may have "held his nose and mouth closed and he was suffocated that way."

Rick Marquardt was sitting in the gallery listening to Smith's testimony. He had wanted to hear the pathologist for himself. He still didn't believe Tammy was guilty. He'd taken a seat in the back of the courtroom with his new wife, the woman he'd divorced Tammy to marry, and they listened as Smith testified about petechial hemorrhaging and asphyxia; his terminology was hard to follow, but his message wasn't.

By the first recess, Rick had heard enough. He and his wife slipped out of the courtroom and headed for their car. As he opened the car door, Rick said Edward Kelly, one of Tammy's lawyers, slammed it shut from behind and shoved Rick hard against it. Kelly wanted to know why the hell Rick had been in the courtroom. Rick screamed back that he had been there to learn the truth. He challenged Kelly to say that after hearing Smith's testimony the lawyer didn't believe his client was guilty as sin. (Kelly declined to speak to me for this book. He is now a judge with the Ontario Court of Justice. Steven Clark also declined my request for an interview. He is now a judge with the same court.)

Edward Kelly took a step back. The two men stood glaring at each other, waiting for the other to take the first swing.

The bailiff and three security guards ran over. Rick accused Kelly of harassment, but before it could go any further Kelly walked away.

When court resumed, Kelly began his cross-examination of Dr. Smith. He noted that Kenneth's diaphragm and epicardium—part of the outer surface of the heart—were both damaged in the process of removing the heart valves, liver and kidneys for donation. "The inability of you to examine these two tissues or organs carefully, did it impact upon your ability to make a proper examination of the child?" he asked.

"I don't think it impacted significantly," Smith replied. "It's more of an inconvenience. The tissues did remain behind and were examined. The inconvenience is simply that I can't know for sure whether or not petechiae were present or absent."

"Is it possible that that could in some way impair your ability to make your assessment?"

"I don't think it affects the assessment in terms of a bottom line. In terms of listing the places where petechiae occur, you know, instead of three sites, it may have been three sites or four sites or five sites, but it doesn't really affect my overall conclusion."

"If it was on the fourth or fifth site," Kelly asked him, "would that alter your opinion about the pattern of the petechiae and maybe lead you to a different conclusion?"

Smith said it would not. "The pattern would be different, but in fact the conclusions would be the same."

Kelly asked if certain types of neurological disorders don't always show up at autopsy.

"Yes. You can have a neurological disorder that doesn't have structural equivalent that I can't see down the microscope. That's possible."

"It's common?" Kelly asked.

"That's a good question . . . I think I would have to say it would be quite extraordinary not to see evidence of it at autopsy, and the exception of course has to do with the whole seizure disorder situation that can cause death in infants and especially in older children, teenagers," Smith said, referring to epilepsy, which he said doesn't always show up at autopsy.

The defence lawyer also wondered if there might be other causes for the petechiae that Dr. Smith found. Kenneth developed pneumonia after he was placed on life support. "Is it not the case," he asked, "that pneumonia can cause some types of petechial hemorrhages to form?"

"Pneumonia . . . can be associated with hemorrhage," Smith agreed, adding that pneumonia would leave a different distribution pattern from what he had seen in Kenneth's autopsy.

Kelly continued. "When we consider the resuscitation attempts that someone would experience and in this type of a situation, is it not also the case that those attempts, which can be quite traumatic for the body, could also cause petechial hemorrhages?"

"They can," Smith said. "More classically they are associated with petechiae in the head and neck region as opposed to the chest."

Kelly also asked if the surgery to remove Kenneth's heart could have been a factor.

"That's possible," Smith conceded. "I examined a lot of the hearts that are removed for . . . heart valve transplantation purposes and certainly petechiae are not commonly seen on those, but I can't rule out the possibility that the trauma of transplantation would cause that."

The defence lawyer continued to push Smith on this point: could he be wrong about what had caused the petechiae? Would other forensic pathologists come to the same conclusions that he did?

"I have often disagreed with other pathologists in the interpretation of petechiae," Smith answered, "and especially in newborn babies or young infants because there are subtle patterns that are apparent, but aren't necessarily recognized by some pathologists . . . I can certainly allow that the patterns of petechial hemorrhage in infants or young children can be misinterpreted."

"Well, my question isn't whether they can be misinterpreted," Kelly said. He wanted to know if other doctors would be as confident in Smith's findings as he was.

"I'm sure you could find other physicians that would not share that confidence, yes."

The lawyer also asked Smith if he could say with absolute certainty that a seizure was not a factor in Kenneth's death.

"No, I cannot, and I can't on two bases. Number one is that it is possible there is some environmental situation that could cause it." And the second possibility was "if someone who is a pediatric neurologist comes along and disagrees with me, I could be convinced by such a person whose knowledge of seizures in young people is obviously much greater than mine."

The problem, from Tammy's perspective, was that her lawyers never found anyone to challenge Smith's opinions. They never found a pediatric neurologist with more expertise on seizures than Smith, or another pathologist to argue against Smith's testimony that the petechial hemorrhages he found were attributable to asphyxia. Nor did they speak to an expert on SUDEP.

The defence did consider calling their own medical experts. Clark and Kelly had approached Dr. Fred Jaffe, a titan of the forensic pathology field in Canada and one of the few experts in the country with the reputation, résumé and gravitas to counter the Crown's star witness. But Jaffe was getting ready to retire when the defence team called in 1994, so he declined. Jaffe also explained that he was a forensic pathologist; he said Tammy would be better served by a pediatric pathologist. But finding one wouldn't be easy. He wrote in a June 1994 letter to the lawyers, "It is a fact of life that, here in Toronto, all pediatric pathologists are associated with the Hospital for Sick Children and are, thus, colleagues of Dr. Smith." He suggested defence counsel speak with Dr. Chitra Rao, a respected forensic pathologist in Hamilton, Ontario.

Jaffe did, though, continue to consult on the case. After reviewing the testimony at the preliminary hearing, he was buoyed. Jaffe found Smith's testimony equivocal and was of the opinion that Dr. Huyer had overstepped his own expertise in opining on Kenneth's cause of death. Jaffe thought an acquittal was possible.

Dr. Rao was less enthusiastic. She considered Smith's autopsy report thorough and reasonable. She didn't believe Tammy's version of events. She didn't believe Kenneth had epilepsy; Rao reasoned that his seizures were caused by fevers, and the anticonvulsant medication he was on was appropriate.

Defence considered calling both Dr. Jaffe and Dr. Rao. But medical experts are expensive, and Tammy was on welfare when Kenneth died. She didn't have money to pay for her lawyers, let alone pathologists' consulting fees. Clark and Kelly were being paid through Legal Aid Ontario, which would provide funding to call only one expert witness.

In the end, they decided to call neither. Nor did the defence seek opinions from any other forensic experts.

It would be up to Tammy.

SIX

AFTER SITTING THROUGH eleven days of testimony from twenty-nine Crown witnesses, Tammy would be the first and last person to testify in her defence. Her lawyers had been pushing her not to take the stand. In fact, they didn't want to mount a defence at all. They never explained their rationale, or if they did, Tammy never understood it well enough to remember.

It is the Crown's responsibility to prove the murder charge. If the defence believed the Crown hadn't proved its case, keeping Tammy off the stand would prevent Crown prosecutors from cross-examining her. But declining to testify could make it look like she had something to hide. The Crown's version of events had been devastating. Tammy felt she needed to get her story on the record; it was the truth, after all.

On Thursday, October 19, 1995, Tammy Marquardt took the stand.

She and her defence team tackled the Crown's case head on. She tried to put her behaviour and the incriminating statements she'd made into some context.

She explained her conversation with Maureen Edwards. She had told the social worker she was worried she might hurt Kenneth; she hadn't meant intentionally. "Parent exhaustion," she explained. "I heard about that, and I was afraid what things can I do, what support can I have around me in case I do—when I become exhausted."

Steven Clark asked her about her conversation with another social worker, Cathy Sorichetti. "Ms. Sorichetti indicated to us you talked about imagining putting your arms or hands around his neck," he said.

"Yes."

"Did you discuss that specifically with her?"

"Yes, I did."

"What did you explain to her about that?"

"That when I was falling asleep, my hands were dropping to his neck and when I jerk awake, they would be around his neck and it scared me," Tammy explained.

"Did you have any concerns about anger towards Kenneth?"

"No, I didn't."

"Were you concerned about how Ms. Sorichetti might react to what you were telling her?"

"No, I wasn't."

"Why weren't you concerned about that?"

"Because I figured it was a support network and that's what they were there for is to support me."

When Tammy was struggling with parenting, when she made a mistake, she felt she should own up to it. She explained how she gave Kenneth a bruise on his leg when they were living at the YWCA in Oshawa. "Kenneth was having a temper tantrum and I just tried to restrain him by holding his legs down, and in turn I ended up causing him a bruise on his leg. It bothered me that I had done that."

"What do you mean it bothered you that you had done that?" Clark asked.

"The fact that I hurt him."

That's why she'd told Marlene Wikaruk, one of the supervisors at the Y, about the incident. "Because I felt bad about it." She understood the information would be passed on to Children's Aid. She was fine with that.

She said Kenneth's seizures worried her. That's why she took him to the hospital so often.

Tammy said it didn't bother her that Rick had fathered a child with someone else. It had happened during one of their off-again phases. She didn't hold it against him, and she didn't hold it against his ex, Jeanine. Jeanine had even babysat Kenneth a couple of times. So when Jeanine went into labour, Tammy felt it was important that Rick be there.

"Why did you want him to go?" Clark asked her.

"I know what it's like to be in labour and alone," Tammy replied.

She said again that she wasn't jealous, she wasn't mad.

"Did Rick have any money to get there?"

"No, he didn't."

"What did you do about that, if anything?"

"I lent him my bank card so he could go to the bank."

She told the story of how Kenneth died, told it as she had told it count-less times before—of finding him tangled in the bedsheet after his nap, of her frantic struggle to get him loose.

"Did you ever grab the sheets or try to rip them away?" Clark asked.

"No."

"Why not?"

"Because I was afraid he would get hurt, because if I pulled them the wrong way, it could hurt him."

Eventually, she said, she got his arms free. "One was behind his back and I pulled it out from behind his back, and the other one was up above his head and I pulled that one down."

"And why did you do that?"

"Just because I thought it was the right thing to do."

Kenneth had been thrashing his legs when Tammy first found him, but by the time she got his arms free, he had stopped moving. "I kept calling his name," she testified.

"Why did you do that?"

"To see if I could wake him up . . . He looked like he was sleeping."

"And what did you say to him, if anything?"

"I said, 'Kenneth, wake up. Mommy is here.' Just kept calling his name."

"Were you calm at that time?"

She said she wasn't.

"How did you feel?"

"I was scared."

"What were you scared about at that point, Tammy?"

"Everything. I didn't know what was happening."

"And how long did this go on for, Tammy?" Clark asked.

"It felt about 20 minutes."

"How do you know that?"

"That's just what it felt like."

When she finally got him untangled, she said, he was like a rag doll.

"Tammy, did you stop him from moving or kicking?"

"No, I didn't."

"Did you do anything to Kenneth to stop him from moving or kicking?"

"No."

"Did you stop him from breathing?"

"No."

"Did you put anything over his face, Tammy?"

"No. I tried to take the sheets off of his face."

"Did you smother Kenneth?"

"No."

"Did you take anything and place it over his face?"

"No."

She said she did forget how to do CPR. She had taken a course and practised on dummies. But in her moment of need, all her training was gone. "I couldn't remember," she testified.

"What do you mean, you couldn't remember?" Clark asked her.

"Everything was just blank."

But she still had hope. The paramedics arrived. They whisked Kenneth off to Oshawa General. Tammy was still frantic, but she started to calm down. She told her lawyer, "I felt that he could sense how I was feeling and if I had been as calm as I possibly could be, it would help him,"

By the time Kenneth was transferred to the Hospital for Sick Children, she had even managed to crack a smile. That's what she needed to help herself cope.

"What is it that allowed you to be calm at certain periods of time, Tammy?" her lawyer asked.

"Mostly talking about the good things that Kenneth did."

"Who would you be talking to about those kinds of things?"

"There was a person from the SCAN team"—the hospital's Suspected Child Abuse and Neglect team—"and they had asked how my pregnancy went with Kenneth, his development, different things he was doing."

Tammy told the court that, to help her cope after Kenneth died, she turned to alcohol. "I was going through a lot of scary stuff. I didn't quite understand my feelings. They were all mixed."

"What were you feeling, Tammy?" her lawyer asked.

"Scared. Confused. Angry. Hurt."

"What were you feeling angry about?"

"That Kenneth died."

Clark asked her why she was angry.

Tammy said because she felt people could have done more. "I was angry at the doctors because I thought maybe there could have been more things they could have done. I was angry at the ambulance attendants . . . because I felt like they could have gotten there faster and could have helped out faster."

"Even though you realize now they probably did."

"I think they did the best they could."

Tammy testified that she saved her greatest anger for herself. "I didn't have to take that nap. I didn't have to lay him down. I should have gone in to check on him instead of going to the bathroom first."

"What else?" Clark asked.

"I forgot my CPR."

The guilt and anger sent her into a free fall after Kenneth died.

"Were you still drinking a lot at this time, Tammy?"

"Yes, I was."

"And were you drunk for many of those days after Kenneth's funeral?"

"Yes."

"Did you have any concerns about being in that condition?"

"No."

"Why not?"

"Because I felt like if I drank enough I'll die."

The guilt and anger were slowly consuming her, until she blew up outside the bar and cemetery a couple of weeks later. "I was outside and I was just screaming at the top of my lungs."

"What were you screaming?"

"That 'I killed Kenneth.' . . . I remember saying that 'It's all my fault. I killed Kenneth. I forgot how to do CPR. It's all my fault.'"

"Who were you screaming that to?"

"Anybody who would listen . . . I wanted the whole world to know how I felt."

"How did you feel?"

"I felt like I had—because I forgot my CPR it was my fault. I felt like I killed him."

"You felt responsible."

"Yes."

She told the court she'd been trying to goad Rick into hurting her. "Behind the bar, he slapped me across the face."

"Why did he slap you in the face?"

"He said it was to try to calm me down, but all that did was make me more angry."

"Did you respond in any way?"

"I pointed at the other cheek and said, 'Even the odds. Hit the other cheek. Kill me.'"

Clark asked her why she had said that.

"I felt if he hit me on the other side, he's strong enough; he could kill me if he hit me hard enough."

The defence lawyer asked her about what she said to Stewart Powell that night outside the cemetery.

She agreed that she told him she'd killed Kenneth. "I felt like nobody was listening to me, and I grabbed him by the scuff of the neck and I remember growling into his face, saying, 'It's my fault. I killed Kenneth. Don't you understand? Because I forgot my CPR, it's all my fault.'"

Crown Lisa Cameron pressed Tammy in cross-examination about her frustrations with Rick. On the day she said she found Kenneth tangled in the bedsheet, Rick had gone to the hospital because his ex was giving birth. But he already had another child with another woman, whom he was continuing to see.

"At first," Tammy explained, "I knew it was because he wanted to see JD [his son], and in order to for him to get weekend visits he needed to see him on a regular basis, and I understood that and I was okay with it."

"Yes, but I'm not asking you about that," Cameron said. "I'm asking you how did you feel? You thought he was cheating on you, right?"

"Yes," Tammy testified.

"How did you feel about that?"

"It hurt." But Tammy said she never spoke to Rick about her suspicions. She said she wasn't sure she was right. But she was sure enough to leave him in June 1993. That's why she went to stay with her sister, Carol— to get away from Rick.

Cameron asked Tammy about a conversation she had had with her sister. "You asked her to watch over you because you had a bad temper and you didn't want to hurt Kenneth. You didn't want to take it out on him."

"I didn't want to be yelling at him, that's what I meant by taking it out on him," Tammy explained.

"So you did say something like that to her?"

Tammy said she did.

"Because this morning you said you never said anything to Carol about hurting Kenneth."

Tammy said she couldn't remember her exact words, but what she was asking her sister for was help. "Getting my life stable, trying to get life back on some kind of track, have Kenneth on a schedule."

"Well, you may not be sure of your exact words, but it's a little different if your position is that you never said anything to her about it."

Cameron reviewed how Rick and Tammy had reconciled later that summer and got an apartment together in Oshawa. Then Kenneth broke his leg and spent the month of September in hospital. Cameron asked Tammy if Kenneth's absence made life better with Rick. "Would it be fair to say the fact that it was just the two of you allowed for the two of you to become closer?"

"No," Tammy replied.

"It wasn't, in a sense, a bit of a honeymoon period, having just gotten back together recently and now having some time on your own, just the two of you?"

Tammy didn't see it that way. "I was mostly up at the hospital with Kenneth."

Cameron asked if she and Rick were back on the outs by October 9, the day Kenneth collapsed. She reminded the court that Rick had left that morning to be with his ex-girlfriend when she gave birth to their child. "Did that not affect you?" she asked.

"No," Tammy said, "because I knew he was going to do that. Him and I had agreed before that that's what he was going to do."

Cameron asked if Tammy had ever done the math and counted back to figure out when Rick's ex got pregnant.

"She got pregnant roughly in January," Tammy answered. That was only weeks before she and Rick got married.

"And did that not kind of have an effect on you thinking, 'Gee, you know, just before we get married he's having a relationship with this other woman'?"

"No, because him and I were broken up at the time that she got pregnant."

The Crown persisted. "And you left Rick in the summer because he was seeing another woman, not Jeanine but Michelle. At least in your mind you felt he was. And then this morning he's off to have another child and it doesn't bring any of your anger or frustration about these other times back?"

Tammy said it didn't. "I knew he would be coming home once the baby was born."

Cameron then pressed her on her statements to social workers and child protection workers. "Isn't it fair to say that your concern was not really so much about parental exhaustion, but the fact that you had contemplated deliberately putting your hands around Kenneth's neck?"

"It wasn't deliberate," Tammy insisted.

The Crown asked about the conversation Tammy had had with Cathy Sorichetti, in which she admitted imagining putting her hand over Kenneth's nose and mouth. Cameron hinted at deception in Tammy's earlier testimony. "You didn't mention this this morning, but you recall telling her that you realize that was dangerous."

Tammy agreed.

"And that you took your hand away," Cameron continued.

"No, because I imagined that I was doing it. I didn't, in fact, do it physically."

"So it was not a situation where you had just put your hand over his mouth, that frightened you and you took your hand away. You imagined all this. Is this your position?"

"What it was that frightened me was the thought that I was imagining myself doing that, and it scared me because I know that you can't do that to a child." Tammy explained that all of her outreach was about being proactive. She was exhausted. She didn't want Kenneth to get hurt.

"What was it about being exhausted that made you think you would harm Kenneth?" Cameron asked.

"Because being exhausted, I could drop him . . . My muscles were really tired and I was afraid he could get hurt."

"So you're saying today that's not a case that, in fact, what your concern was if you were tired, understandably with a newborn, and frustrated, again understandably, that you would lose your temper and do something to Kenneth?"

"No."

"So it wasn't anything like that. It wasn't a matter of your exhaustion making you not able to control your feelings to the point where you might act out your frustrations on Kenneth."

"That's the one thing I would never do. That's why I always had a good support system, tried to have a good support system around me so I could talk to people about how I felt."

"You never wanted to be in a position where you would actually do something to Kenneth because of your exhaustion and frustration or whatever."

"I didn't feel that I would, but I wanted to be sure."

"I'm suggesting that you talked to so many people about this [because] this was a significant concern to you that you might harm Kenneth."

"Not on purpose, no."

"Your position is that you would not, even if you were tired or frustrated or whatever, you would not deliberately hurt Kenneth."

"Right."

The Crown suggested there were inconsistencies in her story. "Are you having difficulty keeping up with all the various things that you've said to people over the time?"

Tammy said she was not.

In her closing address to the jury, Crown counsel Lisa Cameron returned to what she considered inconsistencies in Tammy's story. "She told Dr. Mehra that she was told to do CPR but panicked and couldn't do anything. She told Officer Terry she tried to do CPR. She told Detective Naccarato she tried to do CPR. She told Detective Naccarato again that she got one breath into Kenneth. And at trial, she said [in her direct testimony] she tried, but in cross that she was able to get some air in but only a little bit.

"They may seem like small differences, but added to the catalogue of those kind of inconsistencies and what I would say are manipulations, they create . . . a situation where it makes it very difficult to believe anything that the accused has had to say."

The defence tried to paint another picture of the tragedy. In his closing arguments, Steven Clark characterized Kenneth's death as a "death by accident."

"I'm suggesting to you that the young child died by suffocation on the sheets or by a seizure," Clark told the jury. "Tammy has denied killing her child. She didn't deny it after she had a time to reflect. That's when people decide if they have done something." Instead, he pointed out, she gave a videotaped statement within hours of Kenneth being rushed to hospital.

Clark suggested that Dr. Smith and the other medical experts didn't adequately consider that Kenneth's death may have been an accident. "It's not a cheap shot," he said to the jury. "I'm not suggesting for a moment that Dr. Smith and Dr. Logan, most importantly Dr. Smith, wasn't going about his job the way he would do on each and every occasion. Very experienced and very eminent medical practitioner.

"I'm just asking, was the alternative that we suggest ever considered by the doctors? No one looked carefully at his history. Not because they were being negligent. Not because they were being incompetent. Because it was a stone, ladies and gentlemen, that wasn't turned over. That's what I'm suggesting."

At the end of his closing arguments, the defence lawyer told the jury a story to help them understand how he felt they should approach their deliberations. "When we're looking at things, let's not just look at what is on the face of things. Your function is not to look beyond the evidence necessarily, but when assessing the evidence perhaps this story will assist you," Clark said.

"A man was standing under a light with a stick in the dirt, and he's fishing around with his stick and obviously looking for something. Somebody comes and says to him, 'What are you doing?' And he says, 'I'm looking for my wallet. I lost my wallet.' And he asks, 'Where did you lose it?' And the man says, 'I lost it over there.' And he said, 'Then why are you looking over here?' And the man said, 'Because the light is better over here.'

"I'm asking you to consider that the truth doesn't always lie where it is on the face of things," Clark said. "Don't miss the truth, because the truth could lie somewhere other than where the light is."

The jurors began their deliberations on the morning of Tuesday, October 24, 1995. Later that day, they returned with their unanimous verdict: Tammy Marquardt was guilty of second-degree murder.

A second-degree murder conviction comes with a mandatory life sentence. The question was how long Tammy would have to spend behind bars before she could apply for parole and possibly be released. Six weeks later, at her sentencing hearing, she found out.

The minimum parole ineligibility period for second-degree murder is ten years, and in the end, that's what the judge gave her. Twenty-three-year-old Tammy Marquardt would be spending the next decade of her life—at least—in prison.

Tammy's conviction would not only cost her her freedom. It would also cost her any hope of keeping custody of her son Keith. She had held out hope that if she was acquitted she could get him back.

Tammy was being sent to the Prison for Women, in Kingston, Ontario. She had been able to see Keith at the Children's Aid office while she was out on bail, but he wouldn't be making the trek east with her to Kingston.

Her family lawyer explained that Keith would become a ward of the state after two years in foster care. He was fourteen months old when Tammy was convicted. Once she was convicted, there was no point fighting for custody. She had been trying desperately to find someone to take Keith. Children's Aid will place children with relatives or friends if they're cleared as capable caregivers. But no one in her family would take him. And none of her friends could. Children's Aid said they had a couple eager to adopt him.

SEVEN

BRIAN AND EILEEN Hutton weren't overly concerned. Sure, a murder conviction made the circumstances of the adoption a little strange, and it would make an already difficult conversation about Keith's biological mother even more difficult. But that was years down the road yet; the couple weren't thinking about that. For five years they had tried to conceive a child. When that proved impossible they tried a private adoption, but on the day the young mother gave birth she decided to keep her baby. The next mother who agreed to have her baby adopted by the Huttons changed her mind one month before her due date. After the third failed attempt at a private adoption, the Huttons investigated adopting a baby from overseas. The cost of pursuing that option, however, proved prohibitive for the couple, who had already spent thousands of dollars trying to create their family. They came very close to adopting a young brother and sister through Children's Aid, but their hearts were broken yet again when that adoption fell through as well. Now, their most pressing concern was simply to get Keith, and to be allowed to keep him. And Children's Aid assured the couple that Keith was officially a Crown ward; Tammy no longer had any parental rights. Even if she won an appeal of her conviction, she would not be able to get him back. Keith would be their son forever.

They met him for the first time in December 1995. He was sixteen months old. Brian and Eileen were beside themselves. After a decade of false starts and failures, they were finally starting a family. And in early January, he came home for good. The nursery room was barely finished. After the pain of earlier near misses, the couple refused to finish it until things were official. It was still painted blue from the first go-around; a friend gave them a crib, and they rushed to fill out the room with baby furniture. It was done with only days to spare.

And then they found out that their young family would likely be growing again—and soon.

Once Tammy was sentenced, guards took her from court to the Whitby "bucket," the local jail where she'd been processed after her arrest. Intake involved another battery of tests, and with them another surprise: she was pregnant again.

Tammy couldn't believe it, although part of her wasn't surprised at all. She hadn't been trying to get pregnant. She was just very fertile. She'd been on the pill when she got pregnant with Kenneth. This time she'd been on the pill *and* using condoms.

Tammy had met Clayton John Eric Brown in rehab. He was a recovering heroin addict. And he had a jealous streak. During the run-up to her trial, Tammy spent a lot of time with her lawyers prepping. Brown accused her of sleeping with one of them.

They dated for a couple of months, but by the time her trial got under way, he had started to disappear. After her conviction, she never saw him again.

There was one consolation: this time, she was clean. Keith had been conceived just before Kenneth's death, and Tammy had tried hard to drink her grief away in the weeks after, not realizing she was pregnant. She still worried what the long-term consequences of that might be. But with this baby, she didn't have to worry. Drugs and alcohol had been strictly prohibited under her bail conditions, and she'd managed to adhere to them.

After she was processed, Tammy was placed on suicide watch and sent down to a segregation cell. The guards gave her a "baby doll" sleeper, which was little more than a life-sized rag with holes cut out for her arms and head. Her blanket was small, hard and itchy, more like a rug than something you'd sleep under.

The Prison for Women was a daunting place. Opened in 1934, P4W was Canada's only maximum-security prison for women until its phased closure began in 1995. Madam Justice Louise Arbour, who led a judicial inquiry into the facility after a riot there in 1994, noted the prison had been described as "unfit for bears." Justice Arbour wrote in her final report: "The prison is an old fashioned, dysfunctional labyrinth of claustrophobic and inadequate spaces holding 142 prisoners of all security levels, minimum through maximum . . . It is inadequate for living, working, eating, programming, recreation and administration. Spaces are insufficient, poorly ventilated and noisy. They are not well connected, and frequently can only be reached through narrow corridors, steep stairwells (there are no elevators), and innumerable locked barriers . . . [The entire cell area] is usually very noisy, made as it is of bare cement and metal."

This was the prison Tammy Marquardt was stepping into as a convicted child murderer.

Tammy and the other new prisoners were first taken to Admissions and Discharge. Everyone was strip-searched, then given their prison kit: two pairs of sweatpants, two sweaters, two T-shirts, five pairs of underwear, five pairs of socks, two bras, four towels, four facecloths, two sheets, one pillow, one pillowcase, a blue blanket and some basic toiletries and personal hygiene products. All of her worldly belongings could now fit inside a pillowcase.

After intake, the new inmates were taken to see the OIC, or the officer-in-charge. His name was Barry McGinnis, and he had some words of advice for Tammy. "If you want that child to live," he said, pointing to her stomach, "you don't tell anyone what you're in here for."

It had never occurred to Tammy that none of the other inmates would know what she was in for. She asked McGinnis what she should say if people asked.

"Tell them you killed your husband," he said.

It was good advice, crucial advice; advice he didn't have to give her. She was never sure whether he told her for her baby's sake, for her own safety or to save himself the trouble of dealing with the aftermath if an inmate tried to beat her to death.

P4W was a multi-security prison, since at the time it was the only women's penal institution in the country. The prison was made up of two ranges, called A and B, a segregation unit and a separate area called the Wing. New inmates—the "fresh fish"—were housed in A range; B range was for the troublemakers, the inmates who liked to start fights and otherwise stir up trouble. Protective custody was in the segregation unit; it was for the baby killers and "goofs"—the pedophiles. The protective custody–special needs unit housed the mentally unstable. The Wing— split into North and South sections—was for minimum-security inmates, or lifers. Inmates were given slightly more freedom down on the Wing, where the cells looked a bit more like rooms than concrete boxes. The Wing was the carrot; if you behaved yourself, that's where they'd put you.

Tammy started out double-bunked on A range. A and B ranges were long, two-tier corridors that ran parallel to each other. Though the walls were concrete, sound travelled through them as if they were paper. Each range housed more than fifty cells, tiny boxes that barely measured nine feet by six. Jammed inside each was a metal bunk bed with mattresses that weren't much thicker than a folded-up blanket. There was a tall cabinet for personal belongings, a metal desk, a metal drawer, a sink on one wall. The toilet was mounted on the back wall, behind the bed. It was such a tight squeeze that the front of the toilet was under the lip of the bed, making it almost impossible to sit on the toilet properly. You had to either sit sideways or straddle the toilet and then carefully slide your feet under the bed frame and your knees up against it in order to sit down. Tammy was barely five feet tall and eighty-five pounds and even she couldn't sit on it properly.

And there was no hope of privacy. Prisoners were allowed to hang a blanket across the metal bars of their cells, but the door itself always had to be kept clear. Inmates and guards, female and male, could see inside as a prisoner squatted in the back corner.

And then there was her roommate. Tammy would be sharing the tiny cell with another pregnant inmate. When she couldn't hold it any longer, Tammy would have to shit in the open cell with her roommate within arm's reach.

But that indignity didn't last long. Lifers weren't supposed to be double-bunked. At her first meal that evening, Tammy met the chair of the lifers group, who immediately started petitioning for her to move down to the

Wing, where living conditions were more passable. The cells there had locks on the inside. The guards could still open them, but it gave the inmates some privacy from other inmates. Tammy was transferred down to the Wing after a month.

She'd been living on the Wing just a couple of weeks when another lifer called her into her cell. Her name was Agatha, and she was pushing seventy, Tammy figured. She was a nice woman who'd taken Tammy under her wing. Agatha reminded her of Tweety Bird's Granny: matronly, but fierce when someone she cared for came under threat.

Agatha asked Tammy if she watched the news. Tammy shook her head. Agatha said she'd seen a story that she thought might be about Tammy, and asked her point-blank what she was really in for.

Tammy started to sob. She hadn't meant to lie, she admitted, but she'd been warned she'd have to if she wanted her baby to live. Agatha only cared what Tammy had been convicted of.

"They said I killed my son."

Agatha said she would get the guards to move Tammy into protective custody, or PC, a separate unit that was a sort of prison within the prison, meant for inmates who couldn't live in the general population because their crimes made them targets—crimes like killing your child.

As if on cue, inmates began banging on Agatha's cell door, screaming obscenities. "Get that fucking baby killer out of here!" "She's just having that kid so she can kill another one!" "We're going to fucking kill her! We're going to torture her!" "Let her out, you bitch! You're harbouring a baby killer!"

The screaming continued for several minutes; it felt like hours to Tammy, cowering in the cell while inmates pounded on the bars and threatened to beat her to death. Prison guards finally arrived to clear the hallway and take Tammy away. They took her first to segregation. She was strip-searched again, and that's when she realized she was covered in blood. The baby was in distress.

The guards rushed her to the health care unit, which then rushed her to Kingston General Hospital. There, the obstetrician gave her a quick examination and an ultrasound. The baby was fine, she said. No need to worry, just some spot bleeding.

Back at the prison, Tammy was returned to segregation. Her bleeding slowed but didn't stop. After a couple of days, she was transferred to the protective custody unit. This was actually two units: protective custody, and protective custody–special needs. Tammy ended up in the special needs unit at first. The cell was just outside the guards' office, and she was under constant supervision. She wasn't allowed out except to shower. She was then moved to protective custody.

It would be her home for the rest of her time at P4W, locked away from the other inmates for her own protection.

"Basically, you had a price on your head [in protective custody]. You were targeted the second you walked in there," Tammy recalled years later.

She would be living alongside baby killers and pedophiles, the mentally unhinged and "psychos." She'd be living in the same unit as Karla Homolka.

Tammy remembers watching Homolka bounce down the stairs, her hair pulled back in a girlish ponytail. She reminded Tammy of Marsha from *The Brady Bunch*.

"Hi, I'm Karla," a bubbly Homolka said outside Tammy's cell. "If you need anything, just holler up and I'll get it for you."

Tammy only nodded. She couldn't bring herself to respond.

They didn't become friends. Tammy kept her distance, and the serial killer didn't push it. But some interactions were unavoidable. Karla was the prisoner representative for the protective custody unit. Any complaints Tammy had about life in PC needed to be funnelled through Karla, who would bring them to the inmate committee and eventually the prison administration. So although some conversation was inevitable, Tammy said she did her best to keep it to a minimum.

Despite the close quarters, there weren't that many opportunities to interact anyway. There were no shared meals in a mess hall. In PC, inmates ate their meals alone, locked in their cells. The unit was on almost constant lockdown, not because of disruptions there but because both of the two

PC guards needed to be present if the cells were to be left open. But one of the guards was frequently called away to help quell disruptions in other parts of the prison, leaving only one on duty—and leaving everyone locked in their cells.

Teresa and Lauralie were the only other women in protective custody. Tammy wasn't sure what they were in for, but the talk among inmates was that they had killed their children. Lauralie was tight with Karla, at least when Karla was within earshot. Otherwise Lauralie would complain that she couldn't stand her. Teresa was large, aggressive and moody.

They had occasional access to the adjacent protective custody–special needs unit as well, but it wasn't a place you'd want to visit. That's where the mentally unstable prisoners were housed, the ones who likely should have been in a hospital rather than a prison. They wailed and screamed, banged their heads against the metal bars of their cell doors. Several tried to kill themselves. One woman threw her own feces at other inmates if they got too close to her cell.

And that was Tammy's world: two alleged child killers, Karla Homolka and a ward full of the mentally unhinged.

Moving around the prison was a problem. P4W was a violent, dangerous place—especially for convicted child killers. But Tammy needed to get around—she was pregnant. She had regular pre-natal appointments in the health clinic, plus she had prison-mandated sessions with a psychologist. But getting from her cell to her appointments could be dangerous.

As a convicted child killer, Tammy was always escorted by a prison guard, who would take her down to a basement tunnel to move her about the prison.

"The tunnel was the danger zone," Tammy explained years later. "There were little hidden corners, little breaks in the walls. I had coffee thrown at me. I had shoes thrown at me. I had bodily fluids thrown at me. I had one girl come up behind us and hit me with her coffee cup."

There was a blind corner at the end of the tunnel. The lighting was poor, the shadows were long, and you had no idea who was waiting around the corner. And sometimes Tammy's escort turned away.

"That was the extreme danger zone," she said. "That's where I got jumped more times than I care to remember. The guard would just walk away or turn around." One time, four women were waiting for Tammy. At first she fought back, but she soon realized it was pointless—it was far from a fair fight. So Tammy learned to go down quickly, turtling on the floor, her arms protecting her head, her legs pulled up tightly to protect her abdomen as a torrent of fists and feet pounded her. "It was only after I was down on the ground that I guess the guard figured, 'That's enough. Don't actually kill her.' Then she would step in."

Eric Anthony Steven Marquardt was born on June 20, 1996, at Kingston General Hospital. Tammy gave birth in shackles and handcuffs. The prison guards refused to take them off because she was a maximum-security prisoner. As well, Tammy was appealing her conviction, which made her a flight risk.

The restraints meant she couldn't get her feet into the stirrups for the birth. She pulled her feet up and in, pushing her knees out to the side, her legs contorted into a diamond shape. The obstetrician draped a blanket over her legs and did the best he could. Labour lasted a day and a half.

After the birth, the guards undid her handcuffs so she could hold her newborn. But they kept the shackles on and chained one arm to the wheelchair. She did her best to breathe in her son, to memorize the lines and creases of his face. Then the social workers bundled Eric up and took him away. Tammy shuffled into the prison transfer wagon and headed back to P4W.

Children's Aid workers wouldn't make any promises, but they told the Huttons they expected Tammy to relinquish her rights at birth. The couple could likely take the newborn home shortly after that.

The transition, however, was not going to be as smooth as they had hoped. About a week after Eric's birth, Children's Aid told the Huttons they wouldn't be taking him anytime soon. Tammy had decided not to relinquish her parental rights. She was appealing her conviction, and she didn't want to make any decisions until it was heard. But Children's Aid assured the Huttons it was only a matter of time, they just needed to be patient.

Children's Aid was supposed to bring Eric to the prison each week for a visit, but that didn't happen with any regularity. And no one would tell Tammy when a visit was being cancelled. She would spend all week fixated on the prospect of seeing her baby, only to be told that morning that it wasn't happening. No explanation was ever given. And when the visits did take place, Tammy still had to risk the tunnel and the violence of its blind corners to get to the visitation centre. But it was worth it. The visits with Eric were the only thing that kept Tammy going. The visits and her appeal.

Tammy was furious about her conviction, and did her best to hold on to that indignation; to use it as fuel propelling her appeal. But hopelessness is also a powerful emotion—and hopelessness was all around her, impossible to escape. By the end of the year, she was ready to let Eric go. She was a convicted child killer who risked a life-threatening beating every time she left her cell. What were the chances she'd be able to beat a system so clearly stacked against her? Her appeal hearing was still more than a year away. The thought of Eric being raised in foster care just added to her anguish. He needed a proper family.

Tammy had never had the chance to properly say goodbye to Keith. After she was convicted, Children's Aid had said they would bring him to the Whitby jail for a final visit. Tammy had said no, she didn't want them to bring her son to such a dark, dangerous place. "Wait until I get settled into prison in Kingston," she asked, not realizing that P4W would be just as dark and dangerous.

Her last visit with Eric was in December 1996. The boy was six months old. He was a beautiful baby, chubby and cherub-like sitting in her arms in that concrete tomb of a visiting room. A guard took pictures during the farewell visit, using a camera belonging to Tammy's social development worker. Tammy had bought some photo film from the prison canteen and paid in advance for the developing. It felt like the visit had barely started and suddenly it was over. She watched helplessly as the Children's Aid worker packed up Eric's baby bag, then she waved at his little face from over the woman's shoulder as they stepped through the door.

With that, Tammy Wynne lost another child.

She had told her Children's Aid worker that she would give up custody and relinquish her parental rights on one condition: her boys needed to be placed with the same parents. If Keith and Eric couldn't have her in their lives, at least they would have each other. The Huttons were happy to oblige. Eric was seven months old when the adoption was finalized.

Tammy's pictures never arrived. The worker left the film in the camera and forgot all about it. "The film was used over again with somebody else's pictures," Tammy would tell me almost twenty years later, "so none of my farewell pictures came out."

NICHOLAS I

ONE

BY THE TIME Lianne Gagnon started her first year at Laurentian University, in Sudbury, Ontario, studying English and history, she and her boyfriend, Steve Tolin, had been inseparable for three years. But she knew their lives were quickly diverging. Steve, two years younger, was still in high school, just starting Grade 11. They still lived in the same city, but their needs and wants were suddenly different: Lianne was starting a new phase in her young life; Steve was still finishing his old one. It's an obstacle thousands of high school sweethearts face every fall. Most don't survive the change, but Lianne and Steve promised themselves they were going to try.

Then Lianne got pregnant. Steve didn't want her to keep it. They were too young, he argued. They weren't ready to be parents. He told her that his mother and father had been young and ill prepared for parenthood when he was born, a fact he'd blamed for a less than perfect childhood. Lianne had always thought of herself as pro-choice. And her choice now was to keep the baby. She was going to be a mother.

Lianne told her mother, Angie, first. She wasn't sure how her father would take the news, so she waited nervously at a girlfriend's house as her mother cushioned the blow.

Maurice Gagnon knew his daughter had always been a good kid, responsible almost to a fault. She wasn't a big partier, and when she was out late with friends, she would call home a couple of times just to let them know she was all right. Maurice was proud to see her doing so well at university. On top of her classes, she was the sports editor at the *Lambda*, the English-language newspaper at Laurentian, and she was a volunteer at the SPCA.

So when Angie sat him down at the dining room table, an unplanned pregnancy was the last thing he was expecting. When Lianne got home, her parents were waiting for her on the sofa in the TV room. It looked like both had been crying. Lianne slid into the chair, bracing herself.

Her father asked if she was considering an abortion. She said her plan was to keep the baby. He told her they would convert the basement into an apartment for her and the baby. He also told her she would be finishing university. She would not quit school.

It was a brief, difficult conversation, and *so* much better than Lianne had expected. She knew how hard this was going to be for her parents. That her father was able to keep his frustration and disappointment in check was a minor miracle. And if she had any doubts about her parents, they were dispelled a week later when Maurice came home with a stuffed dog from *101 Dalmatians* for the baby's room. Lianne had a weakness for Disney, and *101 Dalmatians* was her favourite. An olive branch Lianne gladly accepted.

Her due date was December 30, 1994, midway through her second year. Lianne carried a full course load during the first semester. Pregnancy was a breeze: no morning sickness or exhaustion and just a touch of nausea at the very beginning. Lianne worried that she would pay for that good fortune with a long, arduous labour. Her mother had suffered through difficult deliveries with both her and her older brother, Maurice Jr.

Lianne went to see her doctor the morning of January 2 and was induced the same day. In the end the labour was quick, and eight-pound Nicholas Maurice Gagnon was born at 10:37 that night.

He became the centre of the Gagnons' world. A random gas-induced smile had the power to melt three hearts simultaneously. But those first months were not easy. Nicholas suffered from ear-splitting, headache-inducing, sleep-depriving colic. The Gagnons took turns trying to soothe him, walking the hallway from the den at the back of their Greenbriar Drive house through the kitchen in the middle to the living room/dining room at the front, back and forth, back and forth, night after night, for two months.

It was a difficult time for other reasons too. The stress and strain that had been steadily building between Lianne and Steve finally spilled over that winter, and shortly after Nicholas's birth they decided to end their relationship for good. Steve came by the house less and less, until he was largely uninvolved. Lianne had suspected all along that this was how things would go, but the finality of their breakup was still painful and isolating.

Thankfully neither the colic nor the heartache lasted long. At three months, Nicholas found his personality—curious, quick to smile, with a bottomless appetite—and Lianne settled into her new life.

She took Nicholas everywhere, even to university. She'd leave him in the student centre with her best friend, Sophie Laframboise, while she ran off to class. One day she took him with her when she had to take a picture of the men's hockey team for the school newspaper. Little Nicholas ended up sitting in the middle, a miniature team mascot.

Maurice was the most visible man in Nicholas's life, and he started to see the youngster as more of a son than a grandson. He used to love listening to the steady in and out, in and out, of Nicholas's breathing over the monitor as he slept in his nursery downstairs. Maurice showered the baby with gifts. He worked for the Ontario government and travelled regularly, often to Toronto. He always left room in his luggage for the latest plush toys, knickknacks and baby clothes he picked up at the flagship Disney Store in the Eaton Centre.

And then there was the dancing. Little Nico danced almost every night with his Pépère. Two of their favourite songs were "Sleep Walk," an instrumental lament from the film *La Bamba*, and Tom Petty's "You Don't Know How It Feels." Nicholas would lean into the music, listening to Petty's voice and the steady rhythm of the drums, waiting, waiting for the electric guitar to smash into it, almost squealing with excitement. The sight of him jumping when the wail of the guitar finally landed is one of the fondest memories that both Maurice and Lianne have of the little boy.

Five weeks after Tammy Marquardt was convicted in an Oshawa court-room of murdering her son, Lianne's misery began four hundred kilometres away. Nicholas woke at eight thirty. Angie had already left for work, and Maurice was in Toronto on business. Lianne dressed him and gave him a bottle of Pablum for breakfast. A month shy of his first birthday, Nicholas was into everything. At one point that morning in the bathroom, when Lianne turned her back for a second, he got into the cleaning supplies under the sink, but she quickly pulled him away.

They spent the rest of the morning playing. She had no classes that day. Nicholas went down for his morning nap around eleven, falling asleep in her arms in the rocking chair. Normally Lianne would put him down in his crib once he dozed off, but she left him there that morning, a ball of heat on her shoulder.

Nicholas was a good sleeper, and he didn't wake until almost one. After a quick lunch of spaghetti, Lianne nestled him in a pile of blankets in the antique wooden sled she had just picked up, and the two headed out for a sleigh ride.

"Perfect day for it," Lynne Monk, a neighbour from across the street, called out.

"It's his first time," Lianne called back.

Lynne looked over at the youngster. He was barely visible amidst the folds of his puffy snowsuit and the sea of blankets. "Just be careful with that," she said, nodding at the rope that Lianne was tugging on. "He's getting big. You'll throw out your back if you're not careful."

Lianne nodded and headed off down the street. It was a glorious day, everything freshly buried under the first snowfall of the season, front lawns and snowbanks bright in the midday sun. The pair spent almost an hour weaving through the streets of their north Sudbury neighbourhood.

The fresh air and excitement tired Nicholas out, and he went down without a fuss for his afternoon nap. Again Lianne left him to sleep on her shoulder, sitting happily in the rocking chair for more than an hour as he snoozed.

He stirred around four, and she took him upstairs, where he sat on the kitchen floor, playing as she made him Kraft Dinner, his first taste of the classic. Lianne plopped down on the loveseat in the family room and he sat in her lap as she fed him, noodle by noodle—but only for a while. Nicholas had just learned to walk and was now always eager to go, though he was still unsteady on his feet. After a few minutes, Lianne relented, letting him slide off her lap to play with his toys and the family's Lakeland terrier, Winnie, and to explore the room. He would hurry back to her every half minute or so for another bite, and then head off again. He wandered over to the back corner of the room, underneath Angie's sewing machine. It was a favourite spot of his. With its low windows that ran into the corner along both walls, he liked to sit and stare out at the backyard and the in-ground pool.

Lianne heard a scream from the corner, and she saw Nicholas drop down onto his bum underneath the sewing machine. Her first thought: the poor guy had bumped his head on the underside of the machine. But there was something about his cry that alarmed her. It sounded more like a yelp, a half cry almost, as if he was trying to wail but couldn't generate enough breath to power it.

Lianne ran over and scooped him up, pulled him in close to her chest. "It's okay, Nico. It's okay. Mommy's got you," she said as she walked back across the room, rubbing his back, trying to soothe him. He didn't make a sound.

She lifted him off her chest, holding him away from her so she could get a better look. The moment she saw his face, she knew he wasn't breathing.

Lynne Monk was just sitting down to dinner with her husband, Ron, and their two young sons, chili bubbling in the slow cooker, when she heard a dog barking. Before she could consider whose it was and why it was upset, the side door burst open and in rushed Lianne, Winnie at her heels. She was carrying Nicholas, who was limp in her arms. And neither of them was wearing any winter clothes—no jacket, scarves or mitts, so different from a few hours earlier when Lynne had seen the two of them bundled up for their sleigh ride.

"He's not breathing!" Lianne screamed as she handed Nicholas to Lynne's shocked husband, who promptly handed the child to Lynne.

All the neighbours were under the mistaken impression that Lynne Monk was a registered nurse. She wasn't; she had once worked as a lab technologist. Luckily, though, both Lynne and Ron had recently taken a CPR course that had covered resuscitation for young children. And the first rule she had learned was an important one: take control of the situation.

She ordered Ron to call 911 and sent her two boys off to the living room to wait for the first responders.

Lynne gently laid Nicholas down on the cool linoleum floor in the kitchen. Lianne was hysterical, but managed to blurt out the basic details of what had happened: Nicholas bumped his head on the underside of the sewing machine, let out one cry and suddenly stopped breathing. Lianne had thumped him on the back in case he was choking, but nothing came up. She didn't know what else to do, so she squeezed him tight and ran across the street. She pleaded with Lynne to help him.

Lynne pulled open his blue sleeper. He was wearing a light blue shirt underneath. There were no signs of injuries that she could see. His eyes were half-closed, rolled back in his head. The outer edges of his lips were blue but he still had colour in his face. She checked his neck for a pulse but couldn't find one, then rechecked, worried that her shaking hands might be the culprit. Still no pulse.

"Is he breathing?" Lianne screamed.

Too focused to even acknowledge the question, Lynne propped up Nicholas's neck and pinched his nostrils to start CPR, but his mouth was clenched shut. So she gently blew some air through his nostrils. His jaw released, but he still wasn't responding to her efforts. His lips were getting bluer, and the colour was draining out of his face.

Lianne couldn't watch and backed out the kitchen door. The Monks let her go.

Nicholas's airway was blocked. Lynne's first thought was that he was choking on a button he'd picked up underneath the sewing machine. She bent the baby over her forearm and gave him three sharp smacks to the back, trying to dislodge whatever was caught in his throat. But nothing seemed to work.

Lynne Monk knew she was losing him.

Maurice Gagnon wasn't supposed to be home until later that evening, but his last meeting was cancelled and he managed to catch an earlier flight. He'd still had time to stop off at the Disney Store to pick up another stuffed animal for Nicholas.

As he rounded the corner, he immediately knew something was wrong. Lianne was pacing in the Monks' driveway, and she wasn't wearing a jacket. Maurice quickly parked the car and ran across the street.

Lianne could barely get the words out: Nicholas had bumped his head and wasn't breathing. The two of them rushed inside.

Maurice, desperate for reassurances, peppered Lynne with questions as she huddled over Nicholas's body on the floor. But Lynne could offer him no comfort. None of her efforts were working.

Another of the cardinal rules of her CPR training was to never put your finger in a person's mouth because you'll likely only push whatever is stuck in the airway farther down the throat. But nothing else was working, so Lynne carefully flicked her finger down Nicholas's throat. She couldn't feel anything, so she flipped him over and tried banging his back again. This time it brought up a pink froth, but nothing else. His skin was now a pallid grey, his lips fully blue.

Scanning his tiny body for any sign of life, Lynne knew in her heart that he was gone, even if her mind wouldn't grasp it.

"The ambulance is here, Mom!" one of the boys called from the living room.

Lynne stepped away from the body as André Groulx, one of the two paramedics, took over resuscitation efforts. After two quick blows, he suspected something must be blocking the child's airway. Groulx turned the child over and gave him several back blows. He was able to remove a small amount of mucus from his airway.

"It's clear," he said to his partner, Barry Stenabough. Lynne looked up. By now, firefighters had also arrived, and one began helping Groulx with CPR as they rushed Nicholas out to the ambulance. And then they were gone.

Lynne slumped over on the floor. One thought kept circling around in her mind: *Maybe I killed him; maybe it was my fault.*

She went over everything she had done, searching for a sign that would either put her mind at rest or confirm her fears, but her thoughts were racing too quickly, flashing images of tiny Nicholas in his blue sleeper and light-blue onesie lying on the floor beneath her. He was so small, so fragile. When she laid him down, he was still in there. She could see it in his colour, could still feel his presence—he was still alive. He was saveable. And then he was gone.

Angie Gagnon's hairdresser had just started her highlights when Lianne called. There had been an accident—Nicholas wasn't breathing and paramedics had rushed him to Sudbury General Hospital.

"You have to get this stuff out of my hair," Angie said as she hung up the phone. "I have to get to the hospital!"

She was the first to arrive. Nicholas was in the ER, but hospital staff wouldn't let her in to see him. They were still trying to revive him. He had come in at 5:15 p.m. Dr. Miriam Mann led the resuscitation efforts. It had been almost twenty minutes since he'd bumped his head, and he still had no heartbeat. His skin had started to go blotchy.

Angie was shown into a family waiting room where a chaplain was waiting for her. Lianne and Maurice arrived a couple of minutes later. And then Dr. Mann came in, and they all knew the answer before she spoke a word. Her red, swollen eyes betrayed her.

Mann and two other doctors had worked for another nineteen minutes trying to revive the youngster, but it was no use. At 5:34 p.m., on November 30, 1995, Nicholas Gagnon was pronounced dead.

Lynne Monk arrived at the hospital a little later that evening. She had tried to go back to her dinner, but the sense of dread was impossible to shake. Lynne called a friend, who told her the only thing that would slow her racing mind was answers.

She stood for a moment in the doorway of the waiting room, unsure if she should enter. And then Lianne turned and looked at her. No words were spoken. The two women embraced, crying.

Dr. Mann examined Nicholas's body after he was pronounced dead. She could see no sign of head trauma. The neck was still supple; the pupils were fixed and dilated. There was no evidence of retinal hemorrhaging, a sign the child had been shaken or abused. And she could find no evidence of fractures or bruising on the body. Mann wrote in the chart that the child had presented with probable respiratory failure followed by cardiac arrest.

Dr. James Deacon, the local coroner who would head up the investigation into the death, examined the body about forty-five minutes after Nicholas was pronounced dead. Sgt. Robert Keetch of the Sudbury Police, who was leading the investigation, observed the examination. Keetch noticed a cut on the left side of Nicholas's nose and a small bump on the right side of his forehead, but the skin was not broken and there was little swelling. Deacon reported that the child appeared to be well nourished and clean. Like Mann, he found no external signs of trauma or any injuries other than those from resuscitation efforts. The child appeared to be healthy.

Dr. Teh-Chien Chen did the autopsy the next day. Sgt. Leo Thibeault, a forensic identification officer with the Greater Sudbury Police, observed the autopsy and took photographs of the body. Chen found petechial hemorrhages—small red and purple dots of blood—on the membrane that surrounds the lungs as well as on the outer layer of the heart and the thymus. He also found a moderate amount of fluid in the lungs and elsewhere, along with signs of mild, patchy swelling in the brain. None of these findings were indicative of foul play, and subsequent toxicology and radiology reports showed no abnormal findings. In his final autopsy report, Chen noted that "no anatomical or toxicological cause of death has been established. Autopsy findings are consistent with S.I.D.S. [Sudden Infant Death Syndrome] providing all other aspects of the investigation are negative."

Besides examining the body with Dr. Deacon, Keetch spoke with Dr. Mann and the two ambulance attendants. Then Keetch spoke to Lianne, who explained what had happened at the house. She said Nicholas was a healthy baby, although he had seemed to develop a problem with his balance over the past couple of weeks and had stopped sleeping through the night. Keetch visited the Gagnon home and examined the sewing machine table. The house appeared neat and tidy, and he could see nothing to suggest foul play had led to the child's death. He spoke with Dr. Chen, who advised him that the cause of death was attributed to SIDS.

Six weeks after Nicholas's death, Keetch called the Gagnon home. Angie took the call. They talked about the toxicology results that had just come back, and then the officer told her that he had concluded his investigation.

"If you or anyone else in the family, including your daughter, have any concerns, feel free to contact me at any time," he said.

And with that, the investigation into Nicholas Gagnon's death was over.

Angie made the funeral arrangements at the Jackson & Barnard Funeral Home. The director underestimated the number of guests, putting the visitation in a small room at the back of the building. Lineups stretched all the way outside. A constant stream of family and friends, many from Lianne's high school days, stopped in to pay their respects.

Nicholas was in an open casket, dressed in a *101 Dalmatians* outfit Maurice had picked up for him in Toronto. At one point, Maurice rushed home to get Nicholas's matching *Dalmatians* hat. Lianne, Maurice and Angie had each written letters to Nicholas, and they placed them in his casket. Lianne cut a lock of his fair hair.

The graveside service was touching and personal. The priest knew the family well. He had baptized Nicholas and played with him at the Gagnon home. On a clear, cold afternoon, Nicholas Gagnon's casket was lowered into the ground at Sudbury's Civic Memorial Cemetery.

That winter was bitter and long. To cope with her grief, Lianne threw herself into a fitness routine. Every morning, fresh out of bed, she would begin an exhaustive regimen of crunches and squats and lunges, set after set, over and over. From there, it was off to the rink, where she would skate for an hour and a half, then run laps around the top of the arena, then back down to the ice where she would scrimmage with the men's hockey team. She did this day after day. She lost forty pounds that first month.

But her nights were the hardest. Exhausted, Lianne had no choice but to slow down, and then there was no escaping. Flashbacks to the night of Nicholas's death, leaving the hospital, walking out to the parking lot without him. And the same thought, racing around and around: she had failed him and now he was gone.

One night she walked around the house, turning all his photographs face down, then crawled into bed in between her parents. She couldn't bear sleeping alone. Eventually, she moved out to a mattress on the living room floor, but it would be another six weeks before she ventured back into her basement apartment with Nicholas's empty nursery.

Lianne also worried about her father; she had never seen him so vulnerable. He became a man of blank stares and angry glares. His temper rose and sharpened. It could explode instantly, triggered by the most innocuous thing, and disappear just as quickly into a sea of tears. Father and daughter started going for recreational skates at the local arena, bonding in their heartache.

Getting through the Christmas season was particularly tough. One afternoon, Maurice was in Walmart when an irrational anger swept over him. People were smiling, holding hands, laughing with their children, having fun. How could they be so joyful? He felt like grabbing someone and screaming in their face, "Stop being happy! Don't you know he's gone?"

Maurice had put the Christmas lights up early that year, so at least Nicholas had seen those. He used to love standing in the window by the front door, his face barely reaching the bottom ledge as he stared out at the flickering lights, Winnie at his side. After he died, Maurice just couldn't bring himself to turn them back on. And then one night, driving home from work, the darkness hit him. It wasn't just enveloping their house; all the houses on Greenbriar Drive had kept their lights off too.

One ray of light broke through into the Gagnon household: Pete Thibeault. The night after Nicholas's death, the Gagnons had a gathering at the house. Friends and family descended, bringing casseroles and condolences. Pete, a high school sweetheart of Lianne's, was among them. Lianne appreciated the gesture. It was nice to see him again, but she was too lost in her grief to think anything more of it.

A month later, Pete checked in again, wondering if Lianne wanted to go see a movie. Another sweet gesture. Lianne resisted the invitation at first. Others had tried to drag her back out to the world of the living, with mixed results. One friend had taken her out to play pool, then had to take her home early when she broke down. Plus it was her mother's birthday, and her younger cousin Celine was over. Countless reasons to say no.

But Pete persisted, and eventually Lianne relented. Celine joined them for a movie and a bite to eat. It was all a little surreal. The last time Lianne and Pete had been out on a date, they weren't old enough to drive.

The following evening was New Year's Eve. Pete was having a party at his place. Lianne attended, and after that, they were inseparable.

That Thursday afternoon in June 1997 was overcast and cool. Maurice was in Toronto on business, but the Gagnon home was a bustle of activity. Angie, Pete and Lianne, and the couple's best friends were all preparing for Lianne's bridal shower, which was just two days away. She and Pete had got engaged a year earlier, and the wedding was planned for later that summer. It had been eighteen months since Nicholas's death, and Lianne felt she was finally starting to let go of her grief. There was joy in her life again: she had a wedding to plan, and she and Pete were planning on starting a family in the fall.

Sgt. Bob Keetch arrived on their doorstep. His partner, Sgt. Dave West, stood behind him. They were there to see Lianne. And in an instant, she was back at the hospital, the sensation so powerful Lianne could almost smell the place, stale and antiseptic, as she cradled Nicholas's tiny body. She burst into tears.

When Angie asked why they needed to see her now-distraught daughter, West explained that they had a few loose ends to wrap up in their investigation into Nicholas's death. The Chief Coroner's Office was reviewing all of the deaths involving children throughout the province. Keetch said they just needed to ask Lianne a few questions at the station.

Angie accused them of harassment and threatened to call the chief of police.

Lianne retreated back into the living room, into Pete's arms, as the police seemed to grow larger in front of her, filling up the room. Something was wrong. Horribly wrong.

Pointed questions and vague answers flew back and forth for a few minutes more.

It was clear the police were not leaving without Lianne. Pete offered to drive her down to the station, but Keetch insisted that she go with them in the cruiser.

Angie demanded to know why they were treating Lianne like a criminal.

Eventually, the officers relented. Pete could drive her to the police station. As they walked out the front door, Lianne looked back inside, at all the familiar faces who had gathered for what was meant to be a happy occasion.

Lianne had never been inside the police station before. Neither had Pete. His uncle Leo was an officer on the force, but he'd never thought to visit him at work.

"You'll have to wait here," Sergeant Keetch said to Pete, pointing to a chair in the hallway. He nodded solemnly as the two officers led Lianne into an interrogation room.

Lianne tried to listen as Sergeant West began.

"If Nicholas's death was not strictly due to a misadventure or illness or whatever; if it wasn't purely an accident and he came to harm by other means, then that could be considered homicide.

"I just want to be certain that you know what your rights are," West continued. "Do you know what your rights are?" He explained them to her anyway. He talked about the Charter of Rights and Freedoms. He talked about her right to a lawyer, about her right to leave at any time.

The words floated around her, opaque. She felt as if she was in a bad episode of *Law and Order*.

"So, do you understand all those rights?" the officer asked.

"Yes," Lianne said.

"Do you want to contact a lawyer?"

"No."

"Okay," West said. "Now, what we would like is that, and as difficult as it may be for you, we would like you to go back to the day of Nicholas's death, and if you could tell us from the start of the day, through the day, everything you can think of that happened that day. Okay?"

And so Lianne told the story yet again, about their happy day, and then the bump under the sewing machine, the randomness of it, and the chaos that followed. And as she listened to herself recount that tragic day, it struck her that it had been a while since she'd talked to anyone about it. Inside her head, that day was always there; over and over it played, at night, during the day. Pete would catch her sometimes staring off into the middle distance, back in a dark place. But to talk about it out loud? That had been a while. What was the point? She knew that someday she had to move on, but it was a struggle letting go. She felt guilty. She hadn't been able to save him, so she felt that the pain of his death should be her burden to bear forever. And she was scared, terrified that letting go of his death would lessen his life. All the good memories kept him alive for her.

"Okay. Anything else?" West asked when Lianne had finished.

"No."

"Lianne, we've had a conversation with the coroner and the head pathologist in Ontario."

"Yeah."

"And the circumstances that you've given for Nicholas's death do not suit the case here and that leaves myself with no doubt whatsoever that you're responsible for his death."

Lianne had been trying—and failing—to maintain her composure, breaking down repeatedly as she recounted the day Nicholas died. But that was pain. Her tears now were fuelled by confusion and guilt. She had spent the past year and a half second-guessing herself.

Maybe it really was her fault. Had she been too vigorous in her resuscitation efforts? Maybe she'd squeezed him too hard during the mad scramble across the street to the neighbours. Maybe she'd banged his back too hard trying to get him to breathe. Was that what this was about?

"The only thing I can think is when he stopped breathing [I] . . . flipped him over and whacked him on his back, and that's the only thing I ever did to him."

"That doesn't cover what the problem is here," West said. "Lianne, both you and I know that there is more here than what you've told us about."

"Oh God," Lianne said. "What did the coroner say?"

"Well, his injuries aren't consistent with what you've said."

"He had injuries?" she asked.

"When the coroner re-examined the case, there's no doubt in the pathologist's mind that Nicholas did not die of natural causes. And . . ."

"Did I mention in the morning when I take a shower, I put him in the bathroom with me and lie him on his pillows with his bottle after his breakfast?

"Well, that day, I got out of the shower and he had got into the cupboard and was playing with the Spic 'n Span. And I had asked the coroner that day if any had got into his system. Did he poison himself with that?"

"No, this isn't a case of poisoning," West said. "I mean, you're the person who knows exactly what happened here with him, and I think you are the person who can fill us in on the circumstances."

West tried the friendly-cop routine. He mentioned his own children. He talked about Lianne's young age, about the isolation she must have felt as a single parent, about the guilt she must be carrying. "I'm sure that if you could somehow talk to him, that you would want to tell him that you are sorry, wouldn't you? You would want to say to Nicholas, I'm sorry for what I did. And like I said to you, it's not a case that you did this out of a sense of meanness or out of cruelty."

"I didn't do anything. I can't think of anything," she said again.

"That's not true. His injuries are such that . . ."

"What are they? Why can't I know what they are?"

"Well, his injuries are such that the most probable cause of his death was asphyxiation."

"Oh my god!"

"And I think what may have happened is that you became overwrought at his crying."

"No!"

"And made efforts to quiet him down."

"No, I didn't!"

On and on the interview went, with Sergeant West hammering away at her story, searching for some rationalization, some version of the truth that would resonate with her. And all the while, reminding her that the police's suspicions were backed by Dr. Charles Smith, one of the brightest medical minds in the province.

"You have to understand that these people, they're professionals: the head pathologist for Ontario," West told her. "I mean, this is a man who's not making idle speculation. This is a man who knows."

The police kept at it for another twenty minutes, but Lianne's story never wavered. When she stopped asking for her parents and started asking for a lawyer, the interview ended.

TWO

UNBEKNOWNST TO LIANNE and her family, police in Sudbury, along with a team of pathologists and coroners, had been re-examining Nicholas's death for months. Suspicions first arose after the Sudbury coroner, James Deacon, filed the final report for his investigation in September 1996, almost a year after Nicholas's death. The report was unremarkable, although the coroner made one adjustment to Dr. Chen's findings at autopsy: he designated the cause of death as SUDS, or Sudden Unexplained Death, instead of SIDS, Sudden Infant Death Syndrome, as Dr. Chen had originally categorized it.

The difference between SIDS and SUDS deaths is nuanced. SIDS is a diagnosis of exclusion; the coroner only comes to it as a cause of death after a full police investigation and autopsy are completed, and every other possible cause has been considered and excluded. SIDS deaths involve children up to a year old, but usually nine months or younger, and usually occur while the child is sleeping.

SUDS is a slightly broader category. It also covers unexplained deaths in children, but these cases involve some factor that moves it outside the stricter exclusionary guidelines of SIDS.

"I think that the guidelines from the office of the Chief Coroner would place this in the S.U.D.S. category because of the association of the death with the bump on the head," Deacon wrote in his Coroner's Investigation Statement.

Lianne had said Nicholas bumped his head, which could have been a factor in his death. The autopsy and police investigation found nothing to support that it was, but it couldn't be fully excluded. There were other factors in Nicholas's case that made it a SUDS case rather than SIDS: He was awake; SIDS deaths occur while the child is asleep. And he was eleven months old, putting him near the one-year age limit and outside the more widely accepted nine-month time frame.

SUDS doesn't mean the death was intentional or involved foul play, but some aspect of it remains unexplained.

Dr. Elmer Uzans, the regional supervising coroner who received Deacon's final report, noted the discrepancy. He agreed with Deacon that SUDS was a more accurate assessment of the case, and decided to forward the case for further review to Dr. Jim Cairns, the deputy chief coroner in the province and the head of the Pediatric Death Review Committee at the Chief Coroner's Office.

From the very beginning, Uzans was suspicious of Lianne's story. How, he wondered, could a simple bump on the head have killed this child? Uzans had discussed the case with Deacon in the days after Nicholas's death. However, the autopsy and the police investigation had failed to turn up anything else that could have caused this child's death.

In his referral letter to Cairns, Uzans laid out the details of the case, claiming "the death was regarded as suspicious from the beginning." He noted that the underside of the sewing table was 56.5 centimetres high, while Nicholas's "crown-rump" measurement was only 54 centimetres, implying that the child couldn't have struck his head because he wasn't tall enough. However, "crown-rump" measures a child's height while sitting, from the head to the buttocks. Lianne said Nicholas was standing when he bumped his head under the sewing machine. Sergeant Keetch had written in his notes that Nicholas's "crown-heel" measurement—from the top of his head to the bottom of his feet—was 78 centimetres. He was more than tall enough to bump his head if he stood up under the table.

Nicholas's crown-heel measurement was listed in Dr. Chen's autopsy report, right next to the crown-rump measurement that Dr. Uzans noted in his letter to Dr. Cairns.

But beyond the specifics of Nicholas's case, another factor in Dr. Uzans's lingering unease was the pervading mindset within the Ontario coroner system at the time. Coroners were actively encouraged to tackle all cases critically. Make sure every possibility was considered. In the late 1980s and early '90s, there was a growing unease that widespread child abuse was going undetected. The Ontario Chief Coroner's Office worried that coroners, pathologists and police were moving too quickly to conclude that deaths were not criminally suspicious.

Three cases in particular had raised red flags. One involved a baby's death in the late 1970s, but it only became an issue in 1993, when the Ontario Provincial Police received a tip from a father in Barrie, Ontario, who suspected his ex-wife had killed their baby years earlier. The couple appeared to be in the midst of a nasty divorce when the tip came in, so the Coroner's Office was not ready to invest much in the complaint. But when Dr. Jim Cairns pulled the file, he immediately found a disturbing sign: a fractured femur that was still healing when the child died. Cairns understood healed or healing femur fractures among six-month-old children to usually be an indication of child abuse.

Officers searched provincial health insurance records and spoke to the family's doctor. Perhaps the child had been in a car accident, Cairns thought; that would explain the broken leg. But police could not find a reasonable explanation. The Coroner's Office ordered the child's body exhumed and a second autopsy conducted. That pathologist found multiple fractures, and the mother eventually pleaded guilty to assault causing bodily harm.

The other two cases didn't involve children, but the fallout from them significantly changed how pediatric cases were handled.

The first involved the death of Tammy Homolka, Karla's younger sister.

Tammy was with Karla and brother-in-law Paul Bernardo when she died on Christmas Eve, 1990. When she was pronounced dead, doctors noted a strange burn on her face. From the autopsy, the pathologist concluded that Tammy had died by choking on her own vomit. Given that, the toxicology report was expected to show a high blood-alcohol level, but it came back surprisingly low. The burn was examined by the province's chief pathologist, who ruled that it was a highly unusual chemical burn. However, the coroner didn't investigate any further, instead focusing on Tammy's medical history. He ruled that she had died of an asthma attack.

Dr. Cairns, in his testimony before the Goudge Inquiry, in 2007, said, "There had been no case conferences, no integration of anything at that time. That case then vanished until . . . Paul was arrested." At Bernardo's trial for the murders of teenagers Kristen French and Leslie Mahaffy, Homolka testified that she and Bernardo had also drugged and raped her younger sister. She said Tammy died during their efforts to revive her.

Cairns lamented that if Tammy Homolka's death had been more vigorously investigated from the outset, Bernardo may have come under suspicion sooner.

The second case involved a domestic homicide that was staged to look like a car accident.

On June 5, 1992, Graciela Montans and her husband, Antonio Alcaire, were returning home from their office-cleaning jobs in Brampton, north of Toronto. Alcaire was behind the wheel of their van while Montans slept on the bench seat behind him. Alcaire told police that his wife awoke suddenly when another car cut in front of them. In a panic she grabbed his arm on the wheel, sending the van careening off the highway and through a ditch and a chain-link fence. Montans was killed in the accident.

Their two-year-old relationship had been troubled from the start. Montans's older children from a previous marriage claimed that Alcaire was brutal, domineering and abusive. The couple had separated four days earlier. Alcaire had threatened to kill his wife and himself if she left him. Montans, who had started seeing someone else, had told her children that she was going to tell Alcaire that night that the relationship was over for good—which should have made the accident suspicious.

When police arrived at the scene, the accident initially appeared to be just that: an accident. An officer did note that there appeared to be an unusual amount of blood in the van, but he chalked that up to firefighters smearing it around as they looked for other passengers.

Montans was pronounced dead at Peel Memorial Hospital, and the Brampton coroner, Dr. William Lucas, was immediately called in. In the ER, Lucas learned that Montans had suffered massive injuries to her face, head and neck.

The pathologist who did the autopsy found signs that Montans had a broken neck, which would have been consistent with a car accident. A radiologist did X-rays and came to the same conclusion. With the radiologist's report now in hand, the pathologist Dr. Sousa completed his autopsy report. His findings: the cause of death was a fracture of the C2 vertebra. Sousa's report did not specifically address what had caused the fatal fracture, but his opinion was that Montans's head and facial injuries, coupled with the extensive bruising on her body, were consistent with injuries sustained in a car accident.

Montans's body was sent to a crematorium, but the cremation was delayed when her children asked that the name on her death certificate be changed from her married name, Alcaire, to her maiden name, Montans.

Meanwhile, the police investigation continued, and discrepancies in Alcaire's version of events began to emerge. He said that Montans had inadvertently caused the accident when she grabbed the steering wheel. But there were no skid marks on the road, no signs of erratic driving as he struggled for control of the van. In fact, it appeared to have left the road in a controlled manner. As well, a rookie officer thought the pattern of blood spatter in the van was "bizarre." Forensic examination revealed that it did not match the expected pattern in any way.

Police contacted Lucas about their investigation. Concerned, he called the crematorium to ensure the body would not be cremated. Lucas then viewed the van for the first time. He was shocked at the amount of blood in it, and he knew immediately that they were not dealing with a straight-forward car accident.

Lucas asked another pathologist to do a second autopsy. For the first one, authorities suspected a motor vehicle accident caused Montans's death. For the second autopsy, the new pathologist was looking for signs of foul play. And this time, he found them.

Dr. Noel McAuliffe found abnormal signs of blunt force injury to the face, including bruising and lacerations; there was additional bruising to the chest, arms and back. He also found petechial hemorrhages in both eyes, signs of manual strangulation, and abrasions on the jaw that would be consistent with Montans's attempts to remove the hands of her attacker from around her neck. Her larynx was injured, along with the hyoid, a small bone found among the muscles of the neck.

McAuliffe believed Montans had been beaten. The cause of death was manual strangulation. He could find no signs of a fracture in her C2 vertebra.

Antonio Alcaire eventually confessed to killing Montans, then staging it to look like a traffic accident. He pleaded guilty to manslaughter and was sentenced to eight years in prison.

Two autopsies of the same body; two very different outcomes. And the only difference was that one autopsy began with the assumption of a car accident and the other with suspicions of something more sinister. Besides illustrating that forensic pathology is far from an exact science, the investigation into Graciela Montans's death highlighted a key worry of the chief coroner's office at the time: Were homicides slipping through the cracks?

In 1994 a Coroner's Council was set up to examine the case. The three-member panel made a number of recommendations to improve communications between coroners, police, pathologists and relatives of the deceased. It made recommendations regarding training and education. New coroners, the report stated, "should be trained to have a high index of suspicion, to assume that all deaths are homicides until they are satisfied that they are not."

Be more suspicious. It was a recommendation the Coroner's Office took to heart. A month after the Coroner's Council report was released, Chief Coroner James Young issued a directive to all coroners, pathologists and police services in Ontario. It stated: "Everyone should be 'thinking dirty' and not get lulled into accepting the most obvious conclusions at the beginning of an investigation. . . . As a general rule, when there are serious problems with an investigation, the major errors have been made at the beginning of an investigation."

"Thinking dirty." It would come to define the Coroner's Office in the province for the next decade.

THREE

THE PEDIATRIC DEATH Review Committee, or PDRC, was established by the Ontario Coroner's Office in 1989. Its initial mandate was to assist in reviewing medically complex cases, with a special focus on the medical care the child had received before dying. The idea was to make sure care had been adequate and assess whether the death raised any larger, systemic problems. Charles Smith was an early member of the committee, along with Jim Cairns, who became the chair in 1992.

But by the mid-1990s, the Coroner's Office was looking to expand the role of the PDRC. In January 1994, it announced that the review committee would now be reviewing all SIDS and SUDS deaths, which would then be compiled in an annual report that would be circulated to coroners and pathologists. The committee was becoming increasingly concerned about undetected child abuse, and in early 1995 it helped craft Memorandum 631, which was distributed to all coroners, pathologists and police services in the province. It outlined the new protocols for the investigation of the sudden and unexpected death of any child under two years of age.

The memorandum reads, "Unfortunately in this day and age CHILD ABUSE IS A REAL ISSUE and it is extremely important that all members of the investigative team 'THINK DIRTY.' They must actively investigate each case as potential child abuse and not come to a premature conclusion regarding the cause and manner of death until the <u>complete</u> investigation is finished and all members of the team are satisfied with the conclusion" (emphasis in the original).

Nicholas Gagnon's case was an important one. It was one of the first SIDS/SUDS cases referred to the PDRC. Memorandum 631 was less than two years old and still fresh in everyone's mind. Early discussions at the committee focused on the discrepancies between Dr. T.C. Chen's initial SIDS designation and Dr. James Deacon's change to SUDS.

As chair of the review committee, Cairns forwarded Nicholas's case to Dr. Smith. Protocols at the time called for Smith to present his review to the committee for discussion, after which the PDRC would issue a final report.

Smith received fifteen microscopic slides from the original autopsy, along with Chen's autopsy report, Deacon's coroner's investigation statement, post-mortem radiographs, the toxicology report, the police report and the letter from Dr. Uzans requesting the review. Smith also enlisted the help of two radiologists at the Hospital for Sick Children. Paul Babyn was the acting chief of the Department of Diagnostic Imaging; Derek Armstrong was a neuroradiologist in the same department.

Upon viewing the X-rays, Babyn noted that he saw a "mild diastasis," or widening, of the skull sutures that may have been a sign of a skull fracture, although he felt it would be best to consult the original X-rays because the films he was forwarded were of such poor quality that it was difficult to be sure. He also noted a suspected fracture at the back of the child's left mandible, or jawbone. Armstrong, too, suspected a fracture along the left mandible, but he wanted to view the original slides to be sure. Armstrong did not provide a written report.

Both Babyn and Armstrong were careful to use caveats and cautious language in their opinions, noting the poor quality of the film they were reviewing. But most of those cautions disappeared when Smith summarized their findings in his own report. Babyn's "mild diastasis" of skull sutures became "splitting of the skull sutures." The suspected mandible fracture was no longer suspected; it was simply present. And while Smith noted the poor quality of the films, he said it affected only the evaluation of the extremities—implying that more fractures might have been be present on those as well. (Smith's misrepresentation of Dr. Babyn's opinions would continue. In an affidavit the following year, he had elevated his colleague's opinion of the skull sutures from a mild opening to a "marked widening" and "widely split.")

In the end, Smith's review dismissed many of Dr. Chen's original findings, instead stating that the child had died from a head injury. "The autopsy does not conclusively exclude the possibility of pre-existing traumatic injuries," he wrote. "In the absence of an alternative explanation, the death of this young boy is attributed to blunt head injury."

Smith's report was immediately forwarded to Sudbury police. According to Smith, because of the findings in his report, Cairns wanted police to complete their investigation before the file was sent back to the Pediatric Death Review Committee.

On January 28, 1997, four days after completing his report, Smith flew up to Sudbury to meet with the police. Dr. Deacon, the investigating coroner, and Dr. Uzans, the regional coroner, were also present, along with five officers and the police chief, Alex McCauley. The group gathered in Chief McCauley's office to listen as Smith went over his report. His final conclusion: this was not a SIDS death, as Dr. Chen had originally classified it; Nicholas Gagnon had died from a blunt force head injury. Smith explained that he was basing his opinion on five findings from his review: evidence of cerebral edema, or swelling of the brain; an increased head circumference; evidence of split skull sutures; a fracture along the left mandible; and a scalp injury.

Five pillars. For Sgt. Bob Keetch, who was the original investigating officer, it was a solid forensic foundation on which to build a case. Police reopened the file as a homicide investigation. Keetch would be the lead investigator. Sgt. Leo Thibeault was also on the team.

Their investigation began immediately. The two officers took Smith and Uzans to Sudbury General Hospital to meet with Dr. Chen and pick up all the remaining materials from the autopsy. Chen informed them the hospital still had preserved brain samples on file, along with the X-rays. Police also obtained search warrants to recover Nicholas's medical records from the hospital and from his family doctor. It was Smith's opinion that Nicholas had a large head circumference when he died, which could be a sign of brain swelling. But Smith had used a standard growth chart for comparison. He would need measurements from when the child was alive to make a proper assessment.

The pathologist returned to Toronto to review the new material, which would likely take months. In the meantime, he would keep Sergeant Keetch apprised of any developments. They spoke in mid-February. By then,

Dr. Babyn and Dr. Armstrong, the radiologists who had originally reviewed the X-ray copies, had now reviewed the originals, and they both said they no longer saw evidence of a fracture along Nicholas's left jaw. Despite the change in opinion, Smith was still highly suspicious, noting that neither doctor could definitively rule out a fracture.

In April, Keetch followed up with Smith about his review of the brain tissue. The cerebral edema was acute, Smith told him. Something had caused Nicholas's brain to swell: trauma or asphyxia, or the more remote possibility of poisoning, but Smith couldn't say which.

They discussed the radiologists' changed opinion about the jaw fracture, but Smith remained unswayed. He pointed out that a lot really depended on what Dr. Chen had observed in the original autopsy. Smith suggested there could have been contusions caused by a blunt force injury that Chen hadn't noticed. And then there was the brain weight. Smith told him normal brain weight for a child Nicholas's age was 880 grams. His was 1,220 grams. Smith said it indicated swelling severe enough to cause death. But Smith said he still needed to determine what caused the swelling.

"Could he have choked on something? Would that have caused the swelling?" Keetch asked. "The ambulance attendants said his throat was blocked." Smith said no.

He said he would have his report written in a couple of weeks, at which time they would need to discuss their next move in the investigation.

They had lost one of the pillars—the mandible fracture—holding up Smith's opinion that the child had died of a head injury, but the pathologist still sounded confident. To Sergeant Keetch, it seemed they were still investigating from a solid base of suspicion.

It took almost three weeks for Smith to complete his one-page report, written as a memo to Dr. Cairns that outlined his findings. He noted cerebral edema in the brain tissue, some flattening and narrowing of the ridges and furrows surrounding the cerebral cortex (the outer layer of the brain), along with smaller ventricles (cavities) in the brain. Smith also noted some other changes that he found "highly suspicious for hypoxic-ischemic encephalopathy," or damage to the brain and spinal cord from inadequate oxygen, which raised the possibility of asphyxia playing a role in Nicholas's death.

Smith and Cairns flew back up to Sudbury on May 7. Sergeant Keetch gave Smith the child's medical records, including Nicholas's head circumference at birth. His growth chart was normal. It looked like Nicholas just had a very large head.

Dr. Smith remained adamant that he was right. He wanted to disinter the child's body, arguing that a second autopsy was necessary.

It was at that May meeting that Sergeant Keetch started to become concerned. They had started with five pillars to their investigation. The mandible fracture had been ruled out. Now the head circumference had been ruled out. The foundation was getting wobbly.

As well, there was the scalp injury. It was very, very slight, a reddish mark consistent with a bump on his head, which is what Lianne had always said happened. Smith had initially argued a simple bump on the head couldn't explain Nicholas's death; that was the whole reason why they were reinvestigating the case. Yet Smith had a scalp injury among his pillars.

Further, Keetch thought Smith was using inverted reasoning in his consultation: the pathologist noted that Chen's original autopsy did not rule out the possibility of pre-existing traumatic injuries. But Chen never said what those injuries might be or what pointed to their existence. Keetch noted the same logic in Smith's conclusion: death caused by blunt head injury. That put the burden of proof on the suspect to prove her innocence, rather than investigators to prove her guilt.

Still, Keetch was grateful. He had been the original investigator, and back then he had closed the case. If the regional coroner, Elmer Uzans, had not been suspicious enough to order a case review, what now looked like a homicide might have been missed.

But Keetch couldn't see anything he had missed in his initial investigation. There simply wasn't any evidence of wrongdoing: nothing at the scene, nothing in the family history, nothing in Nicholas's medical history, and Lianne's story was consistent and plausible.

In fact, the only evidence of wrongdoing was to be found in Smith's report. Five pillars, now down to three—actually down to two if you put aside the scalp injury, which everyone else said was inconsequential. It was good to be suspicious, Keetch thought. He needed to focus on evidence to make a case stick. He wrote down eighteen issues and questions in his notes that he wanted Smith to clarify at their next meeting.

"Mother described that Nicholas seemed to have a loss of balance for last 10 days, prior to death," the officer noted. "Always falls forward, cranky last couple of nights, didn't sleep through night. Any significance?"

Keetch also wondered if life-saving efforts could have had any effect on the brain swelling. "CPR and attempts to resuscitate child took approximately 34 minutes. 19 at hospital. 15 minutes from time ambulance called until arrival at hospital. Could this have caused some edema to brain?"

And then there was the degree of brain swelling. "Dr. Chen describes patchy mild cerebral edema in autopsy report. Do you agree or disagree with this finding?"

It isn't known how Dr. Smith answered Keetch's questions; no one who was at the meeting took notes. But Keetch found Smith's arguments persuasive. The pathologist was adamant, definitive and emphatic: Nicholas Gagnon did not die a natural death. Dr. Cairns, the deputy chief coroner of the province, who also attended the meeting, was just as convinced of his colleague's opinions.

For Sergeant Keetch and his police colleagues, it was hard not to be won over by Smith's and Cairns's convictions. At the end of Smith's presentation, Cairns announced that the next step would be to exhume the body so that Smith could examine it for himself.

Disinterring an eleven-month-old who had been in the ground for more than a year was not a decision to be made lightly, but the officers agreed that it had to be the next step in their investigation.

Dr. Uzans, the regional supervising coroner, put the request in writing to Sudbury police chief Alex McCauley later that month. It was a hard sell, and like Dr. Smith in his first consultation report, Uzans overstated some of the evidence to help bolster their case. Dr. Babyn's initial consult had referred to a mild opening of the skull sutures; Uzans described them as "skull fractures." He mentioned the potential fracture of the left mandible—which others had already ruled out—and added, "The findings are highly suggestive that the death was the result of a head injury . . . In view of the above, an exhumation and repeat autopsy by Dr. Charles Smith is needed to reach a conclusion in this case."

While Pete Thibeault sat out in the hallway waiting for police to finish interviewing Lianne, he was approached by his uncle Leo, an officer with the Sudbury police. When Pete asked his uncle what was going on, Leo explained that an important doctor from Toronto, the top child pathologist in the province, had reviewed Nicholas's case and believed foul play was involved in the baby's death.

Pete, shocked, told him that was impossible. But even as Pete protested that Lianne was innocent, his uncle counselled that there was still time for him to call off the wedding. Leo was certain Lianne was guilty.

Pete was marrying Lianne, he told his uncle. He knew she couldn't have done the things he accused her of. Rather than continue to argue in the hallway, Leo explained that the matter would soon be settled. They were going to dig up Nicholas's body. There would be another autopsy.

The police hadn't shared that development with Lianne during their interview. It fell to Pete to share that news with her. He went to see her in the interview room. Lianne, caught between sorrow and anger, asked the obvious question in response: If the pathologist was so sure she had killed Nicholas, why did he have to dig her baby up at all?

Lianne hadn't wanted to watch. That's not why she went that morning.

After Pete told her at the police station that they were planning to exhume Nicholas's body, Lianne had stormed out of the interview room, demanding an explanation.

Sergeant Keetch explained to her that they needed to exhume the body and they had a court order to do so. There was nothing Lianne could do.

But Keetch said the plan was to exhume the body very early in the morning, when no one would be around. They would be as discreet as possible, and for that Lianne was grateful.

She and her parents had worked hard to make the gravesite look as pretty and well kept as possible. She had planned on going to the cemetery after the fact, to check on the condition of the gravesite.

It was almost eleven on Wednesday, June 25, 1997, when Lianne pulled into the cemetery. Police cruisers lined the road. And then she saw them: a crowd of people down by Nicholas's plot, and a shiny yellow backhoe digging up the ground. It looked like they were just getting started.

She parked the car and opened the door. It swung closed again, a hand holding it shut. It was Pete's uncle, Sgt. Leo Thibeault. He told her not to get out of the car until they were done. He did not explain why they were running so much later than expected.

Lianne leaned back in her seat. They had told her they were going to be discreet, but the cemetery was crawling with people gawking as they dug up her baby.

And then she spotted him, a young boy kneeling in the growing mound of dirt. He looked to be ten or eleven, wearing a pair of black track pants and a white T-shirt. Lianne squinted into the blazing midday sun. Yes, she was right. There were teddy bears on his T-shirt.

"Who the hell is that, Leo? There's a kid up there?"

Leo wouldn't tell her anything.

For another thirty minutes, Lianne watched in stunned silence, her eyes never leaving the young boy as he kneeled in the dirt that had just held her dead son, playing with a dump truck.

It would take several days of heated questions at police headquarters, but Lianne and her parents finally got their answer. The boy was Dr. Charles Smith's eleven-year-old son, Aaron.

The boy's presence, along with the late start, was too much for Maurice Gagnon, who would make a formal complaint to the College of Physicians and Surgeons of Ontario—the first of many he made about Smith's behaviour. In his complaint, Maurice wrote:

We had been assured that the disinterment would occur at daybreak, between 5:30 and 6:30 a.m., to avoid curiosity seekers and to minimize the impact on the family. However to accommodate Dr. Smith, the disinterment took place at high noon, in the presence of onlookers and the child's grieving mother. Had protocol been followed, my daughter would have been spared this devastation.

In what I can only assume to be unprecedented in the annals of civility, Dr. Smith brought his young son to the gravesite to witness the exhumation, no doubt for the boy's entertainment. Not only did Dr. Smith, the man responsible for the disinterment, trivialize the desecration of our baby's grave, he contemptuously mocked my daughter and the memory of her son by flaunting his "live" son while cavalierly digging up her "dead" son.

What manner of a man can be so callous, so cruel, so oblivious to the consequences of his actions?

Smith later explained his son's presence at the gravesite in a letter to Dr. James Young. He said he had had to make a presentation to a group of doctors the night before and didn't get home until after nine, but still had to drive to Sudbury that night to be there for the disinterment the following morning. His wife was concerned that he might fall asleep during the four-hour drive, so she insisted that he take one of their children for the trip.

Upon their arrival at the cemetery the next morning, Smith wrote,

I gave my son the option of waiting in my car or watching the backhoe in operation. Because of his special interest in machinery, Aaron chose to watch. Aaron, who has previously attended funerals, was aware that the backhoe would remove a steel vault from the ground and knew that there was no coffin or body to be viewed. Neither I nor anyone else present considered his attendance to be inappropriate.

At no time following the arrival of Nicholas's mother did she or anyone else indicate to me that they were uncomfortable with the presence of my son.

Smith was apparently not aware that police had confined Lianne to her vehicle for the duration of the disinterment.

In a letter responding to Maurice Gagnon's complaint, Dr. Young wrote: "It is the policy of the Office of the Chief Coroner that only authorized personnel attend a disinterment and it was not appropriate for Dr. Smith's son to be there. He could have either stayed at the police station or in Dr. Smith's car."

As for the delay in starting the disinterment, Young put the blame on Dr. Uzans, the regional coroner, who didn't arrive at the cemetery until about 10:15, shortly before the backhoe started digging. Dr. Smith and his son had arrived at police headquarters an hour earlier.

That was still hours later than the five-thirty start time the Gagnon family had been told about, but it appears the police had no intention of ever starting that early. Sergeant Keetch, the lead investigator, didn't start on duty until eight that morning, and he spent the first hour of his shift at the courthouse, obtaining a search warrant for the casket. He arrived at police headquarters at nine, shortly before Smith and his son.

Young wrote to Maurice, "Dr. Smith has been apprised of our concerns and is sorry if any of his actions offended your family. It was certainly not his intention to be insensitive or to offend anyone's feelings . . . The Office of the Chief Coroner apologizes for any pain or anguish that the presence of Dr. Smith's son at the disinterment may have caused your family."

FOUR

SERGEANT KEETCH ARRIVED at the coroner's office in downtown Toronto at nine o'clock sharp the morning after the exhumation. The officer didn't look forward to this part of his job. Autopsies were grim work, especially autopsies of children, but Keetch knew that Dr. Smith's work that day would be key to understanding exactly what had happened to Nicholas Gagnon, and he looked forward to having some clarity in the case.

Three people were present: Smith, his assistant Barry Blenkinsop, and Keetch, who would act as the forensic identification officer. The family had purchased a sturdy steel vault for the burial, and it took several minutes to loosen the nuts and remove the lid. The child was laid to rest in a smaller casket inside.

Nicholas Gagnon was wearing a black and white hat, a pair of white socks and hand-knit booties, a yellow *101 Dalmatians* sleeper, a white undershirt and a disposable diaper. He was holding a soother in his right hand and a small bell in his left. A teddy bear sat in one corner of the casket, along with a cross, seven photographs and three letters. Keetch opened the one entitled "To My beautiful lovely Nicholas xo," which appeared to be written by Lianne, and quickly scanned it to be sure. He had obtained a court order to seize it for further analysis.

After eighteen months in the ground, the child's body had started to decompose. The officer watched as Blenkinsop cut the clothing off Nicholas's body. Keetch had wanted to return the body for reburial in as close to the same condition as they found it. The family had clearly taken much care in choosing the boy's final outfit, but it was going to be impossible to put him back in his original clothing, which was now a pile of tattered rags.

Keetch photographed the body, then watched for the next ninety minutes as the body was carefully X-rayed. At eleven thirty he left with

Dr. Smith for the Hospital for Sick Children to deliver the film to Dr. Babyn, one of the radiologists who had done a consult for Smith's original autopsy report. He would be doing the same for the second autopsy. By 12:45, they were back at the coroner's office to begin the autopsy itself.

Keetch took more photographs as Smith carefully examined and dissected the body, working his way through head and skull to the face and neck, and then examining the chest and abdomen. He observed the condition of the skeletal system, studied the eyes and optic nerves for signs of hemorrhaging, and examined all the internal organs, dictating his opinions to his assistant as he went. Hours later, the child was dressed in new underwear, an undershirt and a sleeper. They weren't as nice as what he had originally been buried in, and obviously carried none of the emotional significance, but they would have to do.

Nicholas was placed in a new coffin and his personal effects tucked in around his body: the teddy bear, cross and photos to one side, the soother in his right hand, the tiny bell in his left. The letters were laid on top of the body, except the one written by Lianne, which had been seized as evidence. The coffin was closed and placed back into the steel vault, which was resealed. It was then placed back into the transport vehicle for the return trip to Sudbury to be reburied.

It was a small gathering, just Lianne, Peter, Angie and Maurice. The grounds had been cleaned up for the ceremony. Lianne and her parents had made a stone flower box for in front of Nicholas's gravestone. The box had been broken during the excavation; dirt was strewn across the ground, the flowers dead and crumpled. Some had fallen into the hole. The groundskeepers at the cemetery had tried to clean it up in the days since the exhumation, but it was difficult for Lianne to wipe the sight of it from her memory.

The owner of the funeral home said a few prayers before Nicholas was lowered back into the ground. Lianne spotted a police officer leaning against his cruiser, watching. If she had once felt intimidated by the police and their authority, she didn't anymore. She took off like a bullet, screaming obscenities as she sprinted toward the officer. The cruiser spit up dust and gravel as the cop hightailed it out of the cemetery.

The phone call came out of the blue, and it immediately struck Lianne as odd. She hadn't spoken to Steve Tolin, Nicholas's father, in months. It was late July 1997, less than a week before her wedding to Pete.

Steve told her the police had called him. They'd asked him if he could come into the station the next day. He said he'd find out what he could from them and wondered if Lianne would want to meet after that.

It had been a brutal summer so far. Pete's grandfather had just died. Everyone was devastated. And Nicholas's death was still hanging over her, with no word yet on the results of the second autopsy.

She had landed a job that summer laying railway track for Inco. It was hard work, which she welcomed; inserting the ties, laying the track, hammering the pins in place was gruelling, but it also left her mind with lots of time to wander and worry about what was taking so long. She suffered panic attacks. Sometimes she would get so angry and distracted that she would accidentally shatter sledgehammers on the railway tracks, which was no easy task.

Lianne wanted answers, and the prospect of inside information from the police was enticing enough to overcome any suspicions she had about Steve's call.

Lianne was practically climbing the walls by the time Steve called late the next afternoon. She demanded to know what the police had told him, but Steve wanted to meet in person, not talk over the phone. She invited him over. He suggested they go for a drive instead. He said he'd pick her up. Lianne thought going for a drive was strange, but she didn't seem to have any choice. She started pushing for answers as soon as she got in the vehicle.

Steve waited until they were parked in Bell Park before telling Lianne what he'd learned: Dr. Smith had completed the second autopsy. The police had his evidence. They were going to arrest her.

Lianne was distraught. How was this possible? She had been convinced this was all just a horrible misunderstanding, that it would correct itself after the pathologist had a chance to look at the body himself. It was the only positive thing she could see in Nicholas's disinterment. But the second autopsy hadn't fixed anything.

Steve pushed her to tell him what had really happened. She told him what she'd been telling everyone from the beginning: Nicholas bumped his head, then he stopped breathing.

But Steve wouldn't believe her.

And that's how the next hour went. They didn't leave the car as Steve peppered her with questions, goading her to tell him the truth. He had offered to meet to tell her what the police told him, but all he had were questions. Lianne felt like she was back in the interrogation room.

"Fine," she said. "You want to know if I'm responsible for his death? Yes, I am."

"What do you mean?" he asked.

"I'm his parent. And parents are supposed to be responsible for their children. And that day, it didn't matter what I did. I failed. He was my responsibility and I let him down. He's not here, and it's my fault."

Steve asked her to explain. Lianne said she wanted to go home. Steve pushed her to tell him the truth. "Take me home!" she yelled.

Steve started the car.

When she got home Lianne told Pete and her dad everything. She was going to be arrested.

Lianne watched as her father got up from the table. He was wearing a bathing suit, an old stained T-shirt, knee-high socks and slippers. He disappeared out the front door.

Where was he going dressed like that? she wondered.

Maurice hoped he was wrong. Lianne didn't deserve more bad news, but he had a sinking feeling more was coming. He'd always liked Steve—or at least he'd wanted to. But Steve Tolin had been a disappointment before, so

Maurice wasn't surprised when he pulled into the headquarters of the Sudbury police and saw Steve's car in the parking garage.

The idea had come from Det. Sgt. Jim Van Allen, who worked with the Behavioural Sciences Section of the Ontario Provincial Police.

Sergeant Keetch had sent Lianne's original statement to police to Van Allen in May. He had sent back a damning, strongly worded report in which he said Lianne was concealing information and had played an "active role" in her son's death.

Keetch reread her original statement and found nothing suspicious in it. Yet the behavioural scientist found it deceptive, based on her lack of emotion and use of passive language. He even suggested asphyxia as the cause of death.

Sergeant Keetch was grateful for the opinion, but noted that Van Allen had made one obvious error, arguing that Lianne's statement suggested she had a strained relationship with her parents and a poor relationship with Nicholas at the time of his death. Both the chief and the deputy chief of the Sudbury Police were close friends of the Gagnons and knew this to be untrue.

And asphyxia seemed a stretch, Keetch thought. All the behavioural scientist was reviewing was Lianne's first police statement. It was one thing to deduce deception from her tone and choice of words. But Keetch didn't see how he could accurately deduce the child's cause of death from phrases like "but his breath kept getting cut off."

Regardless, Keetch saw the analysis as a useful investigative tool, and he was keen to see what Van Allen would come up with after reviewing her other statements. After the disinterment, he sent Van Allen a video-tape of Lianne's interrogation, along with the letter he had taken from Nicholas's casket.

Detective Sergeant Van Allen's second review mirrored his first, concluding that there was a "high probability" that Lianne was responsible for Nicholas's death. The new report dissected her letter, finding sinister meaning in a number of seemingly heartfelt statements. Sentences like "There are no babies in the world as beautiful as you are, or as smart and personal and funny" and "Everyone loves your precious blue eyes, golden blond hair, and a smile that could light up a room" appeared to Van Allen "to be written for others to read." And because she used "Everyone" instead of "I," the behavioural scientist felt the sentiments were actually not Lianne's feelings but those expressed by other people.

He also found problems with her use of verb tenses. "It is unexpected that the mother of a deceased child would refer to him in the past, present and future tense," he wrote. "Gagnon refers to her child in two tenses in some sentences, '. . . but I wished you could be here with me,' is past tense, and suggests that she doesn't wish he could be with her at the time of writing."

Van Allen didn't like the structure of this sentence either: "You loved and your love was returned a million times by your mommy and everyone who knew you." He reasoned: "The distance in the sentence between the child and the mother is significant, and is believed to reflect the distance in the actual relationship."

He found the use of affectionate names (phrases like "Nicholas, my darling"; "sweetie"; "my beautiful baby boy" and "my precious Nicholas") to be overused because Lianne hadn't used the same terms in an earlier written statement to police.

Lianne referred to herself as "your mommy" throughout the letter, rather than using personal pronouns such as "I" or "me," which Van Allen felt deflected commitment. And he noted that "mommy" was never capitalized, unlike other words in the letter, such as "Grandpa," "Christmas" and "Tom Petty."

As for her taped interrogation, Van Allen noted that although police were not able to elicit a confession, he felt that was because they were trying to resolve an issue that Lianne had already apparently resolved in her mind. "Gagnon's language indicates deception, lacks sufficient detail, lacks commitment to facts, and evades issues. She avoided telling the truth by stating what usually happens instead of what did happen. She contradicted herself in sentences like 'I put him down for a long nap that was unusually short.'"

He again found deception in the way she used pronouns when describing Nicholas: "the mouth" rather than "his mouth," and "the eyes" instead of "his eyes." And he found it suspicious when she said, "I didn't cover his face and choke him."

"This had not been said by others, and I believe it may indicate the means by which the child died," Van Allen wrote, arguing that the statement was consistent with the forensic findings of asphyxial death.

He went on to consider her memory. "She suggested she had difficulty remembering what she said to police a year and a half ago, rather than relying on the actual memory of what occurred approximately eight months previous. Truthful people are expected to accurately recount details from important events in their life with only some minor discrepancies." Nicholas's death and the initial police investigation occurred a year and a half before the police interrogation, so it's unclear what Van Allen was referring to when he criticized her for not recalling an event that happened "eight months" earlier. And his statement that truthful people have accurate memory recall assumes that she was not being truthful and not giving an accurate account of what happened.

Van Allen's report ends with "Investigative Suggestions." It makes only one: use Lianne's former boyfriend Steve Tolin to wear a wiretap and try to extract a confession from her. "We note that Gagnon planned to marry on 02 August, 1997. The preceding period, in conjunction with waiting for the police investigation to conclude, will be a very emotional time for her. This should be added to, by orchestrated events by police. If the ex-boyfriend continues to be supportive, trusted and a potential source of information concerning the investigation, Gagnon may be inclined to disclose to him."

Sudbury police ran with Van Allen's suggestion. Sergeant Keetch contacted Tolin, who was amenable to the idea. Police technicians installed a listening device in his car and on his home phone and strapped one to his body. Officers would monitor their conversation from an unmarked van that would trail his vehicle.

Maurice went home to share his suspicions about Steve working with the police and to take Lianne back with him to the station. They pulled into the underground parking lot at the Sudbury police station, right next to Steve's car. Lianne couldn't believe Steve would do this to her.

Father and daughter were sitting in the parking lot, stewing, when Lianne noticed the security cameras that lined the ceiling of the garage. She got out of the car and walked up to the closest one. "You might as well bring him out now because we're not leaving," she yelled.

Steve Tolin appeared shortly afterwards. Sergeant Keetch accompanied him to his car. Lianne and Maurice were on top of him before he reached the door.

Maurice confronted Steve with their suspicions, accusing him of wearing a wire and trying to get a confession out of Lianne. Keetch intervened, saying Steve didn't have to answer the charges and urging father and daughter to remain calm. Maurice asked the sergeant directly whether the police had put a wire on Steve. The officer denied that they had. Lianne couldn't contain her frustrations. Letting the expletives fly, she challenged Keetch to tell her why the investigation was taking so long. Keetch admitted they were still waiting for Dr. Smith's second autopsy report, and he wasn't sure when it would be completed.

After a fuming Lianne and Maurice drove out of the parking lot, Steve broke down. He hadn't imagined that Lianne would be able to figure out what he had done. Now he regretted agreeing to help the police. As best he could, Sergeant Keetch tried to reassure Steve that he had done the right thing.

Following the autopsy, Dr. Smith told police it would take two to three weeks to complete his report. Sergeant Keetch started calling for updates after two weeks. And calling and calling and calling. By the end of July, he had switched his efforts to Dr. Cairns; at least he could get the deputy chief coroner on the phone. Cairns told him that he had spoken with Dr. Smith several days after the autopsy: preliminary results showed evidence of fresh hemorrhages inside the skull, supporting the theory that Nicholas died after a blunt force injury to the head.

They discussed setting up a meeting to go over the results in more detail once Smith had completed his report. Cairns suggested mid-August.

He also mentioned that Maurice Gagnon had called twice over the past two weeks, inquiring about the results of the autopsy. Cairns told Keetch the report was not finished yet, and he assured him that he wouldn't release it to the family without first consulting the police.

FIVE

DESPITE LEO THIBEAULT's warnings, Lianne and Pete went ahead with their wedding on August 2, 1997, and then moved into an apartment around the corner from her parents' house. Five days later, the people who would decide her fate gathered in a conference room at the Sudbury police headquarters. It had been six weeks since Nicholas Gagnon's body had been disinterred, and Dr. Charles Smith was in Sudbury to present the results of his autopsy. Much of the police force's senior team had gathered for the meeting: Chief Alex McCauley and Deputy Chief Jim Cunningham were sitting around the table, along with the local coroner, James Deacon, and Crown counsel Greg Rodgers. Keetch had met with Rodgers the day before to discuss the case. He was keen to hear the prosecutor's thoughts after the meeting; his opinion would be key in deciding not just whether but what charges could be laid against Lianne Gagnon.

It had been a tough week. Sergeant Keetch's run-in with Maurice and Lianne in the parking garage was still sitting heavy on his mind. The incident had shaken up Steve Tolin, who was now guilt-ridden about working with police. And for all that work, and all that stress, the wiretap had yielded nothing. Lianne Gagnon had not admitted anything.

Keetch knew that not all suspects confess. The police themselves had failed to get a confession out of Lianne during their interrogation. But it sure would have helped; Keetch was running out of ideas. Every other angle was coming up empty, just as it had during his initial investigation. It looked like the case would have to rest on Smith's autopsy findings.

And Smith's findings were straightforward: Nicholas Gagnon, he told the gathering in the conference room, did not die of SIDS; he did not die from any other natural disease process. It was Smith's opinion that the cerebral edema and the splitting of the skull sutures could not be explained by the child dying suddenly after hitting his head on the underside of a sewing machine.

Smith was still completing his written report, but he and Dr. Cairns encouraged the police to continue their investigation in the meantime.

Keetch knew he had to make the call, but that fact didn't make it any more attractive. The last time he had spoken to Maurice Gagnon was in the parking garage as he and Lianne lobbed expletives and accusations at him and Steve Tolin. He had had to lie to them about the wiretap and surveillance. The officer wasn't happy about it, but neither was he about to jeopardize his investigation. He had also told Maurice that he would keep him up to date on the investigation, and he planned to keep his word about that. The family had waited long enough for Smith's autopsy report. They wouldn't be happy with the results, but they had a right to know.

Keetch showed Maurice into an interview room at police headquarters and closed the door. Maurice asked if Lianne had been cleared. Keetch said the results of Smith's autopsy showed Nicholas's death was not consistent with Sudden Infant Death Syndrome. The child didn't have an underlying disease. It was not a natural death. And Smith felt Lianne's explanation of Nicholas bumping his head on the underside of a sewing machine could not account for the injuries he observed.

Maurice felt the colour drain from his face. He asked what the injuries were.

Keetch said Smith found signs of cerebral edema, or brain swelling. There was no fracture along Nicholas's jaw. But a behavioural scientist with the OPP studied Lianne's police statements and the letter she wrote to Nicholas and found signs of deception and untruthfulness. Maurice asked the detective what he thought. Keetch said he thought Lianne wasn't telling the truth about what really happened.

Maurice searched for another explanation. What about a previous injury? Could that have exacerbated the bump on his head. Keetch said he didn't know but he would ask Smith.

Maurice had other questions: How much time could pass between the time of injury and the time of death? How long would it take for the brain swelling to build up to the levels it was at the time of death?

Keetch said he would get them answered too.

Maurice asked if they were considering other suspects if the timing opened up the possibility of an earlier injury. Keetch said all the information he had showed Nicholas's fatal injury occurred on the day he died, while he was in the care of his mother.

"You don't know my daughter like I do," Maurice said. "There's just no way. I don't believe she could have been responsible. If she was, she would have told me by now. There has to be another explanation."

Keetch said they would be making a decision about charges shortly.

Maurice and Angie sat down at the dining room table with Lianne to try to figure it out. They were an attentive family and had kept a detailed account of Nicholas's short life, including every bump, bruise and scrape the child had suffered.

One thing jumped out in particular. On November 8, about three weeks before Nicholas died, he took a bad blow to the head when he fell against a coffee table at the babysitter's house, leaving a large lump, though it didn't seem serious at the time. Now Maurice began to wonder. Looking back, his wife did pick up changes in Nicholas's behaviour after the fall: his equilibrium seemed to be off, especially while walking. He started falling forward, rather than down into a sitting position as he had before. He had also started zoning out, going into a trance for several seconds before shaking his head and regaining his focus. And he would occasionally close his eyes tightly, contorting his face as he shook his head from side to side, as if he'd bitten into a sour pickle. At the time, Maurice just thought he was trying to be funny, but looking back now, all three behaviours continued throughout the three weeks before his death.

He wrote a letter to Dr. Cairns outlining his theory. When they spoke afterwards, Cairns was dismissive, reiterating that Dr. Smith's findings showed Nicholas's head injury was acute and that it occurred the day he died. Maurice knew what he sounded like: a desperate father making a last-ditch effort to explain away the most obvious conclusion.

As he hung up the phone, he had the distinct feeling the deputy chief coroner's mind was already made up.

Meanwhile, Sergeant Keetch continued digging. He had the Centre of Forensic Sciences examine Nicholas's stomach contents. During the interrogation, Lianne had mentioned that the child had got into some cleaning supplies that morning while she was in the shower. Neither pathologist had seen any signs of a poison in the autopsies, but Keetch triple-checked just to be sure.

Ray Higaki, a forensic biologist with the centre's Northern Regional Laboratory in Sault Ste. Marie, said that twenty months after the baby's death, it was unlikely they would be able to tell if he'd ingested cleaning solvents. Trace amounts would not have contributed to Nicholas's death, Higaki told Keetch, and if the child had ingested Spic 'n Span in large quantities, the post-mortem exam would reveal significant burning in the throat and mouth area.

Keetch checked another possible explanation off his list.

The detective also raised Maurice's questions with Dr. Cairns. The answers came back as expected: the bump on the head couldn't have triggered an earlier injury, and the time of the injury to the time of death meant that Lianne was the only one who'd been around Nicholas.

Then Keetch tried to track down Lianne's best friend, Sophie Laframboise, who had frequently babysat Nicholas while Lianne was at class, but she was now living in Toronto and finding her was proving difficult.

And he waited. Another month passed and he heard nothing from Smith about when his final autopsy report might be ready. He kept calling the pathologist's office but could never get him on the phone. Smith, he was told, was either sick, out of town or working and unavailable. And he never returned the police officer's messages. Another seven weeks passed.

Keetch finally reached him on October 23. Smith was surprised he didn't have his report already. He said it was completed and had been forwarded to the Chief Coroner's Office for review. Keetch said OCCO didn't have the report as of three weeks earlier, when he last spoke to Cairns. Smith promised to send another copy immediately.

Six more days passed with no word from the Chief Coroner's Office or Dr. Smith about the report. Keetch reached Cairns on October 30: he had the report and would be putting a copy in the mail shortly. Cairns said Smith's findings hadn't changed: the head injury was non-accidental and consistent with blunt force trauma.

A voicemail was waiting when Keetch hung up. It was Maurice Gagnon, requesting a meeting. Keetch wondered if Cairns had called Lianne's father with the results as well. He immediately called the Coroner's Office back, but Cairns had disappeared into a meeting. His secretary, though, said he had not spoken to Mr. Gagnon about the results and would not be doing so. He had forwarded copies to the investigating coroner and the regional coroner, with strict instructions not to release the contents without the consent of the Crown attorney's office, the Sudbury police or himself. A copy for the police would be put in the mail tomorrow.

When Keetch called him back, Maurice wanted to know what stage the investigation was at. He scoffed a bit when Keetch told him the autopsy report was in the mail. He then asked if the investigation was otherwise complete. Keetch mentioned that he was still hoping to talk to Sophie Laframboise. Maurice offered to find her contact information for him. Maurice just wanted it all to be over. Then he shared the news with Sergeant Keetch: Lianne was pregnant.

Three more days passed and the autopsy report still hadn't arrived. Frustrated, Sergeant Keetch called the Chief Coroner's Office and asked Dr. Cairns's secretary to at least fax him a copy until the formal version arrived, which she did. In the meantime, he took new statements from Maurice, and then from Angela, who corroborated Maurice's story about Nicholas banging his head badly on a coffee table at a babysitter's house three weeks before his death. Keetch then checked with Children's Aid about the Gagnons' babysitter, Jillian Marshall, who was also a foster parent. Both she and her husband had since passed away, but there had been no allegations of physical abuse during the twenty-eight years they had worked in the system.

The formal copy of Smith's autopsy report finally arrived in the mail on November 10. Keetch added it to the file that investigators had been preparing for the Crown, who would ultimately decide whether and what charges would be laid. Police were suggesting second-degree murder. As well, Keetch sent the brief to Assistant Crown Attorney Greg Rodgers on November 13.

The call came eight days later.

Sergeant Keetch had met with the Gagnons the day before to let them know the Crown was reviewing the case and that a decision on charges was imminent. With the anniversary of Nicholas's death approaching at the end of the month, the officer said the decision would be postponed until early December. The Gagnons appreciated the gesture, but they also didn't want yet more delays, saying at this point they just wanted the matter resolved.

But the Crown, it turned out, had problems with the case.

Keetch, like everyone else on the police force, believed strongly that Lianne was guilty. Had they made a mistake in their investigation, left a hole that she would be able to wiggle through and avoid justice?

But it was Dr. Smith's report that troubled Greg Rodgers. He saw that Smith had left the door open for an accidental cause of death. Smith's evidence as it stood was not strong enough to offer a reasonable expectation of getting a conviction.

It didn't make sense, Keetch thought. In all his discussions with police, Dr. Smith had been adamant that this was not a natural death and that the timing meant Lianne was the only suspect. His opinion had been the driving force for the whole investigation. Keetch offered to set up a meeting so Smith could answer the Crown lawyer's doubts. He had convinced police; surely he could convince the Crown.

"I think that would be a very good idea," Rodgers said. "Because as it stands, I don't feel comfortable moving forward with charges."

That meeting happened on November 28, 1997. It had been ten months since Dr. Smith filed his first consultation report on the case. The force's senior officers were all in attendance: Chief McCauley, Deputy Chief Cunningham, along with several other officers and Crown counsel Greg Rodgers.

Dr. Smith walked the group through his autopsy report: the cause of death was cerebral edema, consistent with blunt force injury. His main findings were discoloration along the skull sutures and the right parietal bone, the large, flat bone that forms the right top and side of the skull. He reasoned that the discoloration was hemorrhagic, or caused by excessive blood loss, which would be consistent with a blow to the head. Dr. Babyn, the radiologist who had examined the original X-rays, also reviewed the new set taken at the second autopsy. His main finding in the first review was a mild opening of the skull sutures, which Smith later characterized as "widely split." His second consult, included in Smith's report, did not specifically mention the skull sutures. Babyn did note that "extensive changes within the soft tissues are seen in keeping with prior autopsy and post-mortem changes." Those changes to "the soft tissues" could be a reference to the skull sutures, although that is not explicitly stated. Babyn also said there were "no definitive fractures of the skull, mandible, ribs or visualized skeleton," definitively ruling out the mandible fracture that had been suspected earlier.

Rodgers pointed to a phrase in Smith's report: "In the absence of a credible explanation."

The phrase was problematic. It made it sound like there might be a credible explanation, investigators just hadn't found it.

Rodgers asked Smith how confident he was in his medical opinion of the case. Smith said he was very confident.

Then why couch it like that, the Crown asked? Why raise doubt? The pathologist said the phrase was standard practice.

The phrase also bothered Keetch. He didn't doubt Smith's findings, but he understood Rodgers's concern. Keetch told the group it was like a reverse onus, demanding the defendant prove her innocence instead of the Crown proving her guilt.

Smith tried to reassure them that he used the phrase in all his reports, and it had never caused problems before.

But Rodgers wouldn't back down. Not only did he think the phrase was a problem, he said it was a deal breaker: he wasn't prepared to lay charges because Smith had couched his medical opinion.

Chief McCauley couldn't believe what he was hearing. He asked if the Crown was really not going to proceed with a murder charge because of a misplaced phrase in a report?

Rodgers said yes; with that wording, he didn't think he had a reasonable shot at a conviction.

Sergeant Keetch broke the silence that followed by raising another issue: Lianne was pregnant again.

It was early December, and Lianne was just wrapping up the last of her exams at Laurentian. Her English/history degree was a four-year program; this was her fifth year, which she considered to be just fine. From Nicholas's unexpected arrival to the devastation of his death, there had been a lot to overcome during the past few years. And with the police investigation, it was incredible she had any brain power left for school. But if she could hold it together for one more semester, she would graduate in the spring.

The phone rang. Lianne answered. It was her father. He invited Lianne and Pete over. He had an early Christmas present for them.

Lianne and Pete made the short walk up the street to her parents' place. And sitting on the dining room table was a tiny Christmas tree. When Maurice urged Lianne to take a closer look at the tree, she noticed a card tucked into its branches. On it, her father had written two words:

It's over.

Tears were already blurring her vision as she looked up at her parents. Her father was grinning from ear to ear. He had spoken to Sergeant Keetch that morning, he told her, and had learned they were not proceeding with charges.

Maurice chose to leave it at that, to not burden his daughter with the other news Keetch had shared. The police were duty bound to inform Children's Aid about the investigation now that Lianne was pregnant.

The police had spent almost a year investigating Lianne, and in the end, they decided there wasn't enough evidence to charge her with anything.

Maurice assumed that would be enough for Children's Aid too.

JENNA I
....

ONE

SHE NEEDED HELP.

It finally hit home for Brenda Waudby that early October morning in 1996 as she stood on her porch, her no-good boyfriend refusing to unlock the front door of her rundown apartment in her rundown neighbour-hood. In that moment, Brenda finally saw herself for who she'd become: a cocaine addict, stuck in an abusive relationship. And unless she got clean, she would no longer be fit to raise her two children.

She had to get her oldest, seven-year-old Justine, to school. The scream-ing had started shortly after the alarm went off. It was a tense household at the best of times. You never knew when Randy's fists would come up, when his rage would boil over. She had called the police a dozen times. It never made any difference. They'd haul him off for a day or two, things would cool off, and Brenda would take him back.

"When you're in that situation, you don't know how to get out," Brenda would say years later. "You don't think you can ever get out."

It was Randy Mellor who had introduced her to cocaine. Marijuana had been a happy friend, but after one taste of the harder drug, suddenly all that mattered was the next hit. Their dealer lived next door, which meant a steady supply as long as they kept the cash coming. And so any-thing that could be hocked went out the front door. The cupboards went bare. The lights went out. And the children suffered.

A summer storm rolled in one night before the hydro was cut off.

Jenna, not yet a year and a half old, was upstairs, asleep in her crib. Justine was downstairs, watching TV, terrified at the first crack of thunder. She quickly switched off the TV, convinced the house would blow up if she didn't turn all the electricity off. Brenda was not there to comfort her; she was next door at the dealer's. The sight of Justine, sobbing and scared, screaming at her mother to come home, was a picture Brenda wished had never entered her head, but that's where her mind went as she stood on her stoop that morning, banging on the door.

She was tired of being an addict, tired of being a negligent mother. She had forgotten her keys inside—that's why she was banging on the door after Randy locked her out. But by the time Randy opened it, her focus had changed. It wasn't her keys she needed. It was the phone. Brenda punched in the number for Children's Aid but hung up before anyone answered, partly because of nerves, partly because Randy lunged at her when he realized who she was calling. But his aggression only steeled her resolve. A second call went through. And when Randy really started raging, Brenda called her father.

Her father phoned the police, who were at the front door in minutes. Social workers with Kawartha Haliburton Children's Aid arrived in an SUV at the same time, there to take away her girls. More screaming and cursing ensued. A police officer called Brenda a junkie, a cocaine addict, a horrible mother. All true, she knew, but didn't *she* reach out to *them*? Didn't that count for something?

When the situation calmed down a bit, the social worker told Brenda to take her two girls out to the SUV and to tell them they were going on vacation. She told Brenda to say goodbye but to try not to get emotional. It would be easier for her children that way. Brenda knew it was the right thing to do, knew it had to be done. The walk out to the van felt like a walk to the gallows, fiery, protective Justine holding one hand, baby Jenna scooped up in the other arm. Brenda did her best to be strong, to show no emotion; she kissed both her girls, told them she would see them soon. She waved goodbye as the van pulled away, then walked back inside, up the stairs into the room the girls shared. She lay down on Jenna's bed, waiting for the tears to come.

Losing the two most important things in her life gave Brenda Waudby strength she didn't know she had. She had heard kicking the habit would be the hardest thing she'd ever do. It wasn't. Losing her children was the bottom. It was the day she stopped. She never touched hard drugs again.

She stopped hanging out with hard drug users; she changed her favourite haunts. She took court-ordered drug counselling and attended Narcotics Anonymous. She volunteered for drug testing. And she went from being a cocaine addict one day to being a former one the next.

Brenda moved out of the apartment she shared with Randy, got a new place in south Peterborough. Her parents lived just around the corner. She hit it off with her new neighbour upstairs: Maggie, a single mom with three kids. JD, who was fourteen, was the oldest, and Angie was twelve. Perfect, Brenda thought—built-in babysitters for when she got her girls back. Kevin was nine, another playmate for Justine. (All this family's names have been changed because of a court order prohibiting their identification.)

Justine and Jenna had been placed in the same foster home. Justine hated it. She ran away once with an eleven-year-old who was living there too. It took police almost eight hours to find the pair. Brenda saw them outside a convenience store that afternoon, but she didn't say anything to Justine. She was under strict orders not to speak to her daughter, even if she bumped into her around town. It wasn't until later that Brenda found out she had run away.

Brenda passed the random drug tests and attended all her court appearances, and the exile finally ended six weeks later. On November 15, 1996, Justine and Jenna moved into their new home with their mother. Brenda and the girls were ordered to remain under CAS supervision for another eight months.

By the new year, Brenda and the girls were settling into the rhythms of life in their new home. Justine chummed around with Kevin upstairs, and JD and Angie took turns babysitting, with Maggie always keeping a watchful eye. They were good neighbours and good friends; the door between their apartments was always open.

Brenda may have been able to break free of cocaine's grip, but breaking free of Randy was even harder. He showed up one night at the new apartment shortly after she moved in, threatening to commit suicide if Brenda didn't take him back. Brenda called police, who advised her to spend the night at a women's shelter for her own safety. If she was ever going to get her life in order, she had to get away from Randy. But making a clean break was difficult. As Jenna's father, Randy had visitation rights, and it was left to Brenda to supervise them.

On Friday, January 17, Brenda asked fourteen-year-old JD to look after Justine and Jenna. She had a Narcotics Anonymous meeting that night. She told him if she wasn't home by eleven, she wouldn't be home until the morning. JD said that was fine. So did his mother. Brenda stayed out all night with her NA sponsor and another friend, talking about how to stay clean.

Randy had another access visit scheduled for that Saturday. Brenda kept putting him off; she didn't want to see him again after the latest assault. She had been late getting home with Jenna for one of Randy's access visits, and he'd been furious about having to wait. Raised voices had turned into raised fists, and she'd called the police, yet again. Furious after he was finally arrested, Randy repeatedly called CAS, complaining that it was Brenda who was a danger to the children. A police officer stopped by that Saturday afternoon to take a statement from Brenda about the assault. She was getting Jenna out of the bath when he knocked. The officer noted that the toddler looked healthy and in good spirits. He didn't see any signs of abuse on either child.

Brenda first noticed a bruise later that afternoon when she was getting Jenna dressed. It didn't look like the kind of bruise toddlers routinely pick up running around, falling down, banging into things. It was on her back, and it looked like four fingertips. Brenda asked Maggie whether JD had said anything about the bruise. Maggie knew nothing about it, but said she would ask.

Brenda went out with Maggie for a couple of hours that night to buy marijuana. She still dabbled in softer drugs like pot and hash. The girls were again left with JD.

By Sunday, Jenna was acting jittery and scared. When Justine's father,

Joe Traynor, dropped by to pick her up that afternoon, Jenna started screaming and ran to Brenda. Joe wasn't around a lot, but he wasn't a stranger either. Jenna had never reacted to him like that before. It took several minutes of soothing talk and reassurances to calm her down. Brenda didn't know what to make of it.

And there was another bruise. Brenda noticed it that morning when she was changing Jenna. It was on the inside of her left thigh, and it looked like a handprint. Brenda asked Maggie about it later that afternoon. Maggie again said she had no idea, that she would check with JD. Something wasn't right, but Brenda let it go.

She had another Narcotics Anonymous meeting Sunday night. Maggie drove her there, while JD and his younger sister, Angie, took turns looking after Jenna and Justine.

Jenna was still out of sorts. She wouldn't stop crying. True, she had been a screamer since the day she was born. She could get riled up by anything at any hour, even in the middle of the night. The girls shared a room, so Justine became a heavy sleeper out of necessity.

Jenna's inconsolable crying jags had worried Brenda enough that she'd taken her to the doctor several times in the spring of 1996. But Donald Thompson, her family doctor, told her the little girl was in good health. A bit headstrong, perhaps, but perfectly healthy.

Brenda told him she'd like to get a second opinion. Would he write a referral to the Hospital for Sick Children, in Toronto? Thompson said it wasn't necessary, Jenna was fine. Around May 1996, Brenda drove Jenna to SickKids anyway. The toddler was admitted for observation.

Doctors found cysts on Jenna's brain. They weren't life-threatening and did not require surgery or medical intervention. But Brenda was still frustrated that Thompson had not taken her concerns more seriously. Shortly after that, she found a new family doctor.

Jenna's crying was so bad that Sunday night, while Maggie was out taking Brenda to her meeting, that Angie called a girlfriend, desperate for advice. But nothing helped. Exhaustion was the only remedy. Eventually Jenna cried herself to sleep.

On Monday morning, Brenda noticed a mark on Jenna's right cheek. It looked like she had a bit of frostbite. Scrapes and scratches were a part of any toddler's life, but Brenda couldn't shake her unease. The bruises looked like handprints. Or maybe not. Maybe they were from Jenna's tumble down the stairs a couple of weeks earlier. The child was always falling over. Just that morning, Brenda had asked Jenna to sit on a stool in the bathroom while she had a quick shower. Jenna missed, scratching her back on the side of the stool, leaving a nasty red scrape.

Brenda took Jenna to see her mother, Gladys, wondering if she should see a doctor about this new mark on her face. Brenda's parents lived barely three blocks away. Gladys didn't think it was anything to worry about. She kissed her granddaughter and sent her off to play. She was right. Jenna did seem to be back to her happy self as Brenda and her mother continued chatting. Brenda told her mother things were over with Randy—it was the best thing for herself and her kids. She wouldn't even let him back into the house to pick up his things.

Tuesday morning, Justine left for school at 8:45. She was an independent kid and insisted on walking by herself. Brenda took inspiration from her daughter's resilience. She gave her stash of pot to Maggie and called Children's Aid. She asked one of her case workers, Sylvia Elgaly, to arrange with Randy to pick up his stuff from a mutual friend, Chris Hogan.

After that, it was a meandering sort of day. Mother and daughter rode the bus downtown to meet one of Brenda's friends for coffee. Jenna had Chicken McNuggets and french fries for lunch. They braved the cold to visit several other friends that afternoon. They stopped by Chris Hogan's place, and Brenda told him she was getting clean.

Brenda's friends would say later that Jenna seemed content, nibbling on a cookie, sipping on chocolate milk or running around playing while her mother visited. The afternoon slipped away, and Brenda ended up rushing home in a taxi to make sure she was at the apartment when Justine returned from school.

When Brenda got home, Maggie told her a woman from Children's

Aid had called. When Brenda phoned her back, she was told Randy had cancelled his next visit with Jenna. Apparently the timing wasn't great—Randy, too, was trying to get clean and was going through withdrawal. He also told CAS that he didn't want to collect his things from Chris Hogan, because Chris was a drug dealer.

"He's lying," Brenda told the CAS worker. Chris and his roommate, Philip Spinks, were not drug dealers, she insisted. Randy was just saying that to make Brenda look bad. Even so, the worker told Brenda she would need to make alternative arrangements for Randy's things.

Brenda hung up. Her head was spinning. What if Children's Aid called the police on Chris and Phil? Would they think it was her fault if they got busted?

She quickly dialled Chris's number. No answer. She tried Phil. Same thing. Jenna had been agitated since they'd got home. Still, Brenda thought she needed to talk to Chris and Phil as soon as possible. She asked Maggie if she could leave the girls with JD, who had been home sick from school that day. Maggie looked at JD, who shrugged his agreement. Maggie said she'd be there to help with dinner.

Brenda kissed the girls goodbye and left the apartment.

It was 4:45 p.m.

Brenda saw the flashing lights as soon as she turned onto her street. Police, fire, paramedics—a phalanx of vehicles blocked the street in front of her apartment.

It was after one thirty in the morning. Her talk with Chris and Phil had gone better than she'd hoped. They told her not to worry about it; what Randy said to CAS wasn't her responsibility. Later that evening, Brenda ran into an old friend, Dave Titus, downtown. The girls would already be in bed; Brenda saw no need to rush home. So she and Dave went out to play some pool. Afterwards, they ended up back at Dave's apartment, where, despite Brenda's earlier resolve, they smoked some pot. The hours slipped away, and before Brenda knew it, it was almost midnight. Freezing rain pelted the car windows as Dave drove her home. The trip should have taken less than fifteen minutes, but it ended up being an hour and a half of white-knuckle driving. When she saw all the flashing lights, Brenda was sure it was Randy. She had warned Maggie he might show up and told her she should call the police at the first sign of him.

But as Brenda opened her front door, she knew she had it wrong.

"Are you Brenda Waudby?" a police officer asked.

Brenda nodded. The house was overflowing with people. She could hear voices upstairs and down as police officers combed through the two apartments. Standing at the top of the stairs with Maggie was Justine, groggy and half-asleep, looking as confused as Brenda felt.

"Where's Jenna?" Brenda asked.

"There's been an accident, Ms. Waudby. She's been taken to the hospital. I'll drive you over."

Brenda took a deep breath, trying to stay calm, but she could taste fear in her mouth. Maggie told her Jenna had bumped her head on the slide earlier that evening when JD took the girls to play in the park.

"We should go," the officer said.

"Don't be mad at JD," Justine said as her mother turned to leave. "It wasn't his fault."

Brenda waited restlessly in the ER waiting room. The nurse said she had to speak to the doctor before Brenda could see Jenna, but the doctor was nowhere to be found. The waiting was making her crazy. Dave Titus sat beside her.

And then the doctor was there.

Dr. Dale Friesen led Brenda into a tiny room, not much larger than an office cubicle. It was packed with people, so many that Brenda felt claustrophobic. There was Dr. Friesen, and Dave, who hadn't left her side since they arrived. There was the police officer who'd driven her over. And her former family doctor, Donald Thompson.

"I'm sorry, Ms. Waudby, but your daughter has died." It was Dr. Friesen who said the words. "She's gone."

Dr. Thompson asked Brenda to account for any marks or injuries on Jenna's body. Brenda hadn't seen her yet. Her former family doctor was now acting as the coroner investigating Jenna's death. She told him about the bruises she had found on Jenna's back and leg on Saturday and Sunday, and said the mark on her face might be frostbite. Then the doctor asked Brenda if she wanted to see Jenna. She wavered; she wasn't sure she had the strength.

He insisted she should, that if she didn't she would regret it for the rest of her life. They led her back through the ER into a trauma room. Dave was still with her. Jenna was laid out on a gurney, covered by a white sheet that was pulled up to her neck. She looked so small, the contours of her tiny frame barely registering under the sheet. Brenda could only see her head.

Her vibrant blue eyes had gone grey and lifeless. They were pointing in different directions. This wasn't the Jenna Brenda knew and loved. This wasn't the little girl who, along with her sister, had motivated Brenda to get clean and to at least try to start acting like a responsible parent. But even hours past death, there was no mistaking her fire-engine-red locks. This was her baby Jenna.

The coroner led a sobbing Brenda out of the room. He never pulled back the sheet. Brenda never saw the dozens of bruises that covered Jenna's tiny body.

The police officer drove Brenda to the police station so she could give a statement. Maggie and JD were just leaving the station. It was after four in the morning, and they both looked it. Maggie glanced at Brenda expectantly.

"She's gone," Brenda said, too tired to cry anymore.

The two women hugged as JD, off to the side, watched quietly.

TWO

IT WAS 5:42 a.m., January 22, 1997. Brenda had been up for almost twenty-four hours.

She was sitting in a standard police interview room. Det. Const. Dan Lemay of the Peterborough Lakefield Community Police Service sat across from her. He was leading the police investigation into Jenna's death. Brenda told Lemay about Randy and the assault charge. She told him about her cocaine addiction, and that Children's Aid had seized the girls for six weeks the previous fall. He asked her what she had been doing the night before. He asked about her babysitting arrangements. And he asked her about any bruises or marks that Jenna might have had. Did the child suffer any injuries before Brenda left her with JD?

Brenda thought for a moment. Her mind was racing. She tried to focus.

Jenna did have a couple bruises, she said. One on her left thigh. It looked a little like a handprint. And another near the middle of her back. That one looked a bit like four fingers, she said.

What had happened to her baby girl? Brenda wondered. And then she asked herself another, more disturbing question: Had someone done something to her?

Jenna had been acting strange the past couple days, Brenda said. She would cling to Brenda when anyone came to the door.

Lemay asked about any other bruises or injuries. Brenda said Jenna didn't have any that she knew of. The doctors had asked her about a bruise around her ankles and her feet, she said, but Brenda didn't know anything about it.

Lemay asked her if she had noticed that bruise prior to giving Jenna to JD.

Brenda said it wasn't there. She had bathed Jenna and didn't see anything around her ankles or feet. She kept notes, Brenda explained. She had to. Children's Aid was monitoring the children.

—

Brenda stepped out into the bitter cold. The street lights did little to illu-minate the darkened parking lot behind the police station. It was just past six in the morning. She asked the detective to wait for her while she had a smoke. Lemay nodded, wandered over to his unmarked cruiser with another officer.

Brenda had already called her mother from a pay phone at the hospital. Her mother had heard the sirens screaming through their neighbourhood. She was home alone; Brenda's father was away in Las Vegas. Now Brenda had to tell Randy. It was a two-block drive from the police station to the rooming house where he was staying.

The red brick building loomed large as Brenda climbed out of the cruiser. She didn't know exactly which room was Randy's, but in the end, the detectives' door-pounding woke up the whole house anyway. Randy led her and the two officers down a hallway to his room.

It was Brenda who told him. The police officers never said a word.

Gladys helped make the funeral arrangements for the coming Sunday and Monday. Brenda talked to her family lawyer, Laird Meneley, about Justine; Children's Aid had seized her again the night Jenna died while police investigated the toddler's death. Brenda would have to go to court to get her back. Justine spent three days with her old foster family before being placed with Brenda's older brother Tom and sister-in-law Kim.

Meneley told her to call him if the police wanted to speak to her again. Everyone was advising her to get a criminal lawyer, but Brenda didn't understand why she should need one. The cause of Jenna's death had yet to be established.

She needed answers. So when the police called the next day, asking her to come in to clear up a few matters, she checked in with Meneley. He advised her not to go, but Brenda couldn't pass up the chance.

Lemay showed her into the interview room she had sat in only thirty-six hours earlier. Only now it felt less like an interview room and more like an interrogation room. The detective sat down across the table. The day before, his all-business attitude had been softened slightly with sympathy. This afternoon, the sympathy was gone.

Lemay began with a caution, explaining that she had the right to legal counsel. Brenda said she understood.

She declined to have legal counsel present.

Brenda said she had remembered another bruise she saw on Jenna: in her groin area. It was out of the ordinary, she said. And the bruises on Jenna's leg and back puzzled her too. Brenda didn't know where they'd come from. Randy hadn't seen her. No one outside the house had spent any time alone with Jenna. Just Brenda, Maggie, JD and the other kids.

She said JD had looked after the girls on the Friday and Saturday night before. She said she always considered him a competent babysitter, plus Maggie was always around if anything happened. But she added that every time JD came near Jenna recently, she cried and screamed. Brenda told Lemay about a bump on Jenna's head after a fall several weeks earlier. She told him about a cutting board that fell off the counter and landed on her big toe hard enough to draw blood. She told him about a red scratch on her back after Jenna fell off the stool in the bathroom. Brenda said Children's Aid told her that Jenna's death may have had sexual connotations, but the detective quickly shot that down, saying they had no evidence of a sexual assault.

He asked if she had a temper. She said sometimes, but it was never directed toward the children. Lemay asked if she had ever hit Jenna or Justine. Brenda said she spanked Justine. But not Jenna.

Lemay asked if Brenda had any animosity toward Jenna because of her relationship with Randy. Brenda said no. She would never harm her child.

How did she die? Brenda asked.

A severe blow to the abdomen that happened within the twenty-four hours before her death, Lemay said.

Brenda began to cry. In the middle of a police interrogation, she had just learned how her daughter had died.

—

Jenna Mellor had arrived at Peterborough Civic Hospital at 1:02 a.m. on Wednesday, January 22, 1997. She was not breathing and had no vital signs. Emergency room staff worked for almost an hour trying to revive the toddler, but were unsuccessful. At 1:50 a.m., she was pronounced dead.

Her thirty-inch frame looked even smaller than it actually was on the adult-sized stretcher. Her body was covered with bruises and scratches— on her feet, ankles, legs, back, stomach, face. And there were signs of possible sexual abuse. Dr. Dale Friesen noted possible rectal stretching and tears in the vulva. Lucinda Loukras, a pediatrician who also treated Jenna that night, noted bruising to the anus. "Probable sexual abuse," Loukras wrote. Friesen noted in his ER record: "Curly hair found in the vulva area? Source." A nurse pointed out to Dr. Donald Thompson, the coroner, a thread she saw in the vaginal area, partially embedded between the labia. Three other nurses also noted seeing a hair in Jenna's vaginal area.

Const. Scott Kirkland arrived at the hospital shortly after seven that morning to pick up Jenna's body from the morgue and travel with it to the Hospital for Sick Children, in Toronto, where he would observe the autopsy. Kirkland was an experienced officer, only a year away from retirement. He'd sat in on forty or fifty autopsies during his career, several involving children, and a couple conducted by Dr. Charles Smith.

At the hospital, Kirkland met with one of his superiors, Insp. Ray Vandervelde, who asked him to take some photographs and a video of the body for the detectives leading the investigation. Kirkland unzipped the body bag. Jenna was wearing a candy-striped hospital gown. The IV needle was still in her arm. Careful not to disturb any evidence, the officer delicately opened the gown and photographed and videotaped the young girl's bruise-covered body. But the officer was not briefed about the hospital staff's observations and suspicions of possible sexual abuse, and so he did not take any special care in documenting Jenna's pubic area, although one of his photographs inadvertently captured what appeared to be a hair in her labia.

Afterwards, the officer met with another colleague, Det. Const. Mark Ballantine, who gave him a more detailed briefing of the case, including a statement from Jenna's babysitter earlier that morning. Kirkland was given an X-ray and ultrasound to pass along to Dr. Smith. But again, he was not told about the possible hair, or about the concerns of possible sexual abuse raised by the ER doctor.

During the autopsy, Smith did find a hair in Jenna's pubic area, but he dismissed it as a contaminant. Hairs often turn up during autopsy, and many are not relevant to the examination or the police investigation. They fall off frantic caregivers or paramedics or emergency room doctors during resuscitation efforts. Dr. Friesen had not identified the hair found on Jenna's body as a possible contaminant. Neither had any of the nurses. That's because even a professional can't definitively tell what a hair is simply by looking at it. Hairs are supposed to be sent for laboratory analysis to determine whether they are contaminants or not.

The autopsy findings read like a shopping list of pain and suffering. Jenna had been severely beaten: cuts and bruises to the small intestine, pancreas, liver, adrenal gland, lungs, heart and diaphragm. Her abdomen was swollen because of severe internal bleeding, and she had at least thirteen rib fractures, running up the left and right sides.

More than a hundred bruises covered her body. They appeared to Smith to be of differing ages. Some were a deep purple, others were yellowish brown. Jenna had a suspected burn on the right side of her forehead that looked like a grille pattern, as if she had been branded. There was bruising inside her mouth and nose. Her left foot had bruises between the toes and on the heel. Her right knee was bruised. There were two scrapes along the vaginal opening. After her organs were removed, Smith found discoloration along her back and inside her rib cage. He also found evidence of hemorrhaging inside her head.

"Dr. Smith concludes that victim suffered a blow from a blunt object," Constable Kirkland wrote. "(could be fist or foot) causing a rupture in the duodenal [part of the small intestine], pancreas and liver. There was no evidence that this injury had begun to heal. It occurred within a few hours prior to death. Obvious evidence as well of continuous abuse."

The most significant development at the autopsy turned out to be what Kirkland didn't photograph: at no point did Dr. Smith identify or ask him to photograph a hair or fibre found in Jenna's vaginal area. The officer said the presence of a hair never came up during the autopsy. He testified at the Goudge Inquiry that he didn't even know about its existence until years later.

But Smith found one. It was in the child's genital area, just as Dr. Friesen had noted at the hospital.

It is the police's job to submit potential evidence for forensic analysis, but Smith said that when he tried to turn the hair over, the police refused to take it. He said police believed it to be a contaminant and therefore irrelevant to their criminal investigation. Since he felt the same way, he didn't push it. Instead, he sealed the hair in a small evidence envelope and filed it away in a cabinet in his office.

Smith also wrote in his autopsy notes that he could find no evidence that Jenna was sexually abused.

He didn't look very hard.

Smith said he did a simple external examination of the body, including the genitalia, during the autopsy. He said he consulted with Dr. Dirk Huyer, a colleague at SickKids who worked with the Suspected Child Abuse and Neglect, or SCAN, team at the hospital. Through his work with SCAN, Huyer had extensive experience with child abuse cases, but he was not a pediatrician; he was trained in family medicine. And though he was a coroner who had worked as a pathology assistant during medical school (he also dabbled in cosmetic surgery on the side) he was not certified in forensic pathology or pediatrics. Many of the cases he consulted on were about potential sexual abuse of living patients at the hospital.

Smith's autopsy notes state that Huyer examined the child's hymen. The two doctors decided there was no evidence of sexual abuse. Huyer did not put his opinion in writing. He did not file a report. He told me years later that he didn't view his participation as being in an official capacity. Huyer said it reflected a personal interest and an opportunity for professional development, not a formal consultation. Huyer testified at the Goudge Inquiry that had he known a hair was found in Jenna's genital area, and that a male teenager was a suspect, he would have recommended that Dr. Smith complete a full sexual assault evidence kit.

So besides his external examination, Smith did nothing to determine whether Jenna had been sexually assaulted. He did not dissect the child's genitalia or anus. He did not take vaginal swabs, anal swabs or oral swabs. He did not do any microscopic examinations.

Pinning down the timing of Jenna's injuries was critical in the investigation. There was a clear dividing line. If the fatal injuries occurred before 5 p.m., when Brenda went out for the evening and left JD to look after the girls, they suggested Brenda was responsible; if they occurred after 5 p.m., they would point to JD.

It was a complicated case, one of the most difficult Dr. Smith had ever faced. He was trying to determine whether Jenna's multiple abdominal injuries had occurred at the same time or if the child had been abused on more than one occasion.

There are some clues that can help a forensic pathologist determine when injuries occurred. It takes time for the body to heal. The body sends waves of inflammatory cells to damaged tissue to repair an injury, but that process stops when the person dies, freezing the healing process in time. By measuring the level of inflammation, a pathologist can assess how long before death the injury occurred.

But accurately pinpointing the time of an injury is a tricky task, and a pathologist must have sound forensic training and expertise to do so. Smith had neither. To complicate matters, his opinions kept changing. He told Constable Kirkland during the autopsy that the injuries to Jenna's pancreas, liver and duodenum had not begun to heal, indicating that they had occurred within hours of her death.

However, when Kirkland spoke with Detective Constable Lemay later that day, that information changed slightly. According to Lemay's notes, Kirkland told him the fatal abdominal injuries had been caused "up to a few hours before but no longer than 24 hours of her death."

Lemay talked to Dr. Thompson, the investigating coroner, who said he had just spoken with Smith. Thompson reiterated that the cause of death was intra-abdominal trauma that had caused lacerations to the stomach, bowel and liver. He said Smith had found evidence of fractured ribs and facial injuries that were a few days old. Older injuries suggested Jenna was abused on more than one occasion, he told Lemay, but Smith had not found any evidence of sexual assault. Most important, Thompson said that at this point Smith believed the injuries occurred before five o'clock.

The next morning Lemay checked in with Thompson's supervisor, Dr. Peter Clark, the regional coroner. Clark told him that Smith couldn't determine, at least on his initial examination of the body, an exact time frame for Jenna's death.

The injuries occurred within hours of her death. The injuries likely occurred within hours of her death but up to twenty-four hours before. The injuries occurred at least seven hours before. And sorry, but we can't say.

The investigation was less than thirty hours old and police had been given four different answers concerning the fundamental question of when Jenna's fatal injuries occurred.

That wasn't necessarily a problem—yet. The investigation was still in its infancy; police were still narrowing down their main suspects; the autopsy results, which wouldn't be complete for months, would likely become more useful as the investigation took shape.

Lemay finally reached Smith himself later that morning. The officer's notes on the call do not mention any discussion of Smith's findings at autopsy. What is implied is that the timing of Jenna's fatal injuries might be too difficult to nail down, failing to point to one suspect or the other. Smith encouraged police to investigate the child's behaviour and habits throughout the day. Someone had beaten Jenna severely, and it would have been obvious in her behaviour; she likely would have started vomiting or lost her appetite or shown signs of dizziness. Determining when that started would help police determine when the injuries occurred.

Brenda knocked on her brother Tom's front door. It was Friday afternoon, barely two days since Jenna's death, and it was time to tell Justine.

Children's Aid had taken Justine into care the night Jenna died, and she was now living with Tom and his wife, Kim. Justine's social worker first told Brenda she would have to tell Justine about Jenna's death over the phone, but Brenda insisted on doing it in person.

Kim opened the door, and Brenda swept Justine up in her arms. She hadn't seen her since that night, standing on the landing at the apartment. Kim led them downstairs where they could talk.

Brenda looked at the big, comfy couch, unsure if she should sit or stand when she shared the news. Kim took a seat nearby, waiting. A case worker from Children's Aid was there as well.

Brenda stayed standing. She reminded Justine about a cat they'd once had. He'd been hit by a car. Justine remembered—he'd gone to heaven. Brenda told her that is where Jenna had gone too. To join Fat Cat in heaven.

Years later, Justine said she remembers that talk, remembers the moment she heard her little sister was dead. It burned, searing hot, as if her organs were on fire. Justine blamed herself. She hadn't been able to keep her sister safe. A guilt, even now, she struggles to keep at bay.

THREE

THOSE FIRST DAYS after Jenna's death, Brenda, JD and Maggie were again interviewed by police. Their statements remained consistent.

Maggie said she'd made dinner for the kids and then went out to visit a friend around six thirty. She took Kevin with her and offered to take Jenna as well since she seemed to be in a cranky mood that evening. JD said he would be fine. She got home a little after eight. JD told his mother about Jenna's mishap on the slide. It didn't sound too serious, but Maggie wanted to check on her just to be safe. They went to the girls' bedroom, and Maggie said she was shocked by what she saw. She scooped up the little girl in her arms. Jenna had a burn on her forehead that looked like a grid pattern. She also had a bump on her forehead that was starting to bruise. She didn't look well. JD told his mother that she had bumped against the hair dryer while he was drying her hair. The burn had been an accident. Maggie fetched a cold cloth for the bump and some vitamin E cream for the burn. Jenna didn't seem to be in pain. Maggie said she thought about taking her to the hospital but then decided she'd be okay. She told JD to keep a close eye on her.

Justine went to sleep in Brenda's bed around 8:45. Maggie slipped Jenna in beside her, hoping that being close to her big sister might calm the toddler. She then went back upstairs, but kept the doors between the apartments open.

JD told the police that Jenna wouldn't go to sleep, and he was worried that he'd soon have two cranky kids on his hands if he left her in bed with Justine. He said he brought Jenna out to the couch to lie down beside him, but she wouldn't lie still. At one point, she rolled off and banged her head on the edge of a plastic picnic table in front of the couch. She was wailing on the floor, and then suddenly she stopped breathing. JD reached for her. She let out a gasp and started wailing again. As he lifted her up off the floor, she coughed and spit up a little on his arm. It was purplish brown, with little bits of macaroni in it.

JD told police he cleaned her up and put her back to bed in her crib. She seemed to be finally settling down, until about thirty minutes later when she started hacking and coughing. She vomited again when JD picked her up. He took her to the bathroom to lean over the toilet while he cleaned up the mess she'd made on the carpet. He put her back in the crib.

At about 10:15, two of JD's friends stopped by. Jenna was still up. Maggie came down to try to soothe her, then put her back in the crib. But she still wouldn't stay down. JD got the toddler up several times while his friends were over, each time trying unsuccessfully to put her back down to sleep. Both friends noticed red marks on Jenna's face and a bump on her forehead, but neither held her. A little before eleven, Maggie came down to tell JD's friends they had to leave. JD put Jenna down again. Her breathing sounded a little wheezy, but he left her in her crib.

Around twelve thirty, when Jenna started another coughing jag, JD said he checked on her once more. He picked her up and she vomited again. Tired and increasingly frustrated, he said he took her back into the bathroom, leaning her over the toilet again. JD said he thought she was okay, but when he let go of her she fell backward and banged her head on the wall heater. When he picked her up, he noticed her wheezy breathing. Something clearly wasn't right. He took her back into her bedroom where there was more room to lay her down on the floor. JD said her eyes then rolled back in her head and she appeared to stop breathing. He grabbed her and sprinted upstairs, screaming for his mother, who quickly called 911.

Someone was lying. The detectives were sure of it. Their investigation quickly narrowed to two main suspects: JD and Brenda. Neither of their stories added up to the injuries that killed Jenna.

Police executed search warrants for Brenda's and Maggie's apartments. Officers canvassed neighbours about anything they may have seen or heard. Brenda gave blood and urine samples. She also agreed to take a polygraph test, but it was postponed after she was deemed ineligible because of the medication she was taking. JD visited the psychiatric wing of the hospital for counselling to help him cope with Jenna's death.

Brenda ended up taking her polygraph test on January 28, 1997. She failed it.

Brenda now knew that her baby had been beaten to death, and the most likely culprit was the babysitter in whose care she had left her. She should have known something was wrong. She had seen bruises on Jenna in the days before she died. One looked like a handprint.

What's more, Brenda knew JD was unstable. Maggie had told her only weeks earlier about a disturbing incident. The teenager had asked his mother for a cigarette. She said no, and Maggie told Brenda JD grabbed a knife and threatened her. Terrified, Maggie called the police, and JD ended up in counselling.

Brenda tried to rationalize her decision to leave her girls with JD. Maggie had told her she would be upstairs. She was supposed to be close at hand if anything happened.

But she couldn't escape the guilt: if she had been a better mother, she would have recognized the signs that something wasn't right, and her daughter would still be alive.

Police gave JD a polygraph test the next day, but it was cut short when the officer decided the teenager didn't have the necessary intelligence to take it. Instead, police questioned him again about what had happened. His story was consistent with his earlier statements: he said he thought her death was an accident.

Police kept digging. They re-interviewed Brenda and Randy, Maggie and JD, over and over.

And then the letter arrived.

Peterborough police received the letter five days after Jenna's death. The handwriting is tall and narrow, tilting slightly forward as it switches between cursive and printing. Fifty-seven words on a single unsigned page of plain white paper: "I'm not sure how this information could possibly help in the investigation of the death of the 18-month-old girl, but I do know that the little girl was woke up out of her sleep at 2:30 a.m. on Tuesday, January 21, 1997 with blows to her midsection, this lasted until 6:30 a.m., Tuesday Jan. 21, 1997." The date was crucial. Jenna had been in Brenda's care the night of the alleged beating.

Police tried to determine who had written it, taking writing samples from everyone close to either of the suspects. They even seized the condolence book from Jenna's funeral. They had matchable DNA off the envelope and the back of the stamp, so they took DNA samples, fifty-seven in all, from family members, friends, acquaintances and professionals who had worked with either family. Investigators determined the DNA came from a female, but could not make a match.

Detective Constable Lemay showed the letter to Brenda and Randy on March 10. "This is such bullshit!" she said. She was convinced Maggie had written the letter. The detective didn't think so; they'd done DNA testing on the stamp and envelope that proved Maggie didn't send it.

The night before Jenna died, she woke Brenda up at two thirty. That wasn't out of the ordinary. Brenda fed her and changed her, but Jenna wouldn't go back to sleep. That wasn't unusual either. Jenna was screaming. Exhausted and frustrated, Brenda admitted that she lost her temper and yelled at the toddler to go to sleep. "But I never did anything to hurt Jenna," she told Lemay. "I never hit her, I swear."

Whoever wrote the letter knew about that incident. But Brenda hadn't told anyone about it besides the police.

And then there was the timing. Lemay said the forensic pathologist, Dr. Charles Smith, believed that Jenna had suffered her fatal injuries within twenty-four hours of her death, which put the nighttime feeding incident just inside his timeline.

Lemay said someone either wrote the letter to falsely incriminate her, or someone had information that was very incriminating against her. Brenda was outraged. She said she was being set up.

The murder was the talk of Peterborough. Everyone had an opinion on who the killer was. Most of the suspicion centred on Brenda. Police faced intense pressure to make an arrest. The detectives were a constant presence in Brenda's life, asking her the same questions, over and over. Lemay and Sgt. Gord McNevan stopped her at least two or three times a week for the next five months; they conducted dozens of interviews with her, but she was rarely advised that she could have a lawyer present. She would be out having a coffee with a friend and see their cruiser pull up to the curb. It felt like it was verging on harassment.

Police continued to investigate JD as well. They rebuilt the hours and days before Jenna's death, searching for evidence of when the fatal injuries occurred. They couldn't find any. By all accounts, Jenna seemed to be healthy well into the night that she died. Which, in a way, was evidence itself.

Brenda knew she needed to grieve for her daughter, but with a murder investigation swirling around her, it was impossible. She had never felt more alone.

And then she met Ramona.

Brenda's court-ordered Narcotics Anonymous meetings were held in a local church basement. They were intimate affairs, barely ten people in attendance each week. There was a core group of six regulars, including Brenda, with new faces coming and going on the periphery, so Ramona Spiegel's sudden appearance wasn't unusual. The meetings were one of the few places Brenda felt safe. Police were circling her outside. Randy was back in her life and as volatile as ever. But in that church basement, Brenda felt protected. She could talk openly about her struggles to get clean and to stay clean amid the horror of Jenna's sudden death, and the police couldn't hold it against her. What was said in those meetings stayed in those meetings. That was one of the core foundations of Narcotics Anonymous. There was a local police officer among the group, but he wasn't there as a cop. He was a recovering addict, just like everyone else. They were equals.

That Wednesday night in late March, people milled around before the meeting, catching up over coffee. Ramona Spiegel mingled with the group, introducing herself, exchanging pleasantries.

When she got around to Brenda, she admitted she was a heroin addict. She'd just moved back to Peterborough with her boyfriend and this was her first time at a meeting. Brenda assured her it was a good group and that Ramona would be safe here.

Over the following weeks, the two women chatted before or after meetings. And it wasn't just at NA. Brenda bumped into Ramona at the Park Street Mission, a shelter where people could go for a hot meal. Randy lived there on and off. Ramona went with her boyfriend, John.

Ramona was struggling to get herself straightened out and Brenda was happy to listen and lend a hand. Ramona was eager to return the favour. The two women became close very quickly, and their talks soon turned to Jenna. Ramona told Brenda she could relate. She had just lost a baby herself. She'd miscarried in December, but she hadn't yet told John. He still thought she was pregnant. Ramona then asked Brenda how she was coping. Brenda said she was barely holding it together. Every time she turned around, Lemay was dragging her back in for questioning. She was fighting Children's Aid to regain custody of Justine. She felt isolated. Most of her former friends now shunned her because of the murder investigation, or because they were potential witnesses themselves. She was living with her grief by herself.

It was mid-April when they first went to the cemetery together. Brenda went to Jenna's grave several times a week, but always on her own. Inviting Ramona to come with her was a big step.

Little Lake Cemetery is one of Peterborough's oldest, sitting on a peninsula that juts into Little Lake. The Otonabee River runs along the cemetery's eastern flank. Brenda kneeled down, pushing back the grass crowding in around the edges of the small, flat headstone, with its picture of baby Jesus and the Virgin Mary. The inscription read, "Our Little Pumpkin Jenna Clare Ann Mellor, April 21, 1995–Jan. 22, 1997." Justine had come up with the name Jenna. It was the name of one of her school friends, and mother and daughter both liked it.

The two women sat quietly for a bit, and then Brenda admitted to Ramona that the police suspected she had done something to Jenna, and after their incessant questioning, Brenda wondered if it might be true. But just as quickly as the words came out of her mouth she dismissed them. There was no way she would hurt her daughter.

Then Ramona said she'd heard of people who suffered memory lapses after horrible events in their lives. She wondered if that had happened to Brenda. If the police were so sure she was responsible, maybe Brenda had done something that her mind just wouldn't let her remember.

Brenda assured Ramona there was no way she could have beaten her daughter and have no memory of it. But Ramona reminded her she had been smoking marijuana the night before Jenna died. Maybe because she was so high she couldn't remember what had happened. Brenda confessed to Ramona that Justine had once gone missing for a few hours. Brenda had been frantic with worry, so when they finally found Justine she was angry and had smacked the little girl on her bottom. But then Brenda had walked out of the room because she didn't want to lose it. She knew she would never hurt either of her daughters. She just knew it.

A week later, Lemay called Brenda back in for another round of questioning. She noticed a white envelope sitting on the table. Her mind raced. What was in that envelope? Brenda didn't want to think about it. Couldn't think about it.

The detective grilled her about her story, the same questions he had asked her dozens of times before, but Brenda couldn't focus. The white envelope was screaming at her.

"We know you did it," the officer said. "The forensics are back and they show definitively that Jenna sustained her injuries before 5 p.m. When you had her. So why don't you just tell me what really happened? You don't have to carry this burden anymore."

He opened the envelope and took out five photographs. Autopsy photographs, of Jenna. He spread them out on the table in front of Brenda. "I'll be back in a minute. Stay put," he said. And then he left the interrogation room.

Jenna was barely recognizable under the grotesque patchwork of bruises and welts. From limb to limb, from head to toe, no part of her tiny body had escaped the violence that took her life. Brenda knew her child had suffered—the police hammered her with that fact over and over—yet she hadn't really known how much.

She could hear Ramona's questions in her head. Could she have done this and somehow blocked it from her memory?

The photographs should have reinforced Brenda's insistence that she was not responsible. Jenna's injuries were so violent that once committed, they could never be forgotten. But the detective was unequivocal: the forensic evidence showed definitively that her injuries happened before five o'clock. JD could not have inflicted them, which left only Brenda. If she had done something so brutal, maybe her guilt-ridden mind would refuse to remember it.

Because, now that Brenda thought about it, she couldn't recall much of the night before Jenna's death. She had gone to see her mother with Jenna earlier in the day. She had put the girls down at their regular bedtimes. Jenna was a bit whiny but nothing out of the ordinary.

Waves of nausea and stress washed over her. Why couldn't she remember?

Jenna woke up around two thirty. Brenda remembered that. She had a leaky wet diaper. Brenda changed her and the sheets, and both of them went back to bed.

But what had she done earlier in the evening? It was a quiet night. She had stayed home. No NA meeting to go to. Had she just dozed off?

Maybe Ramona was on to something. Maybe she *was* blocking something out.

Brenda started having nightmares about the pictures. Nightmares about the questions Ramona asked. Nightmares about standing over Jenna's crib, yelling at her. Horrible nightmares that Brenda Waudby started to believe were true.

Detective Constable Lemay thought the investigation was going well. Brenda still hadn't confessed, but his focus had shifted toward her as the main suspect. He continued to investigate JD, who doggedly maintained his innocence as well. JD's mother took a lie detector test; the results were inconclusive. In particular, the technician felt she was deceptive when asked, "Did you physically cause Jenna's death?" Maggie reasoned later that the machine probably detected the guilt she felt for not looking after Jenna well enough on the night she died. Police used the results to go after JD even more aggressively. Lemay used the same technique he had tried on Brenda: he told JD all the evidence pointed to him.

The detective told JD his mother failed her lie detector test during one interrogation. He said police believed that was because Maggie knew he did it, and she felt guilty for not stopping him. But JD said he didn't do anything to hurt Jenna.

The detectives interrogated JD repeatedly. His story and his denials were remarkably consistent. If he was lying, he should have cracked by now. And frankly, the kid didn't seem smart enough to deceive them. He didn't even have the necessary intelligence to take the lie detector test. His mother was in the house for most of the night. How could he have beaten Jenna so severely without Maggie hearing something?

There were gaps in this logic. Maggie had been deceptive on her polygraph test. Maybe she did know something, or at least suspected. But the biggest hurdle was Jenna's behaviour. She had been severely beaten, yet had shown no signs of it earlier in the day. If Brenda had hurt her the night before, wouldn't there be signs she was in pain? Yet no one noticed anything. JD even took her and her sister to the playground, and she seemed fine.

Still, the boy was sticking to his story. Police felt they were having more luck with Brenda. Lemay kept up the pressure, claiming that the forensic evidence showed Jenna's fatal injuries had happened the night before she died, when Brenda was caring for her. Brenda wouldn't confess, but there was an air of resignation around her, as if she knew police were closing in.

Throughout the investigation, Children's Aid pressured the police to share information. Social workers worried about Justine's safety. Both girls had been removed from Brenda's care before Jenna's death, but Brenda persuaded a judge to give them back. Now Jenna was dead. Social workers were determined to keep Justine safe.

There was little Children's Aid could do on its own. Social workers weren't equipped to conduct their own investigation, but if police had credible evidence Brenda was responsible, the agency could use that information to stop her from getting Justine back. Despite the CAS's petitions, however, the police wouldn't share. Lemay signed affidavits in April and July stating that releasing any information to CAS could jeopardize an ongoing police investigation. Children's Aid was on its own.

A Family Court judge ordered that Justine be returned to Brenda on April 30, 1997. Going home was difficult for Justine. She loved and missed her mother. But she hated Randy—hated his temper, his screaming, his abuse. And she started to sense the whispers—whispers about how her little sister had died, things her mother had done. Justine would catch parents glancing at her, or teachers being overly sympathetic and protective. She had been an outgoing, social child. She had friends. But after her sister's death and another stint in foster care, Justine withdrew.

On July 7, 1997, Peterborough detectives met with Dr. Smith and Deputy Chief Coroner Jim Cairns to discuss the medical evidence. Smith zeroed in on the injuries to Jenna's ribs. It wasn't new evidence; a skeletal survey and CT scan by Dr. Paul Babyn at the Hospital for Sick Children on the day Jenna died had revealed multiple fractures. The CT report noted the injuries were "without evidence of callus formation," meaning they had not yet started healing. That is, they were new. "Findings are in keeping with acute non-accidental injury given lack of defined healing, multiplicity of fractures and fracture location," Babyn wrote.

However, on that July morning, Smith had a different view of Jenna's rib fractures. He now believed they were older than her other injuries— five to seven days older. There's no indication in the police notes of why his opinion changed, but it was a useful shift: Lemay was trying to persuade a judge to sign off on an authorization for electronic surveillance. But he needed new evidence, and now he had it.

By adding that one word—"older"—Dr. Smith attached a new dimension to the case that would prolong Brenda's legal misery for almost fifteen years.

—

In July 1997, the Kawartha Haliburton Children's Aid Society won a court order requiring Peterborough police detectives to share their files on the Jenna Mellor death investigation.

Brenda had been granted custody of Justine in April, but neither she nor Randy was allowed to be alone with her at any time. After Brenda and Randy broke up again, she asked the court to remove the supervision provision. Her request was denied. Brenda's mother was required to be with them twenty-four hours a day.

Dr. Smith's opinion that Jenna had older rib injuries, CAS believed, showed a pattern of abuse in the household. The agency would use this information in Family Court to bolster its argument for continued supervision. Though the police had resisted disclosing information to CAS in the past, they now saw an advantage in it. If Brenda knew the police had more medical evidence against her, it might push her closer to cracking. And if the police had surveillance equipment in place, they would catch her confession.

Linda Mitchelson, the manager of the Child Protection Unit of Kawartha Haliburton Children's Aid, met with detectives on August 15, 1997. On August 20 she swore an affidavit for a Family Court hearing that would be held the next day.

Legally, Brenda had the right to full disclosure of CAS's case, including Mitchelson's affidavit. But the affidavit wasn't filed in court that day. It wouldn't be filed for another two weeks. So Brenda didn't have any knowledge of the new evidence against her until September 5, when the affidavit was finally filed, by which time the police had the necessary equipment in place to capture her reaction.

Ramona drove Brenda to her family lawyer's office to discuss the affidavit. On the ride home, she asked Brenda what the affidavit had said. Brenda was confused and stressed. She told her friend the evidence pointed to older injuries. And not just any injuries, but eleven broken ribs from days before Jenna's death. How could Jenna have been walking around with eleven broken ribs for days before she died, Brenda wanted to know.

And what about the cop who had answered the call when Randy was threatening Brenda that Saturday? He'd said he hadn't noticed anything wrong with the girl.

Brenda also learned from the affidavit that it had taken Jenna seventeen hours to bleed to death. How could she have been playing, giggling, eating at McDonald's, and the whole time been bleeding to death? It didn't make any sense. The medical experts must have made a mistake.

Brenda told Ramona she was done second-guessing herself. She knew she could account for the time. The reason she couldn't remember much from the Monday night before Jenna died was because not much happened. She didn't beat her daughter to death and then forget about it.

The medical report itself had not been included in the affidavit, just Linda Mitchelson's reading of it. Brenda's family lawyer, Laird Meneley, would try to get hold of the report itself. The police would want Brenda to account for the four or five days before Jenna's death—where she was, what she did. Brenda realized she'd been away from Jenna quite a bit during that time. She'd had an NA meeting on the Sunday night and she'd left the girls with JD and his sister. And she'd been at NA on Friday night, and she was out for a while Saturday night as well. On both occasions, the girls had been in JD's care.

FOUR

THE POLICE CAME for Brenda the morning of Thursday, September 18. She and Justine were living at her parents' house. Still in her pyjamas, Brenda opened the door to three police officers: Detective Constable Lemay, Sergeant McNevan and Const. Cory McMullan. In all her dealings with the police over the past eight months, there had only ever been two officers. When she opened the door to three faces, she knew they had come to arrest her.

"Brenda Waudby, you're being arrested for the murder of Jenna Clare Mellor," Lemay said as the officers stepped inside. The words snapped Brenda's mind and body back together. She glanced inside the living room, where her father was sitting. Justine was in her bedroom. So was Brenda's mother. Brenda asked to move outside just as Justine opened her door.

"You are being charged with second-degree murder. Do you understand the charge?"

Brenda nodded as she watched confusion, then fear flash across her daughter's face. Her father signalled for Justine to come sit with him in the living room. The eight-year-old climbed up into his lap.

"You have the right to an attorney . . ." Lemay continued, then reached for his handcuffs.

"Please," Brenda whispered. She glanced at Justine sitting on her father's lap. "Not in here!"

The detective's eyes followed hers and his hand moved away. Constable McMullan, the female officer among them, accompanied Brenda to get dressed.

While the other two officers waited, Justine asked why they were taking her mother away. Lemay explained that Brenda just had to come with them for a while.

Once dressed, Brenda reached for her bottle of lorazepam. She was supposed to take it twice a day for stress and anxiety, but had yet to take her pill that morning. But Constable McMullan insisted she leave the pills behind.

Again Brenda asked to speak with her lawyer and was told she could call him from the station. Brenda asked her father to call him now instead, and reminded her parents of Justine's doctor's appointment and counselling session later that day. She tried to reassure Justine that everything would be all right. She felt a wave of relief roll over as the three officers took her through the kitchen and out the side door. At least they weren't cuffing her in front of her daughter. Then Brenda glanced back in the front window, where Justine was watching. Brenda hung her head, then looked up again and smiled at Justine, mouthing "I love you" as the officers walked her over to the unmarked police car parked out front.

At the police station, another officer booked her. "Do you understand what you've been arrested for?" he asked.

"Yeah, I believe it is second-degree murder."

"And you've been advised of your rights?"

"Yeah, I believe so."

Constable McMullan took her into a small cell, where she was searched. She had no money on her, just a pack of cigarettes, a lighter and a small leather pouch. It was all signed into an evidence envelope and sealed. McMullan led her back out to the booking officer.

"I'd like to call my lawyer," Brenda said.

It was a little after nine when she phoned her criminal lawyer. Jim Hauraney had already left for court, so she ended up speaking to another lawyer in his firm, Alvin Schieck. He told Brenda to tell the police her name, address, telephone number and absolutely nothing else. She wasn't to answer any questions. She wasn't to talk to anyone. Schieck asked her to repeat those instructions to him. He then asked to speak with the detective, but Lemay refused. Schieck told Brenda he would try to reach Hauraney in court.

Brenda had understood the lawyer's instructions, but she wanted the interrogation to end. Although neither of the detectives said so directly, she had the distinct feeling that she wouldn't be allowed to leave until she gave them a statement. She was terrified of being detained in jail as a suspected child killer. And she worried about losing Justine forever. So she talked.

Detective Constable Lemay and Sergeant McNevan began the interrogation at 9:14 a.m. It wasn't recorded, but that was not unusual at the time. Two statements Brenda would give later in the morning were recorded, but the interrogation that preceded them was not.

At one point, there was a rap on the door. "Do you want to speak to a lawyer?" Sergeant McNevan asked. Brenda said no. To this day, she's not sure why. Brenda didn't realize it at the time, but Alvin Schieck had come down to the police station. The lawyer who told her not to say anything to police. He was waiting outside. The detective closed the door, and the interrogation continued.

At 10:30, Lemay walked her into another interview room to give her statement. McNevan went into a different room to monitor the video equipment.

Brenda took a seat in a corner of the room. Lemay sat in front of her.

"Okay, Brenda, I'll cover the legal aspects first, like we do," the detective began, going over the second-degree murder charge she was facing and her right to remain silent and speak to a lawyer.

Brenda declined both.

"Okay. We've just spoken about what took place pertaining to Jenna, who's your daughter. I know this is very hard, but what I would like to do is for you to explain to me what happened."

Jenna was crying; Brenda was frustrated that she couldn't get her to stop. "I remember picking her up and my back was hurting and I dropped her on the crib rail. I didn't think she was hurt, and she fell back in the crib," Brenda said, tearing up. Jenna seemed fine, though, and Brenda left her to cry herself to sleep. That was it until two thirty, when she woke up. Brenda changed her in the living room and put her back down without any problems.

Brenda admitted to smoking some marijuana, a particularly potent blend, after the kids went to bed. But she maintained that she was clear-headed when she was dealing with Jenna's tantrum.

"Are you sure that's how it happened, Brenda?" Lemay asked.

"Yes. Yes." She was crying harder now.

"Are you sure you didn't get angry and maybe toss her?"

"No."

"Because you know how badly hurt she was. Now you know, you didn't know then. Are you sure something else didn't hap—?"

"I didn't throw her," Brenda said. "I didn't. Honestly. I remember her falling into the crib. And I remember my back cracking . . ."

"Do you remember everything that happened in that room or are there things you don't remember?"

"I'm not sure. I'm really not sure."

The detective asked about the height of the railing, how high she would have been holding Jenna when she dropped her back into the crib. He asked her about the extensive bruising on her feet and toes. The problem for Lemay was that what Brenda was admitting wasn't enough to cause Jenna's severe and extensive injuries. Not even close.

"Did something else happen there?" Lemay asked.

"No."

"'Cause you know as well as I do, when you lift a little one out of the crib, and I have a little one too, you're still relatively close to that rail."

Brenda nodded in agreement.

"So she would have fallen, but not very far to the rail. So for you to react to the point where you thought, 'Oh shit, something's wrong here . . .'"

"I don't know."

"You obviously knew there was a problem," the officer said. "Something must have happened other than that."

"No. I can remember dropping her."

"Did you throw her?"

Brenda looked at the officer. "Nope. No!"

Brenda knew the police were convinced she had killed her daughter. *Someone* killed her little girl, and the police said JD couldn't have done it. It had to be her. It had to be. That fact had been pounded into her for so long, she was starting to believe it. The accusation was embedded in the detective's questions. It was there, in the wayward glances of her family and friends. She even wondered what Ramona thought.

But hearing Lemay's questions now, Brenda realized that she hadn't done the math. She hadn't thought through what killing her daughter would have entailed. She knew she was a poor mother. She was a pot-smoking former cocaine addict trapped in an abusive relationship and barely providing the basic necessities for her children. She had failed her girls. It was easy to conflate that failing with being directly responsible. And so accidentally dropping Jenna on the crib rail became a deadly mistake.

But Brenda realized now how ridiculous that was. Children don't die from a one-foot fall onto a wooden railing followed by a tumble into a cushioned crib. That doesn't cause bruises from head to toe. She would have had to have done more.

"Look at me, Brenda. Did you throw her?" the detective asked again.

"No."

"But you knew there was something wrong and for dropping her just that far . . ."

"I'm overprotective. She's my baby," she said defensively.

"I know she's your baby, but you made a mistake, Brenda. You made a mistake. It doesn't mean you love her any less," Lemay said, as if reading her thoughts. "You made a mistake. And it's something we've got to deal with. But you've got another one to look after. You've got another one to think of, you have to deal with it. It's been eight months and you've wanted it to go away, I know you have. But it's not going away. You have to face up to the guilt and that's what you're doing."

"I know," she agreed.

"I know it's hard. All along these eight months you knew we would come to this day. You knew you'd have to fess up to it."

The video statement ended after another fifteen minutes of questioning, but Brenda didn't confess to anything other than dropping Jenna on the crib rail. She hoped the interrogation was finally over, but they took her into another interview room, and then left.

McNevan thought Brenda wasn't telling them everything. She admitted to having a twenty-minute gap in her memory He thought more had to have happened in that period. Dropping Jenna on the railing didn't explain the extent of her injuries.

Lemay agreed. Brenda had admitted she did something wrong. She was just having a hard time admitting the whole story. But he sensed she was ready to talk.

The two men stepped into the interview room. Brenda was slumped over in her chair. She had finished her cigarette.

The officers told Brenda they had more questions for her. They took her back to the interrogation room and questioned her for another eighty minutes or so. They didn't give her any food. They didn't let her have her anti-anxiety medication. They didn't ask if she wanted to speak to her lawyer, and Brenda didn't ask to.

What they did tell her was that there had to be more, that she wasn't telling them the whole truth about what happened that night.

Brenda was exhausted, physically and emotionally. She wanted— needed—the interrogation to end. And she believed it wouldn't until she told the detectives what they wanted to hear. She couldn't go to jail charged with murdering her daughter. She didn't think she would survive the night. She needed to get home to her parents, to Justine.

Brenda couldn't remember hurting her daughter, but at that moment, it didn't matter. She was ready to fill in the blanks. She agreed to continue her statement.

Detective Constable Lemay once more established that Brenda understood her rights. "I just want to make it clear that there's no inducements on our part, you were not forced in any way to do this. Is this correct?"

"Yes," Brenda replied.

"Okay. We conducted an interview in here earlier today. We, since then, went into room 224 and we discussed it a little further."

"Yes."

"As a result of that," Lemay said, "there's some new stuff has come to light, and you've expressed to me that you wish to talk about this, as hard as it is. So we'll go back to that evening and I'm going to let you do it at your own pace here."

The words cascaded out of her.

"Okay. There was a lot of confusion. I was mad. I was angry. I remember dropping Jenna into the crib. Then it got confusing. I was telling her to go to sleep. I laid her down, I put my hand on her back to hold her down. She kept standing up. She . . . It's just confusing, I remember swinging my arms.

"I don't know. I probably hit her once or twice. I don't remember actually striking her but I remember swinging my arms. The possibility that I hit her is . . . it's there. I can remember her lying in the crib and I was thinking to myself, 'Oh shit, I've done something. I can't tell anybody.' And I didn't realize I caused any injuries.

"I never meant to hurt her."

"I know you didn't," Lemay said. "What was Jenna's reaction during this confusion?"

"She was crying. That's all I remember. She was crying."

"After you swung your arms and stuff what was she doing? You say she was standing, you started swinging your arms."

"She was laying in the crib. And I knew I'd done something wrong."

Lemay asked her where Justine was—whether Brenda was alone at the time. She said her older daughter was in the living room. It happened between eight thirty and ten o'clock. There was no one else in the apartment.

"Did you tell anyone about this?" Lemay asked.

"No."

"How long do you think this rage where you were swinging your arms lasted?"

"Not very long," Brenda replied. "Not very long. I wasn't mad at her. I was mad at everybody." She started to cry.

"Why were you mad at everybody?"

"CAS was pressuring me and Randy was pressuring me. He was making my life a living hell."

"Once Jenna laid down in the crib, what happened?"

"I don't remember."

"Was she still crying?"

"She cried for about five to ten minutes after that and then she went to sleep. So I thought she was fine."

"Had this ever occurred before this?"

"No. No. I don't lose my temper," she said, her words garbled amid her tears. "I talk to my counsellors. I'm frustrated."

"Is there anything else you want to say?"

"No."

"This concludes the interview. It's 12:31 p.m."

That second interview had taken seven minutes. The two detectives had their confession.

Lemay shepherded Brenda into yet another small room. There, leaning against the only table in the room, was Ramona. Lemay introduced Brenda to Const. Maja Schlegel of the Metropolitan Toronto Police Force. Brenda looked from Ramona to Lemay, uncomprehending.

"I'm an undercover officer," Schlegel said, as if on cue. She explained that she had been working with the Peterborough police since the spring to help them figure out what had happened to Jenna. Schlegel understood that Brenda had made a statement. She said that must be a huge weight off Brenda's chest. It was over now, she soothed. She sounded just like a friend.

But Brenda knew she was not.

The undercover operation was new terrain for Schlegel. She was a fifteen-year veteran with the Toronto police, but had only started doing undercover work the year before, with the drug squad. Brenda's case was a major leap, her first undercover work on a murder investigation.

"It looked like it would be an interesting case to work on," Schlegel would tell me years later. "I was nervous too, but you're always nervous. Nervous is good. If you are scared, it keeps you alive. But I was definitely interested in doing it."

She knew little about the investigation, and that was on purpose. "You don't want to know anything," she explained, "because if you go in there convinced that she is the one, what are you going to find? It's the tunnel vision that coppers can get."

She knew the Peterborough police were investigating a baby homicide, and the target of her undercover operation was the child's mother. She knew Brenda had another young daughter and was in an on-again, off-again relationship with the father of the dead child. She also knew Jenna had been in the care of a teenage babysitter at the time of her death, and that he was a possible suspect. But her information went no further than that. She didn't know why Brenda was a suspect, and she didn't want to know. It wasn't her investigation. She was just another tool the detectives could use.

She would be working with another undercover officer, who would pose as her boyfriend, but Maja would be the point person. The idea was to befriend Brenda in the hope that she might open up to her as the police investigation continued to unfold.

She slowly started circling in on Brenda. She knew that she and Randy sometimes ate at a soup kitchen downtown, so Schlegel hung out there. Brenda went to the shopping mall, so Schlegel made sure Brenda saw her there. She started attending Brenda's Narcotics Anonymous meetings. By the second one, she was confident that Brenda recognized her. She went over to say hello.

The fact that Schlegel went to the NA meetings would become a contentious issue for Brenda. Participants are supposed to have anonymity and confidentiality. It's right there in the name—Anonymous. That's the only way they'll speak freely. But starting—and continuing—the undercover operation from inside NA didn't bother Schlegel. "I mean, we were talking about a homicide investigation. It's not like I was taking notes on other drug users. What was said in there stayed in there, apart from what Brenda said."

For the first few months of the operation, Schlegel wasn't convinced Brenda was guilty. She could see that she *felt* guilty, but it didn't appear to be over anything she'd done to Jenna herself. It was over her decision to leave the toddler with JD. But Schlegel's opinion started to shift after they went to Jenna's grave.

"We were hardly there thirty seconds and she wanted to go already," Schlegel recalled. "And I asked her, 'Why? We just got here.' And she said, 'I don't know. You remember that movie *Carrie*? It's like in that movie, where a hand comes out of the grave.' And I'm thinking, 'This is your child. Why would you even go there?' It was bizarre."

The undercover officer said she understands that people grieve differently, but she felt Brenda's comment was a sign that she was struggling with her own guilt. Schlegel started looking at the suspect in a new light.

Brenda made another off-hand comment, before a visit to a psychiatrist she was seeing. In the Narcotics Anonymous twelve-step program, step four requires a person to acknowledge his or her mistakes, and step five requires them to confess those wrongs to someone else. Schlegel remembers, "She said to me something like, 'Well, I guess I can do my step four and step five at the same time.' It was the way she said it. To me, that was the other clincher." (Police would later seize Brenda's records from her therapist, Dr. Mark Ben-Aron, but found nothing incriminating.)

Over a six-month period, Schlegel popped in and out of Brenda's life. Eventually, she felt she was spinning her wheels—she had got everything she was going to get from Brenda. Brenda wasn't going to confess to her, and the officer didn't feel comfortable pushing the issue. So the detectives pulled her out. Smith's autopsy report was released September 8, and Brenda was arrested ten days later. Schlegel remembers when they brought Brenda in.

"She was in shock. I remember her saying, 'I never said anything to you [about killing Jenna] and you were my best friend.' And I said, 'Well, I think you did the right thing. I think you've done it.' And then she surprised me. She said, 'I don't really know. I don't think so.' Which I thought was really odd because they just finished telling me that she confessed."

Brenda said it was during their initial visit to Jenna's grave that Schlegel first mentioned memory lapses to her. Brenda had never considered that possibility, and it took root. When I asked Schlegel about this later, she said, "Hm. Maybe, now that you say it that way. I'm gonna have to dig out my notes. It would be awful if I gave her that, the memory lapse. If she is telling the truth and I planted that in her, I would feel horrible."

"Do you think it's possible?"

"Sure. I have to say that it is possible I said that. Probably something like 'Sometimes it's too traumatic, maybe people can't remember' or something like that. That is possible. But whether I actually did say it, I would have to look at my notes."

But when I followed up with her, Schlegel wasn't interested in revisiting the issue. She said she didn't want to deal with the stress. But passages from her notes were filed in court during Brenda's trial, and they do suggest that it was Schlegel, not Brenda, who, during the gravesite visit, first raised the issue of a memory lapse.

The idea that Brenda had suffered a memory lapse reshaped the police investigation. It provided an explanation for why she couldn't remember what happened. And it influenced what Brenda told Lemay during her interrogation.

Maja Schlegel won a policing award for her undercover work investigating Brenda Waudby.

FIVE

CONFESSIONS ARE WIDELY considered the most powerful and persuasive form of evidence for juries. Studies using mock juries have shown that confessions have more influence on verdicts than eyewitness accounts or character testimony. They tend to overwhelm alibis and other forms of evidence that support a defendant's innocence. And even when the tactics used to garner a confession are known and challenged in court, the strength of the confession itself is hard to overcome. Studies show that when told a confession came out of a high-pressure, coercive police interrogation, the mock juries say they will not let the involuntary confession affect their verdict. Yet those same mock juries are more likely to convict the defendant than a control group not given a confession at all. The U.S. Supreme Court once opined that a "defendant's own confession is probably the most probative and damaging evidence that can be admitted against him."

That's why Brenda Waudby's lawyer, Jim Hauraney, was so furious with his client. Hauraney had told her for months: do not say anything to police. His partner had been unequivocal: do not say anything to police. And yet she did. And when he showed up at the police station to speak to her, she wouldn't meet with him.

Brenda lied to the two detectives. Not to deny her guilt or to protect herself—she lied to incriminate herself. She was not in a rage the night before Jenna died. She did not flail her arms around when Jenna wouldn't go back to sleep. She did accidentally drop her on the crib rail, but Brenda never hit her. Yet she admitted to doing all of that to police.

Brenda immediately took back what she'd said, in a three-page letter she wrote to Hauraney before she even left the police station.

Dan Lemay and Gord McNevan pressured me into giving the second part of my statement. The pressure of looking at Jenna's pictures and no food and

without my Lorazepam . . . they convinced me if I didn't give a statement
I would not be released . . .

I was convinced by them that it would look better coming from me than
it would coming from them. I was just tired and wore out from the investiga-
tion trying to figure out what actually did happen that evening . . . I was not
in my right frame of mind when I was arrested. I was so terrified of what
Randy was going to do rather than the statement I was giving. I deny giving
and delivering any blows to Jenna.

Her desperation screams from the pages, yet the damage was done.
Brenda Waudby was facing a charge of second-degree murder. Her confession could mean a life sentence. It made no sense. If she hadn't hit her
daughter, why on earth would she confess?

Brandon Garrett, a professor at the University of Virginia School of
Law, reviewed the first two hundred wrongful convictions overturned by
DNA evidence. What he found: 16 per cent of the cases contained false
confessions and another 9 per cent involved self-incriminating statements.
The Innocence Project made similar findings: DNA exonerations swelled
to more than three hundred cases by mid-2013; one-quarter of those
involved innocent defendants making outright confessions, incriminating
statements or pleading guilty. The U.S. National Registry of Exonerations
reviewed 873 exonerations in the United States between 1989 and 2012.
False confessions were a factor in 135 cases, or 15 per cent.

Scholars point to a number of coercive interrogation techniques as the
main culprits for false confessions. In fact, the very tactics that Detective
Constable Lemay used during his interrogation of Brenda Waudby have
been criticized for inducing innocent people to falsely confess.

The Reid Technique, a method for interviewing and interrogation,
was developed in the 1940s and 1950s by two American lawyers, Fred
Inbau and John Reid. It grew out of an honest effort to address the often
brutal "third degree" tactics police used during interrogations: threatening and beating suspects to obtain confessions, or stripping them and
withholding food and water for hours, sometimes days. The Reid

184 - JOHN CHIPMAN

Technique was heralded as a more civilized interrogation process that was just as effective at eliciting confessions as beating them out of suspects.

Reid was an early developer of an electronic lie detector, or polygraph. In essence, a lie detector tracks involuntary changes in a person's heart rate and blood pressure to determine whether the person is lying. On the same principle, interrogators using the Reid Technique are trained to read a suspect's body language and behavioural tics, on the theory that such things as tone of voice, posture and eye contact are involuntary signs of deception or truthfulness. For example, leaning forward and maintaining eye contact are viewed as signs of truthfulness. Changing posture and averting the eyes are seen as signs of deception.

But research shows that physiological changes such as heart rate are not reliable indicators of deceptive behaviour—an honest person may be nervous when answering truthfully—such that today the results of lie detector tests are inadmissible in Canadian courts. Likewise, the Reid Technique has faced similar scrutiny, with critics arguing that a person's body language or behaviour indicate nothing reliably—an innocent person may shift in her chair just as much as a guilty one.

While parts of the Reid Technique are ubiquitous in police investigations across North America—careful analysis of the evidence and witness statements, an analysis of each suspect's normal verbal and nonverbal behaviour, an assessment of their response to "behaviour-provoking" questions to determine whether the suspect is being truthful—it is not followed as gospel. Most detectives develop their investigative techniques through a combination of training and experience. They use what works for them. It's common sense to consider each potential suspect in relation to the evidence, potential motives and opportunity. But many detectives have already decided a suspect's guilt or innocence based on the evidence and their investigation, so they jump right to the interrogation stage. That's what Lemay and McNevan did with Brenda Waudby. They may have done some behaviour analysis during one of the previous times they talked to Brenda, but when they walked her into that interview room after booking her, there was no more interviewing. The interrogation began.

And it was an almost textbook Reid interrogation, step by step, designed to extract a confession. The first step is the positive confrontation: the investigator leaves the room, then returns with a file. It can be the actual case file, or it can be empty; it is meant to convey authority. The investigator then tells the suspect that the investigation is finished and the evidence is clear: the suspect is guilty. This confrontation should be brief and unequivocal. It should also be done from a position of authority: standing in front of a sitting suspect, with a confident manner and tone of voice.

In Brenda's case, Lemay was unequivocal. His notes state that as the interrogation began, he told her that for investigators, it wasn't a question of whether she did it. They had no doubt she was responsible for Jenna's death. The police weren't there to argue over the facts with her. They were there to help her deal with the tragedy.

Investigators study suspects' reactions to the accusation. Do they drop their eyes, shift in the chair and offer a vague denial? That is, the thinking goes, the behaviour of the guilty. Or do they lean forward, maintain eye contact and voice forceful, even angry protestations of their innocence? These suspects are more likely innocent. Regardless of the response, investigators are to continue the interrogation undeterred. They should repeat the accusation, just as forcefully, then sit down across from the suspect. This helps investigators transition from adversary to ally just looking for the truth.

It's impossible to know how Brenda responded to Lemay. The police didn't videotape the interrogation, and none of the notes from either Lemay or McNevan make reference to her responses. But Lemay did move on to the next stage of a Reid interrogation.

The second step is developing a theme that will minimize guilt. The idea here is to help suspects justify their behaviour, to provide a reason for their actions that shifts responsibility away from themselves. No matter how disturbing or repellent the crime, the Reid Technique advocates finding a way for the suspect to justify it. For example, if the suspect is believed to have murdered his wife, the investigator should blame the victim for nagging the suspect too much.

Lemay told Brenda police knew she was not a bad person. They knew how difficult her life with Randy was. Lemay didn't think she was a monster. It was just this overabundance of problems she was facing that led her to lose control and make a mistake. In a Reid interrogation, the information-gathering ends with the earlier interview; the purpose now is to get a confession. So the third step is handling denials. The Reid Technique says ignore them. Or better yet, cut suspects off before they even have a chance to voice them. Proponents of the Reid Technique maintain that guilty suspects will preface their denials with phrases like "May I say something?" or "If you just let me say one thing." Interrogators should cut them off and continue talking. If suspects do not preface their denials, if they are unequivocal in their claims, then they may be innocent. Innocent suspects won't ask for permission to state their innocence. According to the thinking, an innocent suspect's denials will strengthen in time, not weaken like those of a guilty suspect.

Without a videotape or audio recording, it's impossible to know for sure how Brenda responded to Lemay's accusation, but his notes make no mention of a denial. They say Brenda appeared receptive to what he was saying. Discussing what happened that night was obviously painful for her, and she became very emotional, more emotional than the detectives had ever seen her before.

If the suspect begins to cry, the investigator should appear sympathetic. A gentle hand on the shoulder will help move the suspect toward acceptance and a confession. Another useful tool: the investigator will offer an alternative motivation. If the crime is theft, did the suspect do it to pay for prostitutes, or to feed his hungry children? Both involve admissions of guilt, but one is much easier for the suspect to justify.

Lemay repeatedly minimized the significance of Brenda's alleged crime, referring to it as a mistake, and he also used his own indiscretions to try to seem empathetic toward her. Lemay told her that three years earlier he had made a serious mistake. It was embarrassing and difficult, he said, but he knew that he had to own up to it. He told the truth about what happened, and in the long run everything turned out fine. He came back to the incident again later in the interrogation, imploring Brenda to do the right thing, just as he had, and tell the truth about what happened to Jenna.

(Years later, Brenda would learn what Lemay had been talking about. According to press reports, Lemay and another off-duty officer, Const. Mark Elliott, were returning from a party three years earlier, in 1994. Lemay lost control of the vehicle, which rolled onto its hood and hit a utility pole. Neither man was seriously injured. The pair called two other off-duty officers, Sgt. Ted Boynton and Const. Marc Habgood, to the scene to help try to right the car, but they all fled before on-duty police arrived. Lemay phoned his wife and told her to call police and say she had been the driver. She was charged with careless driving. Boynton and Habgood corroborated her story. However, civilian witnesses told investigators that there was no woman at the accident scene. Lemay eventually told senior officers what had happened and admitted he had been drinking at the time of the accident. He pleaded guilty to public mischief and was fined $1,000 and temporarily demoted for discreditable conduct.)

Once the suspect confesses, the investigator should start digging for details of the crime. According to the Reid Technique, questions at this point should be open-ended, but if the suspect's answers contradict physical evidence or eyewitness accounts, the investigator should confront him on those contradictions to create a uniform narrative of the crime.

Brenda did not confess during her first statement. She would only say she was tired and frustrated and accidentally dropped Jenna on the crib rail when changing her during the night. Lemay continued to grill her about her statement, saying it couldn't account for the severity of Jenna's injuries. And then Brenda's admission began to shift. "It's just confusing, I remember swinging my arms. I don't know. I probably hit her once or twice. I don't remember actually striking her but I remember swinging my arms. The possibility that I hit her is . . . it's there."

This was as specific as Brenda would be about what she did that night. "Swinging my arms" and "probably [hitting] her once or twice" could not explain the more than one hundred bruises and multiple injuries Jenna suffered, but the detectives didn't pursue a better explanation.

Once the narrative is fleshed out, the investigator should get the suspect to put the confession in writing. It can be a statement the suspect writes and signs; it can be a statement the investigator writes out for the suspect to sign; or it can be a videotaped statement. Whichever form it takes, this statement should be witnessed by another officer, who may ask further questions based on the statement to test its veracity. The goal is to create a confession that could be understood and accepted by someone who knows nothing of the crime.

Brenda's videotaped statement was her only confession. The only signed statement she would write that day was a letter to her lawyer recanting that confession.

From a law enforcement perspective, the main question about the Reid Technique is: Does it work? Does it lead to confessions? The research is clear: yes, it does. From a civil liberties perspective, the question is different: Does it produce false confessions or false self-incriminating statements? And the research is just as unequivocal: yes, it does. And the biggest problem with the technique is that it has no mechanism to differentiate between the two.

Study after study shows that the non-verbal cues interrogators are trained to look for are unreliable markers of truthfulness or deception. Leaning forward in your chair is not a reliable sign that you are being truthful. And averting your eyes does not mean you are lying.

What's more, studies show that police are no better at reading these non-verbal cues than anyone else. Officers with Reid-style interrogation training are no better at differentiating between truthful and deceptive suspects, but they do exhibit a greater degree of confidence in their ability to do so. One study, conducted at Florida International University, enlisted forty-four officers, nearly half of them from police agencies across Ontario. Roughly two-thirds of the officers had received formal training in interrogation and deception detection. Yet after viewing eight interrogations, in which they'd been told some suspects were lying about their involvement, they were able to properly identify the deceitful suspects and the truthful suspects only 50 per cent of the time—no better than chance odds. Of the truthful suspects, two-thirds were incorrectly identified as being untruthful. Despite these poor results, the officers scored their decisions high on a confidence scale: the average score was 7 out of 10.

So Reid-method interrogators are great at eliciting confessions. But they're also good at eliciting *false* confessions. And they're lousy at telling them apart.

Saul Kassin, a professor of psychology at Williams College, in Williamstown, Massachusetts, and John Jay College of Criminal Justice, in New York, is a leading voice in the study of false confessions. In a seminal 1996 study exploring how easy it is to induce a false confession, he asked seventy-nine students to type a series of letters into a computer as they were read out to them. The subjects were explicitly told not to hit the Alt key because it would crash the computer and all the data would be lost. After a minute of typing, the computer crashed. None of the subjects had anything to do with the supposed crash, but the experimenter accused the subjects of hitting the forbidden Alt key. The experimenter then turned to a witness, who either said she had seen the subject hit the Alt key or said she had not seen what happened.

The subject and the experimenter then left the room, where a third person reinforced that the computer crash had occurred by asking the subject what they did to make it happen. The subject was then taken back into the room, where he was asked to reconstruct how or when he had hit the Alt key. Thus, his guilt was forcefully affirmed. As a consequence, even though none of the subjects had actually touched the Alt key, 69 per cent signed a confession saying they had, 28 per cent exhibited signs of internalized guilt, and 9 per cent offered details to support their belief in their guilt.

The results were even more pronounced under high-stress circumstances. In a fast-paced scenario, with a witness claiming to have seen the subject hit the Alt key, *every single one* of the subjects signed a confession, 65 per cent showed internalized guilt, and 35 per cent came up with supporting details.

Kassin's experiment, of course, bears little resemblance to reality. Its test subjects are random students, not suspected criminals; hitting the forbidden key could have been accidental, and carried little serious consequence. Kassin argued that these shortcomings should not be overstated. "The more important and startling result," he wrote, was that "many subjects privately internalized guilt for an outcome they did not produce, and that some even constructed memories to fit that false belief."

To address the noted shortcomings, in 2005 Kassin teamed up with a group of academics led by Melissa Russano from Roger Williams University, in Rhode Island. To test for both true and false confessions under circumstances closer to a real-world scenario, roughly three hundred students were given tests to be completed in part on their own and in part with a partner. During the individual portion of the test, the partner (who was in on the experiment) would become upset and ask the subject for help. Some subjects helped (guilty of cheating); others didn't (innocent).

After the test was completed, the experimenters would separate the subjects from their partners. Each subject was told that they had the same wrong answers as their partners on the individual portion of the test and was accused of cheating. The subjects were also told that the professor overseeing the test had been informed of the situation and was upset. The experimenters said they did not know how the professor would handle the situation or whether the university would be notified about suspected cheating. The subjects were then told that the professor wanted them to sign a written account of what they had done.

During this interrogation, with some of the subjects the experimenters used minimization tactics—"I'm sure you didn't realize what a big deal it was"—popularized by the Reid Technique. In a police interrogation, this technique is perfectly legal. To other subjects they offered leniency in exchange for a signed confession (although Brenda was not offered leniency). Interrogations that offer outright deals have been dismissed by most courts as inadmissible on the grounds that they are egregiously coercive.

Almost half (46 per cent) of the guilty subjects confessed without minimization or leniency tactics being used, and a small number (6 per cent) of innocent subjects gave false confessions without any coercion. But confession rates rose for both guilty and innocent subjects when subjected to either tactic. Minimization persuaded four out of five guilty subjects to confess, and 18 per cent of innocent subjects gave false confessions. Offering a deal alone garnered false confessions from 14 per cent of subjects. But fully 43 per cent of innocent subjects gave false confessions when interrogators used both the minimization tactic and the offer of a deal.

Critics of Reid-style tactics say there is a more open-minded, objective alternative called PEACE, which stands for Preparation and Planning, Engage and Explain, Account, Closure and Evaluation. PEACE was developed in the United Kingdom in the early 1990s after the overturning of several convictions involving questionable police interrogation tactics and their resulting false confessions.

PEACE interviews are built around objectivity and open-ended questions. Whereas the Reid Technique and its offshoots teach investigators to bully, berate and break down suspects by refusing to listen to their explanations or denials, PEACE encourage investigators to listen carefully while suspects give an uninterrupted account of what happened. Once the suspect completes his account, the interviewer leads him back through the details, probing for clarity and more precise details. Detectives can challenge a suspect, but they don't do it in an aggressive or accusatory manner. Discrepancies are pointed out, and the suspect is given the opportunity to clarify or explain them. The detective remains objective, professional and respectful throughout.

Research shows that despite the stark differences between PEACE and more aggressive, accusatory methods like the Reid Technique, both are equally effective at garnering confessions. But because suspects are not coerced or manipulated into confessing, confessions obtained through a PEACE interview are less likely to be deemed inadmissible in court. And the police themselves benefit: officers conducting PEACE interviews are less likely to be disciplined or subjected to civil lawsuits for conducting negligent investigations. There is even evidence that PEACE reduces the "boomerang effect," in which a suspect is prepared to confess but decides not to because he feels manipulated or mistreated.

Proponents point out that PEACE's end goal is not necessarily a confession; it's to find out exactly what happened during a crime. By taking the emphasis off getting a confession, PEACE interviews are better equipped to allow investigators to discover the truth. PEACE is gradually being adopted by police forces across North America. In Canada, the Royal Newfoundland Constabulary was the first to make the switch, in 2008.

Brenda achieved her goal. She would not spend the night in jail. After giving her second statement, a bail hearing was held and she was released later that day on a $30,000 surety bond. Brenda was responsible for a third of it; her mother and father put up the rest. Her bail conditions included: living with her parents, checking in with police twice a week and refraining from being around anyone under the age of eighteen unless accompanied by another adult.

She drove home with her parents and brother. They picked up some Kentucky Fried Chicken for dinner. The social worker allowed Brenda ten minutes that night to say goodbye to Justine. She would be returning to her foster family until after the trial, at least.

Brenda kissed Justine on the cheek. She could taste the salt of her own tears that ran onto her daughter's face. She looked so tiny, standing there in the front hallway. So small in her new jacket and shoes. She was too young to be dealing with this. Brenda had failed her again.

NICHOLAS II

ONE

THE DAYS SLIPPED by, and as each one passed with no word, Maurice Gagnon became more and more hopeful that Children's Aid would not take any action against Lianne. Not that he wasn't angry. Involving Children's Aid in his daughter's life struck him as a vindictive move by police; they couldn't nail her with criminal charges, so they would leave it to someone else to punish her.

In a letter of complaint he wrote in December 1997 to Bob Runciman, then Ontario's solicitor general, he said:

> It has always been my understanding that a basic premise in our system of criminal justice is a presumption of innocence until proven guilty—the burden of proof being on the Crown. Since the Crown admittedly could not prove the allegations, simple logic would dictate that my daughter was and still is innocent. She was never charged.
>
> I would then like to know under what statute your office is able to "black-list" an innocent person, as the police are doing to my daughter with the CAS. Is this not defamation of character or perhaps even criminally libelous?

It wasn't. As Runciman pointed out in his response, section 72 of the Child and Family Services Act requires that police report suspicions of potential abuse to child protection services, regardless of the criminal culpability of the suspect. In fact, this "duty to report" extends to many professionals, including doctors, nurses, teachers, social workers, lawyers and police who have reasonable grounds to suspect a child may be facing abuse. So even though the evidence police had collected did not warrant criminal charges, officers still believed Lianne was responsible for Nicholas's death and were therefore required by law to inform Children's Aid. Cairns told Maurice that he would have notified CAS himself had police not done so first.

At the time, Maurice Gagnon felt a kinship with the deputy chief coroner, a fellow senior manager within the provincial civil service. The investigation into Nicholas's death had been misguided, but it was Smith who had done the second autopsy and Smith who was giving the opinions. Maurice was convinced that Cairns was only doing his job. When the police investigation ended, Maurice was elated, but he was no closer to knowing what, in fact, had killed Nicholas. And he still had questions about how Smith had arrived at his opinions.

Maurice set up a meeting with Cairns in early February 1998 to review the results of both autopsies. The pair discussed Nicholas's increased head circumference, the suspected jaw fracture that turned out to be nothing, and the shifting theories about how Nicholas died, from Lianne smothering him to Lianne hitting him on the head.

Maurice had read that someone who suffers a brain injury—as Nicholas may have done when he fell against the coffee table at the babysitter's house—might later develop frontal lobe epilepsy. Could Nicholas have suffered a seizure on November 30, during which he banged his head against the sewing machine table?

Cairns had no answer. (This exchange is based on Maurice Gagnon's recollection and notes of their conversation. Dr. Cairns declined to speak to me for this book.) In fact, whenever he did have an answer to one of Maurice's questions, it was often frustratingly brief, echoing what Smith had said in his report and offering no insights into the underlying reasoning or the medical literature that supported it. Maurice didn't fully appreciate it at the time, but that was because Cairns had no expertise in pathology. Although he'd studied forensic medicine at medical school in Northern Ireland in the mid-1960s,

Cairns had specialized in obstetrics and began his career as a family physician and emergency doctor before becoming a coroner. He was ill equipped to explain Smith's opinions or to judge their quality. It was becoming clear to Maurice that he was not going to get any answers from Cairns.

Nevertheless, he asked Cairns why Smith hadn't concluded that the cause of Nicholas's death was unknown. Autopsy reports routinely state that the pathologist has not been able to resolve the exact cause of death. In fact, "undetermined" (along with "natural," "accident," "suicide" and "homicide") is one of the five official categories for cause of death in Ontario. It would have been completely acceptable for Smith to state that he couldn't determine the exact cause of Nicholas's death, and for Cairns to accept that. But Cairns said nothing to put this all to rest.

Sudbury police sent their case file—two binders full—to the Children's Aid Society of Sudbury-Manitoulin in late February, 1998. The next month, the agency provided notice to St. Joseph's Health Centre that they were planning to apprehend Lianne's child upon birth. The notice was sent out before case workers had reviewed the file with either the police or the Chief Coroner's Office or spoken with Lianne or Pete.

Cairns, Sgt. Robert Keetch, a social worker and a Children's Aid lawyer attended a case conference on April 8. Cairns told the CAS officials that Dr. T.C. Chen's original autopsy findings were flawed, explaining that his SIDS characterization was incorrect, and claiming the pathologist had made other mistakes during the procedure. After doing a second autopsy, Dr. Smith had concluded that the child had died from cerebral edema caused by a blunt force head injury and that Lianne's version of events was not consistent with the medical evidence he found.

One of the social workers asked Cairns to define blunt force head injury, according to notes taken about the meeting.

The deputy coroner said it is not a trivial injury. It is dispersed over a wide area of the head. Brain swelling takes time. The child would not have died instantaneously after bumping his head, as Lianne said happened, Cairns told the group.

Dr. Cairns was asked about the lack of a significant external injuries. Why wasn't there one if the child was hit hard on the head? Cairns said it was very common for a baby not to show any signs of external trauma to the head even when a serious head injury has occurred.

Cairns stressed this was not a shaken baby case. The second autopsy had ruled out asphyxiation as a possible cause or death. He explained that in asphyxiation cases, cerebral edema is noticeable, but there would not be bruising of the right parietal bone—the right upper portion of the skull—which is what Smith found during his autopsy.

The Children's Aid workers wanted to discuss the evidence with Smith directly, so a second case conference was scheduled, for May 8, this time at the coroner's offices in Toronto. Two CAS lawyers and Gisele Haines, another social worker from the agency, flew down for the meeting.

Cairns and Smith were clear and unequivocal: No one in the Gagnon family had provided an adequate medical explanation for Nicholas's death. Despite the Crown's decision to not lay charges, the Chief Coroner's Office still supported Smith's findings at autopsy. Cairns and Smith both said Smith's medical opinions were correct.

The CAS team had much to consider during their flight home. Time was of the essence. Lianne was due in less than two months. All three agreed that there were grounds to make an application for a temporary custody order to protect the well-being of Lianne's baby after the birth. They started the paperwork.

Julie Boivin, the supervisor of the francophone child protection team at the Sudbury CAS, asked to meet Pete and Lianne. Pete wanted to meet at Maurice's home, so he could be present too. Boivin, though, insisted that the first meeting be conducted in private at the CAS office. It would be informational, she said, for their benefit. They wouldn't have to answer any questions.

Maurice was having no part of it. After the interrogation his daughter had endured eleven months earlier, when police coerced her down to the station to clear up some "loose ends," there was no way he was allowing the young couple to go into the CAS office alone. He called the family's lawyer, Berk Keaney, to fill him in on the latest developments.

There was little doubt about Berk's place in Sudbury's legal community. "If you got a case that can't be won," Maurice would say years later, "you go see Keaney."

Maurice had put Keaney on retainer during the criminal investigation. Keaney didn't fault the police for their investigation; they had one of the most prominent medical experts in the country telling them Nicholas's death was a homicide, a homicide they had initially missed. But to Berk Keaney's eyes, things just didn't add up, and when he saw Dr. Smith's final autopsy report, that one phrase—"in the absence of a credible explanation"—screamed out at him. The Crown's burden is to prove its case "beyond a reasonable doubt." Smith's seven-word caveat left a truck-sized hole in their case that he would have been able to tear open even wider in court. So Keaney was not at all surprised when police announced they wouldn't be laying charges, and he figured the case was finished. He hadn't known Lianne was pregnant. And he had no idea CAS had launched their own investigation.

Keaney accompanied Pete and Lianne to the CAS office the next day. "Do you mind if I record this conversation?" he asked, placing a mini-recorder on the table.

"Uh, no. Go ahead," Boivin said.

"Thanks. Mr. and Mrs. Thibeault won't be having any meetings with your agency without legal representation."

"Oh. Well, then, we'll have to reschedule so our own legal counsel can be present."

"That's fine."

And with that, the meeting was over before it began.

Keaney knew the small victory at the CAS office was just that. He was very troubled by this latest development, not only because he thought the allegations against Lianne were baseless but because it would be much harder to disprove them in a Children's Aid case. The initial threshold for laying a criminal charge is "reasonable and probable grounds," which is not a particularly high bar. It is much lower than "beyond a reasonable doubt," which the Crown would have to prove in court. And yet the Crown had decided Smith's evidence didn't even meet that low standard.

Children's Aid would use the same evidence as the police had relied upon, and the custody case would turn on the exact same question: Did Lianne cause the death of her son? However, the CAS application wasn't a criminal matter; it was governed by the Child and Family Services Act, which has a much lower threshold—proof "on the balance of probabilities"—than the proof "beyond a reasonable doubt" required for criminal charges.

"There's the rub," Keaney would say years later, his head still shaking at the thought of it. "Eventually there would be a trial of the issue, which is whether or not she was culpable for the death of her child in accordance with Smith's theory, but on the balance of probabilities as opposed to proof beyond a reasonable doubt."

And while the stakes were different, they were no less terrifying. If Lianne lost, she wouldn't be facing prison time, but she would lose custody of her new child.

"Of all the trials I've done before," Keaney said, "there's never been as many sleepless nights as there was in that case. Not only the consequences, but what are we going to do about Smith?"

The lawyer knew he had little time to build his case. It was already the middle of May. Lianne was due on June 24. They needed to find specialists to refute Smith's medical opinion, and they needed to find them fast. Keaney specialized in criminal matters, so he brought in another lawyer, Roy Sullivan, who knew family law and had done work for CAS in the past. And then he went digging for medical experts.

Keaney reviewed other cases involving children's deaths that had turned on medical evidence, especially ones that ended in acquittals. If medical experts had been able to disprove the Crown's theories in those cases, they might be able to refute CAS's in this one. And he looked into other cases in which Dr. Smith was involved; he would need to find someone confident enough to take him on, with a CV that carried the same weight.

Maurice was also digging. He had already immersed himself in the latest medical literature in an effort to understand how his grandson had died.

Neither man can remember exactly who stumbled across it, but the case against Samantha McIntosh, in the Northern Ontario mining town of Timmins, turned out to be a pivotal one for Lianne, and eventually for Smith. (Samantha McIntosh is not her real name. She was a minor at the time of the incident that follows, and has never been identified publicly. Court and legal documents refer to her by her initials, S.M.)

TWO

IN THE SUMMER of 1988, Samantha McIntosh was settling into her burgeoning career as a babysitter. The twelve-year-old had taken a three-month course, diligently sitting through three-hour classes after school, reading books, taking notes and honing her diaper-changing skills on a volunteer three-month-old. So when her neighbour Faith Sheridan (also not her real name) approached Samantha about looking after her sixteen-month-old daughter, Amber, over the summer, Sam felt she was ready.

The two families had been neighbours for four years, but this would be a big responsibility, and the Sheridans did not take it lightly. Faith checked with other neighbours whose children Sam had babysat. She talked to relatives whose children played with Sam on the same Little League team. And she quietly observed the girl for months, watching her out the front window as she played with her friends, studying her temperament. Everyone she spoke with had nothing but good things to say about the Grade 7 student. She seemed like a conscientious, responsible young woman. Faith felt confident she would be a good fit.

And it was. Amber loved Sam. She would rush to greet her, squealing at the window as Sam walked up to the house. She would cry when Sam left for the day.

The plan was for Sam to look after Amber three days a week that summer, either full days from seven till four or just mornings until one. Faith checked in by phone every hour and a half most days.

The arrangement was working well. Amber was always clean and content when Faith got home. Not that everything was perfect. The toddler still picked up the odd scrape and bruise while being cared for by Sam. During the first month, Amber smacked her forehead on the coffee table, leaving a bruise that lingered for two weeks. And she picked up a small bruise on her cheek toward the end of July, although neither her parents nor Sam could recall exactly what caused it. But the Sheridans didn't see either incident as anything more than evidence of the inevitable tumbles every toddler takes.

On July 28, Sam arrived at the Sheridans' at 7 a.m. sharp. Amber was still asleep, and the Sheridans soon left for work. Amber started to stir around nine, her normal time. Sam got her up and took her downstairs to eat. She wasn't very hungry, though, and seemed listless and warm to Sam. The toddler wasn't far into the soup Sam was feeding her for breakfast when she threw it up. Several new teeth were coming in, so the child had been vomiting regularly for the past week. Sam took her upstairs for a bath.

The pair spent the rest of the morning playing, dancing, watching a little TV. Around noon, Sam served more soup for lunch. Amber kept it down initially, but threw up later while Sam was changing her. When Sam picked her up, she vomited again, this time more extensively than before. Sam phoned Faith to let her know, then took Amber upstairs for another bath.

Around one that afternoon, Sam and Amber accompanied Sam's mother, Paulina (not her real name), to the animal pound—Paulina was taking a kitten in. It took about an hour to make the trip to the pound and back. It was a nice, leisurely walk. By the time Sam got back to the Sheridans', it was pushing two thirty and time for Amber's nap.

Just after Sam put her down, Faith called to check in. Sam told her the vomiting had stopped and that they had enjoyed a walk with her mother.

Amber woke around three. Sam changed her, and held her hand as the two of them approached the five stairs down to the living room. What happened next would be the central issue in a police investigation and criminal trial that dragged on for the next three years.

Sam would give five slightly different versions in the coming days, weeks, months and years. Initially, she told a doctor at the hospital that she had been holding Amber's hand, but the toddler was vigorously pulling her along as they got to the top of the stairs and Amber's hand suddenly slipped out of her own. The child catapulted down the stairs, missing all the steps before landing at the bottom. In her second account, made to her mother, Sam said Amber had pushed her hand away before she fell down the stairs, hitting all the steps on her way down. In her first statement to police, she said Amber had tripped and tumbled down the stairs, hitting her head several times at the bottom, with one hard strike to the top of the head. She was unsure whether her head hit any of the steps. A later police statement was slightly different: this time Amber had still tripped and fallen down the stairs, but she had hit her head hard in the front and once more less severely in the back. She also said Amber struck her jaw on the third step from the top. Her final statement was given at trial: Amber tripped and fell head first down the stairs. Sam wasn't sure whether she had hit her jaw on the third step, although she did hear a bang before the child hit the floor at the bottom. She said Amber hit her forehead at the bottom of the stairs. Her head bounced off the floor as she rolled over, and then she hit the back of her head. Sam explained away the minor differences in these accounts by saying it had all happened so quickly, and was so horrifying to witness, that it was difficult to recount the exact details.

Sam raced down the stairs. Amber was moaning on the floor. Her eyes were open, but her body was limp, her breathing pinballing from quick and shallow to slow and lethargic. When a cold cloth didn't revive her, Sam placed the child in her crib and called her mother. Paulina McIntosh came running but could do nothing to revive the child. They phoned 911. Blood was coming out of Amber's mouth. Her upper lip was bleeding. There were two large red marks on her face, one on her right cheek, another above her right eyebrow. The child's breathing was now so shallow, Paulina could barely hear it.

The extent and severity of bruising on the child's face and body would become a crucial point at trial, but initially, none of the professionals paid the bruises much heed as they tried to resuscitate her. The paramedic may have noticed a bruise on the cheek, but couldn't remember any marks on her forehead. An ER doctor noticed the red mark over her right eyebrow, but felt it was a few days old. Another noted a reddish-purple forehead bruise, but didn't think it was recent or a factor in the brain injury. A pediatrician found no swelling or bruises. X-rays found no sign of skull fractures.

The pediatrician suspected cerebral hemorrhaging and ordered an air ambulance to the Hospital for Sick Children, in Toronto. In the meantime, Amber was rushed into surgery to halt rising pressure inside the skull. She was flown to Toronto that evening.

Geoffrey Barker, a pediatrician and intensive care specialist, was in charge of Amber's care at SickKids. Dr. Fred Keeley assisted. Both men thought that a fall down five stairs could not account for Amber's grave condition, so they notified the hospital's Suspected Child Abuse and Neglect, or SCAN, team.

Meanwhile, Amber continued to deteriorate and was pronounced dead at 11:10 a.m. on July 30, two days after her fall. Because Sam's story of the fall did not seem to account for her death, an autopsy was ordered. Katy Driver, a pediatrician with the SCAN team, initially suspected a non-accidental cause, likely whiplash.

The doctors suspected this might be a case of shaken baby syndrome, or SBS. As the name implies, SBS involves violent shaking of a child that leads to a fatal head injury. Pathologists have traditionally looked for three findings at autopsy to establish SBS. As Justice Stephen Goudge lays out in his final report, this triad of conditions includes: hypoxic-ischemic encephalopathy, which is often associated with brain swelling that affects mental functioning; subdural hemorrhage, or bleeding between the brain and dura, the thick membrane that surrounds the brain and spinal cord; and retinal hemorrhaging, or bleeding in the retinas. Pathologists also looked for a fourth condition: diffuse axonal injury, or shearing of nerve fibres within the brain, which often causes a loss of consciousness. The presence of axonal injury was useful from an investigative standpoint because it occurred during the shaking: only people who were in the presence of the child at the time of collapse could be responsible since the axonal injury was immediate.

That was the generally accepted view of SBS within the medical community in the late 1980s and early 1990s, but some people were starting to question the validity of the diagnosis, wondering whether it was even physically possible to shake a child violently enough to cause the triad of conditions. Despite the general acceptance of SBS, little empirical data existed about the syndrome at the time, and the research that had been done compared the condition to adult whiplash in traffic accidents, without taking into account the huge acceleration forces those victims would have experienced.

In 1987, the year before Amber's death, Ann-Christine Duhaime, an American pediatric neurosurgeon, did an experiment that involved shaking models of one-month-old infants fitted with accelerometers. Duhaime found that the velocity and acceleration forces created by even violent shaking of the models were still well below what was needed to cause injury.

Debate ensued. Some doctors argued that the full triad wasn't needed, that the presence of retinal hemorrhages alone was enough to diagnose SBS. Other researchers went in another direction, arguing that the triad of conditions traditionally associated with SBS may, in fact, be caused by something else, such as injury to the head from an accidental fall.

But at the time of Amber's death, shaken baby syndrome remained a legitimate and widely accepted diagnosis.

Dr. Charles Smith was tasked with doing Amber's autopsy. By 1988, Smith had been working as a pediatric pathologist for seven years, but as the Goudge report pointed out, he had no formal training or certification in forensic pathology. Nor did he have much experience in doing the more complicated criminally suspicious autopsies, of which Amber's was certainly one.

Mistakes were made, before, during and after the autopsy. First, during Amber's first night at Sick Kids, a pediatric neurosurgeon removed a subdural hematoma, or blood clot, from her brain, but it was never sent to the pathology lab for analysis and measurement. In shaking cases, such bleeding is usually thin, but the surgeon who removed the hematoma in Amber's brain said it was very large and extensive—an atypical finding for an SBS case. (Justice Goudge noted that at Sam's trial, Smith used the absence of an exact measurement of the clot to downplay the surgeon's observations.)

Next, after a mix-up at SickKids, Amber's body was released for burial without the autopsy being done, so like the Gagnons in Sudbury, the Sheridans in Timmins had to go through the traumatic experience of an exhumation three weeks after their daughter was buried.

Lastly, a skeletal survey—X-rays of all the bones in the body—was not done during the autopsy, even though, in Ontario, one is required in cases of suspected child abuse.

Smith was looking for evidence of blunt force trauma to the head, such as a skull fracture. Along with Dr. Barker and Dr. Driver, he felt such a finding would be necessary if Sam's story of Amber's fall was to be believed. Smith did find the triad of conditions associated with shaken baby syndrome: subdural and retinal hemorrhages, along with hypoxic-ischemic encephalopathy. But he found no evidence of a skull fracture or of bleeding between the scalp and the skull. He found no congenital malformations. He found nothing to suggest an accidental death. He found four bruises, on Amber's forehead, right cheek, left hip and leg, but dismissed two of them as predating her fall and all of them as trivial.

Shaken baby syndrome is most common among young infants. Amber was sixteen months old. Whether a twelve-year-old female would have the strength to shake a sixteen-month-old toddler violently enough to kill her was not a question Smith considered.

Smith completed his autopsy report in late November 1988. Two weeks later, he and Deputy Chief Coroner James Young met with police and the Crown in Timmins. The two doctors said Amber Sheridan had died of a head injury caused by severe shaking. Two days later, twelve-year-old Sam McIntosh was charged with manslaughter.

The trial, before Mr. Justice Patrick Dunn, involved twenty expert medical witnesses and lasted thirty days, spread out over thirteen months (while Sam was in Grades 8 and 9). Intentionally or not, it became a microcosm of the growing debate over shaken baby syndrome that was then taking hold of the medical community. Dr. Ann-Christine Duhaime, who had written the influential paper in 1987 that kicked off the debate, testified for the defence. So did Dr. Ayub Ommaya, whose work on adult whiplash in car accidents was often cited by proponents of SBS.

The defence's case hinged on a simple but controversial argument: that Amber's fall down five stairs could, and did, kill her. It wasn't a long fall. The height of the steps was about five feet; the floor at the bottom was carpeted. But the defence's medical experts argued that, although rare, it was possible. Most of the Crown's experts argued that it was not. Smith was particularly dogmatic, testifying that there was "no possibility whatsoever" that a fall that insignificant could have killed the child.

"You have to drop children from three storeys in order to kill half of them," he told the court. He said his own children had "bounced down more steps than those [five], and they are still happy and healthy children. But that's personal, you can discard that if you want." Justice Dunn did.

As for the variations in Sam's five statements, Justice Dunn found her testimony credible. He noted that several of the medical experts testified that it can be very difficult for witnesses to recall exact details of catastrophic events because of the trauma involved in witnessing them.

In the end, Justice Dunn found the defence's arguments more persuasive. He acquitted Sam.

But it was the reasoning he used in setting aside the Crown's case that really interested Maurice Gagnon. It was clear that the judge was unimpressed with the work and testimony of several of the specialists from the Hospital for Sick Children who testified for the Crown, especially that of Charles Smith. Dunn noted that the defence had asked Smith to send his autopsy report, pictures and slides to Dr. Lucy Rorke, one of its expert witnesses. When Smith sent the materials to Rorke, he told her that it was standard policy at SickKids to have two neuropathologists review the case material of anatomic pathologists such as himself. However, Smith testified at trial that only one neuropathologist had reviewed his case material. And he said he didn't know who did the review, or when it was done or whether there was a written record of its findings.

The judge also pointed out the complaints several of the defence witnesses had about the lack of thoroughness in Smith's autopsy report. They felt important information was missing and that key areas had not been investigated.

Dr. Jan Leestma wanted to know about the subdural hematoma: whether it was acute, subacute or chronic together with its location and extent. There was little documentation in the autopsy report about that either. He said if the pictures did not exist, one would have difficulty referring the location of anything in the autopsy report to Amber's body.

Dr. [Floyd] Gilles believed the report should have stated the distribution of contusions and their location in the frontal and occipital lobes.

I think Dr. Rorke best described the reasons for the need of a thorough autopsy report. She said: "The purpose of the post-mortem report is to describe as precisely as possible everything that the pathologist sees and does, so that somebody who is not present at the time will have a perfect mental picture of exactly what was seen."

She went on to say: "In this regard, the post-mortem report that was prepared on this child falls far short of that standard."

Dr. Smith had the time to do a thorough autopsy report. He knew that this case would likely be coming to court and he would be a witness. There is little in the report even to indicate a shaking diagnosis. He does not say he followed a protocol on autopsies, whatever the standards of that might be.

Maurice Gagnon couldn't believe what he was reading. The ruling was nothing less than a professional excoriation of the very man whose opinions on the cause of Nicholas's death had led Sudbury police to investigate and were now leading Children's Aid to attempt to seize Lianne's new baby.

The criticisms went on and on, page after page.

Dr. Smith went so far as to say even if he did find a linear fracture, he still would have said that Amber died from shaking. That is an inconsistent statement, in the opinion of Dr. Rorke. What she meant is once there is a clinical evidence of impact, that removes the case from the pure shaking syndrome. Perhaps the problem is, as Dr. Gilles said, Dr. Smith's definition of the aspects of shaking keeps changing.

Dr. Smith said twice in his testimony that an autopsy was not needed to confirm the clinicians' diagnosis of shaking. He thought the purpose of the autopsy was to try to find another cause of death. I do not understand that statement at all. Surely an autopsy is required before a clinician can have any certainty in a diagnosis of shaking. How else can a clinician be sure there are not fractures or subcutaneous bruising? . . .

Dr. Smith was apparently of the view that there was "ample clinical evidence" to support a diagnosis of shaking . . . He believed this to be the case, even before he began his autopsy. When asked by [defence attorney] Mr. [Gilles] Renaud, "What was that evidence?" he said he did not know and Drs. Driver and Barker would have to be asked. I do not understand how he can state to Dr. Rorke, another professional, that there is ample clinical evidence when he does not know what it is. Certainly none of the defence witnesses was aware of it. What is troubling . . . was that [Dr. Smith's] belief might colour his approach to the facts as well as his medical opinion and perhaps even affect the way he would undertake the autopsy.

Charles Smith found evidence only of his own preconceptions. Indeed, Dunn's most pointed remarks were about Smith's closed-mindedness.

Other medical experts called by the defence testified that they could consider the possibility of shaking because there were elements of the case that suggested it. On the other hand, Dr. Smith would not consider the possibility of a subdural hemorrhage and brain swelling from a fall, but even then he admitted that he is not current in the biomechanical understandings of falls.

There is an expression lawyers use, "Justice must not only be done, it must seen to be done." It would behoove Dr. Smith in making such an important decision as a diagnosis of shaking that would lead to a manslaughter charge, to show he seriously considered possibilities other than shaking.

Maurice Gagnon was floored. All his concerns about Dr. Smith were validated in Justice Dunn's ruling. He knew the pathologist was wrong about his daughter, but Maurice thought there had to be a reason. Smith was too well trained, too important, too highly regarded to simply be wrong. But he was wrong in Samantha McIntosh's case. Now Maurice believed even more fervently that he was wrong in Lianne's case too.

A line from the decision jumped out at Maurice. It wasn't as powerful or damning as some of the judge's other criticisms, but it was just as telling: "When first presented, the Crown's case appeared quite plausible," the judge wrote. "But after the evidence of the defence experts, it is riddled with reasonable doubts."

If you wanted to win, you had to launch a vigorous defence. Samantha McIntosh's parents had flown in expert witnesses from Los Angeles, Philadelphia, Chicago, Washington, Winnipeg and Ottawa. Maurice figured it must have cost them a small fortune. But it only solidified his resolve to do whatever it took, pay whatever it cost, to find experts to counter Smith's opinions.

The other thing that struck Maurice about Justice Dunn's decision was the timing. It came down in May 1991. It was now May 1998. How could Smith still have a job? Wasn't anyone paying attention? He wished the McIntosh family had complained back then. Maybe Smith would have been reprimanded, or demoted. Maybe the case against Lianne never would have happened.

Maurice Gagnon didn't know it at the time, but Sam's father had complained.

The case had been financially devastating for the McIntosh family. Sam's parents emptied their retirement savings and sold the family home to pay for all the expert medical witnesses to prepare reports and testify at the trial. Total costs reportedly ran north of $150,000. At one point, the family moved in with their lawyer.

Dave McIntosh (not his real name) had watched his daughter, his whole family, suffer through this hellish ordeal for three years, all because of the overzealousness and incompetence of Smith and other doctors at SickKids. Not only had Justice Dunn acquitted his daughter, but his scathing ruling had given Dave a weapon. And he intended to use it.

On November 6, 1991, Dave McIntosh first wrote to the College of Physicians and Surgeons of Ontario to complain about the conduct of the team of doctors from SickKids in his daughter's case. McIntosh included a copy of Justice Dunn's decision. "Our case has been a tragedy but let's not have this repeat itself," he wrote. "My fear is that many of the problems arising in our case are endemic to the SCAN and quality control programs at [the Hospital for Sick Children]."

The College of Physicians and Surgeons is the regulating body for doctors in Ontario. Membership for all practising doctors is mandatory. And the College is mandated, by law, to monitor and maintain standards of care in the province, which includes investigating complaints against doctors and disciplining any found to be incompetent or to have committed professional misconduct. Accordingly, the College launched an investigation in the McIntosh case.

The complaint couldn't have come at a worse time for Charles Smith. His career was just beginning to take off. He had recently been appointed the staff pathologist in charge of autopsy services within the Department of Pathology at the Hospital for Sick Children. Dr. M. James Phillips, the pathologist-in-chief at SickKids and Smith's boss and mentor, was pushing to create a specific unit within the hospital to focus on pediatric forensic cases. Smith had helped him develop the proposal, and Dr. Ross Bennett, the province's chief coroner at the time, was receptive. The Ontario Pediatric Forensic Pathology Unit was created in 1991 with a grant from the Chief Coroner's Office, and Dr. James Young, who was then a deputy chief coroner, put Smith's name forward to be its first director.

In the midst of that, Justice Dunn rendered his decision and Dave McIntosh filed his complaint. The SCAN team held a meeting to review the judge's decision. Smith claimed he had consulted with an American expert on the case. A consult would certainly bolster his now discredited opinions—at least they wouldn't be his alone. But it was the first anyone had heard of such a consult. Smith had not referred to it in his autopsy report, nor had he mentioned it in his testimony at trial. In fact, the Crown prosecutor said that had she known about it during the trial, she would have liked to have called the expert as a witness.

On April 1, 1992, the College's investigator, Duncan Newport, wrote to Smith and the SickKids doctors named in the complaint requesting a response. Smith came out swinging. In his defiant three-page letter, the pathologist said that he remained "as convinced as ever" that Amber's death was not an accident; that despite several days of vigorous cross-examination by the defence, his opinion never wavered. He hinted that a motivating factor in the complaint might be a desire for compensation, and he warned that complaints like this could have a chilling effect. "At the best of times," he wrote, "physicians are reluctant to testify in court. Should it become commonplace for physicians to be investigated by the College when their medical opinion is not upheld in a court of law, there will be an even greater disincentive for physicians to participate in important medico-legal matters."

But that thinly veiled threat wasn't Smith's most remarkable statement. This was: "On two occasions during my week of testimony, the judge, Patrick Dunn, discussed my evidence with me at length. He repeatedly indicated to me that he believed [the defendant] to be guilty, and that he believed the opinions provided by Drs. Barker, Driver and me."

Dave McIntosh didn't believe it for a moment. He wrote back to the College: "In light of Judge Dunn's strong criticisms, I submit that Dr. Smith is fabricating this point to mislead the reader. I am of the opinion that Judge Dunn should be asked to comment on Dr. Smith's remarks. In my opinion, Dr. Smith cannot be trusted."

Duncan Newport did not take McIntosh's advice to seek clarification from Justice Dunn. In fact, it appears that not much of anything happened on the file. Months passed, then years. On October 30, 1995, Newport finally wrote to Dave McIntosh to apologize for not getting back to him sooner. "As you know, the investigation in this matter seems to be dragging on," he wrote. "I hope to have all the information soon so that I can get this matter proceeding as quickly as possible toward either a discipline hearing or some form of mediated settlement."

Almost four years had passed since McIntosh had sent his first complaint to the College. While the file languished, Smith's star had continued to rise. He became the pre-eminent expert on pediatric forensic pathology in Canada. And he continued to work on complex, criminally suspicious cases. In fact, five days before Newport wrote that letter, Tammy Marquardt was convicted of second-degree murder in the death of her son Kenneth.

THREE

WHILE MAURICE AND Keaney continued digging into the McIntosh case, Tammy Marquardt languished behind bars. But at least she still had some contact with her boys. The adoptive parents had agreed to keep a line of communication open, and sent her a letter about the boys once a year. Tammy was allowed to send the boys a single letter back. And at Christmas she could send them each a gift through the prison chaplain.

It wasn't much, but it was all Tammy had. Living in the chaos of prison, that single letter was the only thing keeping her alive. That, and the hope of her appeal. She didn't know where her boys were living, and she knew nothing about their adoptive parents, not even their names. She wasn't even sure what the boys' names were—their adoptive parents could have changed them. She addressed her letters to Keith and Eric; for her, those would always be their names.

In her first letter, she told her boys she was their birth mother. She told them she missed them. She said she hoped they were happy, and that their new parents were good to them and gave the boys what they needed but didn't spoil them. She said she hoped she would see them again one day when they were all grown up. She told them that she loved them, and she always would.

The gifts and the letter were sent at Christmas. In the new year, she received her one allowed letter from the adoptive parents. Their words were awkward but heartfelt. The boys were adjusting well; Keith was obsessed with Thomas the Tank Engine. They promised to raise them in a caring, loving home. They wished her well.

Tammy could send her boys only one letter a year, but that didn't stop her writing to them. She started keeping diaries for each boy, and she wrote in them almost every day. They were juvenile diaries, with little locks to keep out prying eyes. Some days she tried to be profound, to pass on life lessons that she had learned, but most of the time she wrote about how much she missed and loved them. Always how much she missed and loved them.

Tammy cross-stitched bibs for them; she made them blankets and teddy bears. She bought them cards in the canteen for every occasion: birthday cards, Easter cards, Valentine's Day cards, Christmas cards. She packed everything up and stored it away. Once she got out, she would find the boys, she told herself. She would give them everything she'd been holding on to for them for so long.

Tammy was transferred out of the Prison for Women in April 1997, after 16 months. Correctional Services was slowly closing down the prison, gradually moving the inmates to five new facilities across the country. Tammy was sent to Grand Valley Institution for Women, in Kitchener, Ontario, which had opened that year. Inmates lived in a series of dormitories arranged around a central courtyard. There was green space on the grounds, and trees. Even though she was still in a protective custody unit, the arrangement of the courtyard dormitories made it much harder to avoid contact with the general population. Security between the dorms was not stringent. Tammy slept even less than she had at P4W, terrified that someone was going to sneak into her cell and knife her in the middle of the night. Getting across the prison grounds meant walking across the courtyard. Tammy found herself almost longing for P4W's labyrinth of tunnels, dangerous as they were.

In mid-January 1998, Tammy's annual letter from the boys' adoptive parents arrived. Tucked inside it was a photograph. The boys are in the bath. Keith is on the right, squatting, his ash-blond hair smushed against his forehead as he smiles up at the camera. A smiling Eric is looking up too. Eric's hair is darker, but other than that, they look like twins, even though Keith is almost two years older. It had been more than a year since Tammy had said goodbye to Eric, and even longer since she had laid eyes on Keith. She couldn't believe how much they'd grown. They looked happy, content, safe.

Months later, during a head count, Tammy was called out to meet the prison chaplain. The chaplain did not call for inmates, especially during a head count. Unless there was a death in the family.

As Tammy was led into the chaplain's office, she demanded to know which of her boys was dead. Nobody was dead, the chaplain said. But there had been an incident involving her boys.

The chaplain explained that when a volunteer delivered Tammy's Christmas gifts to Eric and Keith, their adoptive mother had been very upset. She told the volunteer that the boys weren't Tammy's children and that she didn't want Tammy having anything to do with them anymore.

Tammy pleaded that they were her kids. But the chaplain explained they were someone else's children now. Tammy begged him to talk to the parents, to remind them of the promise they had made to send her updates. But the chaplain would not. He told her Keith and Eric had good parents who were just doing what they thought was best for their children.

Tammy sank into a depression. Her appeal was heard later that month. It was dismissed. By the summer, she was suicidal. She hoarded pills, mostly Tylenol. One July night, Tammy Marquardt huddled in her cell and swallowed pill after pill.

FOUR

DAVE MCINTOSH HEARD nothing from the College for another year after Duncan Newport's letter of October 1995. Newport left the College in 1996, and the complaint was handed off to another investigator, Michelle Mann.

Of the twenty cases involving Charles Smith that the Goudge Inquiry reviewed, eleven of the children's deaths occurred between the time of Dave McIntosh's initial complaint, in November 1991, and when Mann took over the file, in October 1996. Kenneth Marquardt's was one of them. And of those eleven death investigations, nine ended in convictions, including Tammy's.

Mann started a fresh review, and arranged a meeting with James Young in February 1997 to discuss the file. Mann would later tell the Goudge Inquiry that when she reviewed Amber's case with Young, she reminded him that several medical experts called by the defence had contradicted Smith and that Justice Dunn's decision was highly critical of Smith's role in the case. While Young agreed that defence witnesses may have criticized Smith's opinions, he told Mann that it didn't change his impression that the case was "hard fought" and the verdict swung on the defence convincing the judge that shaken baby syndrome didn't exist.

The conversation with Mann didn't prompt Young to read Dunn's ruling for himself. In fact, it would be another decade before Young finally read the decision, in preparation for his testimony before the Goudge Inquiry. (That's what Young said during his Goudge testimony in November, 2007. He also told the inquiry he was unaware that a number of expert witnesses had testified for the defence, and that Justice Dunn was sharply critical of the Hospital for Sick Children and the methodology Smith and other SickKids witnesses used in the case. However, Young was later called back to testify after Mann told the inquiry how she had discussed the Dunn decision and the McIntosh case with Young during their 1997 meeting. Young told the inquiry that after reviewing Mann's notes, he agreed that he had been made aware of the Dunn decision in greater detail than his earlier testimony suggested.)

Based on Sam McIntosh's trial, Maurice Gagnon knew there were plenty of pathologists out there who would challenge Smith's opinions. He and lawyer Berk Keaney focused on the Canadian experts who had testified against Smith, but in the end, they settled on a pathologist who hadn't been directly involved in the Timmins case.

Dr. William Halliday was a professor of neuropathology at the University of Manitoba and had a practice at the Health Sciences Centre in Winnipeg. He was a consultant to the chief medical officer in the province and had worked on more than fifty shaken baby cases. He was an experienced witness in court. And when it came to Nicholas Gagnon's death, he thought Smith had the pathology all wrong.

Halliday had worked at the Hospital for Sick Children in the early 1980s and knew Smith well. In his affidavit in the Children's Aid proceedings to take custody of Lianne's newborn, Halliday said he had consulted for Smith, noting that he was an anatomical pathologist, and like other anatomical pathologists at SickKids, Smith regularly farmed out neuropathology to specialists in the field. Neuropathology focuses on the ways the nervous system can be injured or damaged, which was one of the main areas of inquiry in Nicholas's death. "It is not uncommon in major pediatric centres for the neuropathology to be done by someone with expertise in this field, ideally a trained neuropathologist," Halliday wrote. His implication was clear: Smith was out of his depth.

Halliday argued that Smith's finding that Nicholas had died from brain swelling consistent with blunt force injury went "far beyond the boundaries" of the scientific and forensic evidence. He noted that Smith had taken Nicholas's large head circumference to be evidence of brain swelling, but had not charted out his actual circumference in life. It turned out the child had always had a large head.

Halliday also found it unlikely that Dr. Chen would have missed a large area of discoloration along the skull that Smith found in his second autopsy. It was more likely, Halliday said, a "post-mortem artifact," or a change in the body after death. "In the first autopsy the scalp was reflected [folded back] and the scalp removed," Halliday wrote. "During this procedure, a plane would be established between the scalp and the skull. Blood-tinged fluids could accumulate post-mortem in this plane and cause the discoloration noted by Dr. Smith in the right parietal bone. It is highly unlikely that Dr. Chen would overlook hemorrhagic sutures."

Similarly, Halliday had difficulty with the heavy reliance Smith placed on the opinions of the two radiologists he consulted, who found evidence of split sutures, while dismissing that of the original radiologist in Sudbury, who found no abnormalities. "The assessment of sutures is a common and important part of the radiological investigation of these cases and it is highly unlikely that [the radiologist] would have overlooked split sutures."

Both points speak to an important foundation of pathology: initial findings are given the most weight because the original specialists are working with the body closest to the time of death. Second autopsies are not as reliable: bodies deteriorate over time and artifacts can be created depending on how specimens are stored. That's not to say review is not warranted and necessary, or that mistakes aren't made the first time round. But dismissing the work and opinion of the original pathologist has to be justified. Smith thought Chen was incompetent, missing crucial signs of blunt force trauma. Halliday thought it was more likely that those signs were never there.

Halliday completed his affidavit on June 16, 1998. Time was running out. Lianne was due in eight days. The next day, a lawyer for Children's Aid, Réjean Parisé, sent Jim Cairns a copy of Halliday's affidavit, along with an excerpt from Justice Dunn's ruling in Sam McIntosh's manslaughter trial. That judgment was pointed in its criticisms of Smith, but one charge stood out: that the pathologist had refused to consider any other cause of death. The pathology in the two cases was different—Smith argued that

Amber was a shaken baby case and that Nicholas was a case of blunt force trauma—but the criticism of Smith's closed-mindedness in his testimony at the McIntosh trial was echoed in the criticisms now being levelled against him by the Gagnon family.

That excerpt was the first Cairns had read of the judge's decision, but it didn't come as a complete surprise. Smith had mentioned it to him earlier, but assured him that he had subsequently spoken with the judge, who confided in him that he had got the decision wrong. As well, the SCAN team at SickKids continued to support Smith's findings in the McIntosh case, so Cairns didn't give Dunn's decision much weight now. He made no effort to review the entire judgment. In fact, two days later he wrote up his own affidavit in support of Smith's autopsy results for Nicholas Gagnon.

Children's Aid had Smith's second autopsy report, and his unequivocal "99 per-cent certain" position on blunt force trauma as the cause of Nicholas's death. The agency also had the affidavit from Cairns supporting Smith's position. The Gagnon family, on the other hand, had Halliday's affidavit refuting Smith's findings. They also had a similar affidavit from Dr. Chen. But Smith's opinions had effectively neutered Chen's; Chen had been removed from the region's roster of pathologists doing autopsies of children under two because of the fallout from the Gagnon case.

The CAS proceedings were still not settled when Lianne went into the hospital for the delivery. CAS had made it clear that Lianne would not be leaving the hospital with her child. Maurice and Angie subjected themselves to a humiliating vetting process by CAS to qualify as foster parents so the baby could at least go home with family members. But a settlement had yet to be reached.

Lianne thought about running. She thought about it a lot. "I just remember thinking, they're going to take the baby away," she told me years later. "And I knew what CAS had said to Pete, that he could keep her without me. So in my head I'm thinking, he's going to take her away. I would if I were him. I mean, if somebody was going to take my baby away but I had a way of keeping her? I would do it. I think a mother would pick her kid over her husband any time," Lianne said with a laugh.

"I had this fear that I was losing my family all at once. I was going to lose my daughter. I was going to lose my husband. And I wasn't going to be allowed to go anywhere near her."

These were not ideal conditions for a stress-free birth.

Lianne's doctor, Miguel Bonin, was most concerned about the effect a seizure at the hospital would have on mother and child. No one from CAS had spoken to him about their specific plans. All he knew was that an apprehension notice had been sent to the hospital. Lianne was feeding him information as she learned it. Protocol at St. Joseph's at the time had expectant mothers labouring in one room, delivering in another and recovering in yet a third before returning to their bed on the ward. "My concern at that point was bonding of the child with the mother," Bonin told me years later. "The word that we had was, as soon as she comes out of the delivery room, they were going to apprehend. That was my assumption because we had heard nothing official." So Bonin made arrangements with hospital administrators to let Lianne recover in the delivery room, just to keep mother and child together as long as possible. "That's what I didn't want," he said later, "to get into a wrestling match with the baby in the middle."

Nicole Melanie Thibeault was born on Saturday, June 27, 1998, at 8:37 p.m. The moment she was born, she went on Lianne's chest so bonding between mother and child could begin. It was standard procedure, but in this case, it was also ammunition. Bonin would later argue that the bond between mother and daughter had already begun, and it would be unfair and unhealthy to break that bond; plus, Lianne needed access to the baby so she could breastfeed.

Usually, the doctor's job ends with the delivery, but Bonin stayed for the recovery, letting Lianne breastfeed Nicole while he kept watch in the hallway to see if anyone was coming.

Just the night before, Angie and Maurice had reached an agreement with CAS: they could have temporary supervision of the child, so long as the newborn had twenty-four-hour supervision. Failing that, the baby would have to spend the night in the hospital's nursery, so Angie and Pete's mother, Carolle, took shifts in Lianne's room. Dr. Bonin kept Lianne in the hospital an extra day to allow her constant access to her newborn. Once she left, her access would be down to three hours a day.

Mother and daughter checked out of the hospital on June 30. "It should be a happy day going home with the baby, but I was just constantly crying," recalled Lianne. "I was just constantly crying and completely upset. The CAS workers were there to make sure I didn't get in the car with my parents, that I was in a separate vehicle from Nic."

The caravan of cars snaked through Sudbury's streets back to Angie and Maurice's home. Lianne wasn't allowed in the house with the baby without someone from CAS present to supervise. Lianne gritted her teeth and did as she was told. She was allowed three hours with Nicole that first afternoon. At one point, she asked to excuse herself to breastfeed the baby. The CAS worker insisted on joining her to make sure she didn't suffocate the child.

Day-to-day parenting fell to Angie. They were on their own with the baby twenty-one hours a day. It had been more than two decades since Angie had had that kind of responsibility. The sleep deprivation, the constant feedings, the diaper changes were a shock to the system.

Lianne and Pete lived in an apartment just up the street. Lianne didn't want Nicole bottle-fed, so she pumped breast milk, and Pete ran it over to her parents every day. "He was just running back and forth, back and forth. And he never stayed. He didn't want me to feel that he was having more time with her than I was. If I wasn't allowed to be with her, he wouldn't stay."

The second night home, Maurice went over to Lianne's apartment and snuck her and Pete back to the house to be with their daughter. They stayed until three in the morning. That was the beginning. Everyone knew they were taking enormous risks, but it didn't matter. It was worth it. And each time Lianne snuck over and didn't get caught, it emboldened her even more.

"By four weeks into it, I'd finish my three-hour visit and walk down to our apartment. CAS had barely turned off the street and I'd turn around and walk back," she said with a laugh. When Nicole was about three weeks old, Maurice called Lianne one afternoon to say he had some errands to run with her mother. He wanted to drop Nicole off with Lianne. By now they were feeling confident about breaking the rules, but Maurice still drove around the back of the building and went up the stairs, out of sight.

Lianne's parents had helped them build an elaborate nursery in their apartment, with new carpet and Winnie the Pooh wallpaper. Mother and daughter didn't leave the nursery that afternoon. Lianne burned through an entire roll of camera film.

Once during that first month, Lianne was at her parents' place with Pete and Nicole. Maurice and Angie were out. There was a knock at the door. She was sure it was CAS making an impromptu check. Lianne sprinted into her parents' bedroom and hid in the closet.

It turned out to be Pete's sister. She had just bought a new car and had come by to show it off. Pete was so excited for her that he forgot to go and get Lianne. She spent twenty minutes cowering in the closet before he finally remembered.

Such was Lianne's life for Nicole's first month—taking big risks to be a mother and then worrying about the consequences. With good reason: CAS wasn't backing down. The agency had immediately moved forward with an application for Crown wardship of Nicole—a permanent seizure that would end with a formal adoption.

Maurice took the lead in fighting Children's Aid. He had managed to get Lianne through the police investigation, and he had the money and the know-how to take on the agency. Pete's parents, Louie and Carolle, had neither. As first-time grandparents, they felt helpless and cheated, pushed to the sidelines by a system unconcerned about what they were losing. The case had driven an irrevocable rift through Louie's family. His police officer brother, Leo, continued to believe Lianne had killed Nicholas. What's more, he was chairman of the board at CAS. Louie's relationship with his brother never recovered.

Nicole's birth was quickly followed by a series of new, and conflicting, affidavits. Smith swore the first of these, two days after Nicole was born. In it, he reiterated many of the findings he had made in his autopsy the year before: that Nicholas died as a result of cerebral edema, consistent with a blunt force injury, that the fatal blow occurred while he was under the exclusive control of his mother and that her explanation of what happened did not jibe with the medical evidence. Smith added that he could not rule out asphyxia as a cause of death.

As evidence of the edema, he pointed to, first, the split sutures and discoloration along the suture lines and, second, Nicholas's brain weight.

Once again, Smith categorically dismissed Dr. Chen's original autopsy, saying that the pathologist's opinion that Nicholas's edema was mild was "absolutely and clearly wrong." He was equally dismissive of the opinions William Halliday had outlined in his affidavit two weeks earlier: Halliday said it would have been more ideal for a trained neuropathologist—which Smith was not—to perform the neuropathologic aspects of the autopsy. Smith claimed that a pediatric neuropathologist named Venita Jay had reviewed the case, although she had not written a formal report.

In March 1999, Berk Keaney followed up with Dr. Jay, who said that she had no recollection of giving Smith a verbal consultation of the case. The autopsy had been completed less than eighteen months before.

While Halliday's opinions had little sway with Smith or Cairns at the Coroner's Office, they did cause some reflection at Children's Aid. The agency received Halliday's first affidavit calling Smith's findings into question on June 16, 1998, almost two weeks before Nicole was born. Concerned about the conflicting opinions, CAS arranged a conference call with Smith and Cairns that afternoon. Agency officials had one simple question: Was Halliday's theory medically reasonable? If it was, Children's Aid would stop its intervention in the case.

Louise Huneault, a CAS lawyer, wrote in a later affidavit: "Dr. Smith and Dr. Cairns were extremely clear . . . that the theories put forth by Dr. Halliday were not sustainable and that the position of the Coroner's Office had not changed relative to the cause of death."

Halliday followed up Smith's criticisms with a new affidavit of his own. In it, he used even stronger language to criticize Smith's opinion, saying that while Smith admitted in his first affidavit that he "cannot be absolutely certain as to the cause of the fatal injury," he was of "the opinion, to a high level of certainty, that the death . . . was due to a non-accidental injury." Halliday wrote: "I repeat, in my opinion this conclusion goes far beyond the boundaries that can be supported by the presenting scientific and forensic facts. If Dr. Smith cannot be absolutely certain as to the cause of the injury, how can he be so certain as to the nature of the injury (ie. non-accidental)?"

Halliday had similar concerns about other aspects of Smith's findings. He pointed out that Smith contradicted himself. For example, in one place Smith noted he found "no evidence of subarachnoid or intraparenchymal hemorrhage." Then, in another, he states that there was some evidence of intracranial hemorrhage present at the time of Nicholas's death, writing, "It would appear that a very small amount of subarachnoid hemorrhage was present, but it does not appear extensive."

Halliday argued that not only were such statements indicative of Smith's inconsistencies, but the bleeding itself was also key evidence of post-mortem artifacts created during the autopsies. "A microscopic amount of subarachnoid blood could be consistent with the removal of the brain, which necessitates the cutting of vessels," he wrote.

Post-mortem artifacts were an issue Halliday came back to again and again. Differentiating between changes that occurred at the time of death and those that occurred after death or during the autopsy is one of the primary challenges facing a pathologist. Halliday argued that Smith had misread these changes on several occasions. For instance, he argued that the discoloration of the right parietal bone Smith saw at the second autopsy was actually created when the brain was removed for examination during the autopsy.

And then there was the issue of Nicholas's heart. There wasn't one. It's unclear what happened to it, but it appears that Nicholas was not buried with his heart after the first autopsy by Dr. Chen. In his second autopsy report, Dr. Smith notes that "no cardiac tissues were found." He does not appear to have made any efforts to locate them at the hospital in Sudbury or from Dr. Chen. In his affidavit, Smith states, "there was no evidence at autopsy of a natural disease that could account for Nicholas's death." Yet he also admits "there are a number of disorders which present as sudden and unexpected death and which may be associated with cerebral edema. This may include the cardiovascular system."

Halliday argued that Smith's finding that there was no evidence of a natural disease was misleading, since he hadn't been able to examine the heart, which he admitted could show signs of just such a disease. "This means that Dr. Smith's opinion on the heart is based solely on the slides prepared by Dr. Chen and the first autopsy observations of Dr. Chen, which he doesn't appear to trust." In other words, Smith was interpreting Chen's findings only in ways that supported his theory of blunt force trauma. Where Chen's findings contradicted that, Smith disregarded them. But when Chen said he found no signs of a natural disease, Smith accepted it. Without having been able to examine the heart firsthand, Halliday argued, "Dr. Smith is not in a position to assess the full gambit of cardiac causes of sudden unexpected death."

Halliday went on to outline a scenario that he believed might explain Nicholas's tragic death. Three weeks before his death, the toddler had smacked his head on a coffee table, leaving a large bump on his head. "I believe that Nicholas developed a symptomatic degree of cerebral edema after this event . . . On the morning of his collapse, this boy could already have had a swollen, edematous brain. When he stood up under sewing machine, he re-injured himself . . . Unfortunately, Nicholas may have already been in a precarious situation and the added intracranial volume precipitated his collapse, which was associated with the onset of severe neurogenic pulmonary edema." Halliday said Smith's theory that asphyxiation may have been a cause of death would fit this scenario.

But Smith wasn't done. He swore yet another affidavit ten days later. In it, he stressed that after considering Halliday's comments, he still believed that Nicholas had died of a non-accidental blunt force trauma. And if asphyxia was a factor, it too was non-accidental and caused by Lianne. He also dismissed Halliday's theory that Nicholas's head injury three weeks earlier could have been a factor, arguing that the forensic literature shows that cerebral edema dissipates in less than a week.

Children's Aid was in a quandary. It had the strongly held opinions of two esteemed pathologists: Dr. Smith, who believed that Nicholas was purposefully killed, and Dr. Halliday, who argued that the evidence didn't support that conclusion. Smith had done one of the autopsies. Halliday had not. Smith's opinion was backed by a similar affidavit from the deputy chief coroner of Ontario, and Jim Cairns was esteemed in his own right. Halliday had the original pathologist in his corner, but Dr. Chen's work had been so thoroughly dismissed by Smith and Cairns that it was difficult to give his opinion much weight.

After considering the flurry of competing affidavits, the agency decided it was still on strong ground, and continued with its application.

The next court date was scheduled in July. A judge would decide whether the CAS application had enough merit to continue to a full hearing and whether the terms of the temporary custody order were appropriate. Lianne and her family had no idea which way things might go. The judge could throw out the CAS application, or allow Lianne more access to her daughter. Or it could go the other way: Maurice and Angie's custody could be revoked, and Nicole could be placed in foster care.

Justice Louise Gauthier made her ruling on July 28. Lianne, Pete and her parents listened in amazement as the judge took aim at Smith's work on the case.

"The most compelling criticism relates to Dr. Smith's description of the split skull sutures," Justice Gauthier said. "In his affidavit, Dr. Smith states that Dr. Babyn indicated 'marked widening of the skull sutures.' In fact, when one reviews Dr. Babyn's report . . . it does not speak of marked widening of the skull sutures. Rather, it uses the adjective, mild. Dr. Smith's statement, then, is somewhat misleading." The judge had similar concerns about Smith's claim that a number of doctors at the hospital noted a bruise on Nicholas's head when he was admitted. In fact, both the emergency doctor and the investigating coroner said at the time that there was no evidence of trauma on his head or anywhere else on his body.

"It is my conclusion that despite the weaknesses in Dr. Smith's material . . . the Society does establish a concern about the death of the first born child," Justice Gauthier said. "There is the fact of the unexplained death; the fact of the head circumference after death; the elevated brain weight; the possible association of discoloration to the parietal bone with head injury."

Maurice understood that much of the case came down to a difference in opinions, but some things were just facts. Dr. Halliday had charted Nicholas's head circumference and determined that he'd always had a large head, and the circumference at his death fit almost perfectly on his natural growth curve.

The judge concluded, "It will be determined at trial whose theory is the correct theory, but, for the purposes of this proceeding, the evidence is sufficient in my view to meet the risk test."

But as the judge turned to the issue of custody and supervision, her reasoning took another decisive turn in Lianne's favour.

From all accounts, Lianne was a devoted mother to Nicholas . . . It is said that she was completely dedicated to the child's well-being . . . There is no evidence that Lianne has a temper or anger problem. There is no evidence that she has violent tendencies. There is no evidence that she suffers from substance dependency. There *is* evidence that she has been reared in a loving supportive family; that her parents are happy healthy individuals with great strength and courage. They are people who are dedicated to family and who have provided in their home a foundation of love, affection and security.

Nicole is a very young infant, barely one month old . . . It could be some time before the trial of this matter occurs. Based on the evidence before me, I cannot conclude, firstly, that this infant should be taken from the home of her grandparents and placed in foster care. There is no risk posed to this child by her grandparents or her father. In fact, it would be contra her interests, in my view, to remove her from this nurturing, loving home. I also cannot conclude that there is a reasonable basis for the belief that Nicole could suffer harm at the hands of the mother if another person is present.

It is my conclusion, therefore, that the least restrictive plan of care for Nicole is as follows: That Nicole be placed in the care of her mother and father subject to supervision by the Society.

The judge went on to list various conditions: the child would continue to live with her grandparents; she would reside in a bedroom upstairs while Lianne and Pete would sleep in the basement apartment; Children's Aid would still have access to the home but they would now have to give advance notice of a visit; and Lianne's contact with Nicole would continue to be supervised.

Lianne and Pete were free to be parents to their child without someone constantly standing over them.

Their elation was short-lived. Two days after the hearing, Lianne was notified that her name had been added to the Ontario Child Abuse Register. She had known since before Nicole was born that it was coming, but the letter was devastating nonetheless. Lianne had planned to go to teachers' college. Now labelled a child abuser, she had no hope of a teaching career.

Meanwhile, Berk Keaney was keen to talk to Smith about his affidavits to better understand his differences of opinions with Halliday. He also needed to get the slides and physical specimens from Smith's autopsy (and Chen's original examination). Halliday's first two affidavits were based on a paper review of the case, which would likely not carry as much weight as Smith's findings since Smith had done a physical examination of the body. It was crucial that Halliday review the specimens to buttress his opinions.

But Smith was impossible to track down. The doctor refused to return his phone calls. Weeks of trying turned into months; Keaney was convinced that Smith was actively avoiding him. So, like many defence lawyers, police officers and Crown attorneys before him, Keaney turned to Jim Cairns to act as a conduit to Smith. In late January 1999, seven months after CAS had launched its custody application, Smith finally provided Cairns with various samples he took at autopsy. The hospital in Sudbury provided samples from Chen's autopsy around the same time. After reviewing the physical specimens, Halliday wrote a third affidavit, reiterating his earlier opinions that Nicholas did not die from blunt force trauma to the head. But now he had a new theory about the cause.

"I am pleased to have had the opportunity to examine the material," Halliday wrote, "for all it has confirmed to me is that Nicholas did not die from the result of a cranio-cerebral injury and resultant cerebral edema. The skull X-rays do not show widely split sutures. I believe them to be normal." He added that he found the brain swelling to be mild or moderate, not extreme as Smith was contending. "In summary, I believe Nicholas, having just finished a meal, hit his head beneath the sewing machine. This was painful and when he forcefully cried, he aspirated stomach contents and choked to death."

In tracking down the autopsy exhibits for Dr. Halliday, Keaney also had a chance to speak to Dr. Cairns about his own affidavit. And as the two men discussed the case, a troubling realization started to dawn on Keaney: Cairns may have been the deputy chief coroner of the province, but he wasn't qualified to review the case directly.

Keaney asked Cairns what qualifications he had in pathology. It was an innocent question. But the answer shocked him: Cairns said he was not a trained pathologist.

"Then how did you write your affidavit?" Keaney asked. Cairns said he simply wrote it to support Smith. They had worked together for many years. Both he and the Coroner's Office had complete confidence in Smith's opinion.

I wholly agree with the specific and crucial findings of Dr. Smith that the cerebral edema suffered by the infant was severe rather than mild as characterized by Dr. Chen.

I agree with the conclusions of Dr. Smith that the infant did not die of SIDS . . .

The essential variables that lead to the conclusion that the child was harmed by an unexplained intentional use of force are: the findings of Doctor Smith . . .

I am aware of the contents of Doctor Smith's affidavit. I share the opinions stated in the affidavit.

In short, Cairns never based any of his findings on the autopsy or forensic evidence themselves; all his opinions simply supported Smith's. At first and even second glance the affidavit gives the impression that Cairns had independently reviewed the case file and come to his own conclusions. Keaney had missed that subtlety earlier. He was mad at himself for overlooking it, but he was also incredulous. This man had signed a sworn affidavit. Was he even qualified to write it?

Keaney suspected that if he'd missed the nuance of Cairns's affidavit, Children's Aid likely had as well. And he was right. Keaney wrote to CAS lawyer Réjean Parisé about his discussion with Cairns and calmly explained that Dr. Cairns was not a trained pathologist. He never made any of his own findings. The agency was being misled.

On March 8, 1999, Parisé wrote to both Smith and Cairns. "I have been advised by Mr. Keaney, by correspondence, that Dr. Cairns has indicated he is not, himself, a person who can provide opinion evidence as to the cause of death of Nicholas Gagnon . . . In light of the fact of opinions proffered in earlier meetings and in the affidavit material, it was somewhat surprising to have such a comment being made. By the same token, if [Keaney's position] is an appropriate comment, then certainly it is one which I would wish confirmed as soon as possible."

The realization was a blow to CAS's case, but it wasn't necessarily a death knell. Months earlier, the agency and the Coroner's Office had decided to seek another expert opinion to buttress Smith's findings and to counter the evidence of the Gagnons' own expert witnesses. At the time, Parisé believed he already had Cairns's opinion as backup to his star witness; another expert would be further insurance. But now that the legitimacy of Cairns's affidavit had been brought into question, Parisé needed another second opinion.

The Coroner's Office settled on Dr. Mary Case, a well-respected forensic pathologist at St. Louis University Health Sciences Center and the chief medical officer for St. Louis. She completed her four-page report in March 1999. Case agreed with the initial findings of Smith (and Dr. Uzans, the regional coroner) that Nicholas's death should not be classified as SIDS. But that was where her agreement ended.

"I would not attribute this death to a head injury as there are no findings on which to make such a conclusion," she wrote, explaining that the brain swelling, or cerebral edema, was based on higher brain weight and some "mild" splitting of the skull sutures. Case said that this level of brain swelling is not uncommon in many deaths. "For teaching purposes, I often demonstrate such brain swelling in photographs in non-traumatic deaths to illustrate how the terminal event of dying from many causes can result in rather marked swelling . . . Certainly, brain swelling or cerebral edema should never be used as an isolated finding to make a diagnosis of head injury."

Case dismantled many of Smith's other findings as well. She noted that abusive head injuries in children usually have a set of distinct markers, including subdural and subarachnoid hemorrhages in at least 95 per cent of cases. Even Smith could find no large-scale evidence of either type of hemorrhage, and she felt the microscopic evidence he did find was a post-mortem artifact, most likely caused during the autopsy, as Halliday had contended. Similarly, she said the discoloration of the right parietal portion of the skull was not a sign of injury but was more likely caused during the exhumation. Finally, she said there was insufficient evidence to suggest asphyxia played a role in Nicholas's death. "There is no cause of death that I can find in either autopsy and I would consider both the cause and manner of death to be undetermined," she concluded. "Children of this age do die without our always being able to determine the cause of death."

On March 23, 1999, a day after receiving Dr. Case's report, officials at Children's Aid called an emergency meeting. There was Dr. Chen's original autopsy report that found nothing untoward in Nicholas's death. There were Dr. Halliday's affidavits thoroughly repudiating Smith's findings. There was Dr. Cairns's misleading affidavit for which he had not done any physical review of the slides or specimens. And now there was the report of Dr. Case, an independent forensic pathologist commissioned by the Chief Coroner's Office, who had also dismissed almost all of Smith's findings. There was only one thing to do.

"The instructions I have received," Réjean Parisé wrote in a letter to Berk Keaney, "are to request the court to vacate all temporary orders, withdraw the present application and withdraw the registration under the child abuse register.

"At this time, on behalf of the Society, we are of the view that the death of Nicholas Gagnon was an unexplained tragedy. We express our sympathies to the family. We express to the whole of the family unit our confidence in their ability to provide a good life to Nicole."

ONE

IN SOME WAYS, the second-degree murder charges laid against Brenda Waudby on September 18, 1997, came almost as a relief to her. For months she had known that charges were inevitable, but she didn't realize how heavily the stress of waiting and worrying had been sitting on her. And now that weight was gone.

Life was still hard. The charges were front-page news, and the *Peterborough Examiner* printed every detail of her bail conditions, right down to her living arrangements and her parents' address. People had whispered about her before; they whispered about her now. At the supermarket, on the street, at the mall, Brenda saw the disdain, the hatred in their eyes.

Her life now revolved around the two visits with Justine she was allowed each week. A CAS contract worker would bring Justine to Brenda's parents' house for the two-hour visits. Brenda would take her daughter to the park or for dinner. She'd ask about school, about friends, about her favourite TV shows and pop stars. They wouldn't talk about Jenna. Some places were still too painful to go. Brenda tried to fill their hours with the ordinariness of life. She wanted their time together to feel as normal as possible.

Justine appeared to be content. The eight-year-old hugged and kissed Brenda at the start of every visit, hugged and kissed her at the end. She said she missed her mother. She did ask about coming home. Sometimes Brenda lied, told her soon. But Brenda knew she was facing the prospect of life in prison. Would Justine ever be coming home? She had no idea.

Months passed. Christmas came and went, then March break and Easter.

Brenda's criminal lawyer, Jim Hauraney, continued prepping for her preliminary hearing, which was scheduled for the fall of 1998. There was little he could do about Brenda's statement to police. She had retracted it, but the damage was done.

"Retractions to a lawyer really don't mean much," Hauraney would say years later. "If she said something and then retracted it to the police, that may have some weight, but what she told me wouldn't have."

Hauraney considered Brenda's letter self-serving and wasn't sure it would be admissible in court, since it was protected by lawyer-client privilege. To introduce the letter as evidence, Brenda would need to waive that privilege, and then Hauraney might be compelled to testify as well. However, even though Brenda alleged the police had coerced her to make her statement, Hauraney never instructed her to rewrite the letter directly to the police. The retraction faded into the background.

The case, however, still seemed far from lost. For one, the case against Brenda didn't quite add up. Jenna had been severely beaten, her tiny body a grotesque patchwork of multicoloured bruises. And yet Brenda had paraded her around to friends throughout the day on Tuesday, *after* the alleged beating, and no one noticed any sign of it, either in her appearance or in her behaviour. Even Maggie and JD said they didn't notice anything unusual about the toddler when JD started babysitting just before five that afternoon.

Brenda's preliminary hearing was held over three days in late October 1998. Det. Const. Dan Lemay, Charles Smith, Maggie and JD testified. Hauraney was anxious to question Charles Smith about the timing of Jenna's injuries. The pathologist had a reputation as a commanding witness at trial. He carried himself with the authority one would expect from someone in his position. So his testimony at the preliminary hearing was surprising.

Smith was vague about the timing of Jenna's injuries. In response to questions asked by Crown prosecutor David Thompson, Smith said the medical literature suggested that life-threatening injuries could take time to manifest themselves, especially in cases of child abuse, which is how he characterized Jenna's case. "In the child abuse cases," he said, "frequently there was not a day that went by—but, you know, three, four days—that kind of thing—and so a child who seemed initially well and became ill over a period—or increasingly over a period of several days has died." That testimony suggested Jenna's fatal injuries were days old, implicating Brenda Waudby as the perpetrator. Yet only moments later, Smith widened his time frame to "anything from hours to several days," suggesting JD could also have been responsible. He stated, "There's not the degree of science that allows us to be extremely specific and I end up in ranges."

Smith also said the number of injuries Jenna suffered made determining when exactly they occurred even harder. "It is easy to assume that all of the injuries in Jenna occurred at a given point of time, but I can't prove it. I mean, she could have been injured on a single given point in time; she could have been injured on two occasions, you know, two minutes apart or two hours apart; or three occasions, three minutes apart and three hours apart. I can't answer that."

Smith suggested the injury to Jenna's liver was six to twelve hours old. And yet the injury to her mesentery (a fold of tissue just below the liver) appeared to be older. "The problem there is that we have, you know, we have obviously vital reaction in the liver [but] we have none in the mesentery, and yet the two are side-by-side, so presumably whatever caused one injury also caused the other, but we have this discrepancy here. Can we explain the discrepancy? Well, we may have to use the idea of a delayed reaction to that."

When he examined the small intestine, he said, he saw evidence that suggested an injury that was anywhere from six to twenty-four hours old. He assigned different time estimates to Jenna's rib injuries as well. He felt they were definitely not more than five to seven days old. As for a lower limit, at least three of the fractures appeared to be twenty-four to forty-eight hours old. "Some of the information says we're dealing with six hours—12 hours minimum—others, you know—other observations say it could be a day or two, you know," he testified. "I mean it could be more than a day or two but, if we're much more than a day or two, then other observations should have been apparent here. This is not something that occurred in just a few hours—it didn't occur in one hour, or two hours, or three hours or four hours. It occurred in, you know, half a day—a day—maybe two days. You know, I must tell you I'm very, very reluctant to push it in terms of several days."

The Crown asked him, "Given those observations, then, and assuming the life-threatening injuries that were caused to Jenna, is there anything inconsistent in your observations with those injuries having been caused about 28 hours prior to the time death was pronounced?"

"Sure. Yeah, that's consistent," Smith answered. "Is it 12 hours? Yeah, some of the observations don't fit. [But] at 12 hours, some fit it really nicely. Is it 48 hours? You know, I'm reluctant. But 24, 28 hours. Certainly in my opinion, it's consistent with that."

Hauraney zeroed in on other contradictions in Smith's opinions. During the autopsy, Smith had told Const. Scott Kirkland that the injuries to Jenna's liver, pancreas and duodenum had not started to heal, which suggested that they happened within hours of her death. But during Hauraney's cross-examination, Smith dismissed these initial opinions as unreliable because they were based on "naked-eye observations," which were not as accurate as what he later saw under the microscope.

And then Smith raised another possibility—Jenna's rib injuries might have happened at different times. "Some could have occurred an hour before death and some a day before death," he testified under cross-examination. "Some of them, you know, I can look at it down the microscope and say, if I ignore everything else and just look at this one fracture, could this one fracture be a few hours? Sure."

He said that nailing down the timing of the injuries was made difficult not only by their number but by the differences in how they were healing when Jenna died. "I can show you rib fractures and say this could have occurred an hour prior to death, and at the same time it could have occurred six or eight or ten hours prior to death. And I can look at other things like the adrenal or the liver and say it looks like it's six hours but it could be 24 hours. And so the problem [is] . . . I have evidence which says injuries occurred, because of their concentration in the body, it seems reasonable that they all occurred at about the same time. And yet, if you look at each one individually, there's no absolute concordance in that, and that's the frustration here. Some can be interpreted as being early, some can be interpreted as late. If they all occurred at the same time, then I have to go to the later observations but I cannot assure that they all occurred at the same time. Could she have been injured 24 hours prior to death, and then 12 hours, and then six hours and then two hours, and then an hour prior to death? Sure, she could have."

Hauraney then asked if, given that the forensic analysis of the timing of Jenna's injuries was so inconclusive, there were other things to consider in determining when they occurred. "So, I take it then, doctor, what we have to look at is perhaps the child's behaviour? The next best thing, I take it, would be the child and how she reacted over [her last twenty-four hours]. Is that fair?"

"Yeah. If you have good observations of that, that can help. Yeah."

"And so, if we have observations that the child was generally happy and played around, etc., in the afternoon, would that tend to lead to an opinion that maybe the injury occurred after that period of time?"

"Well, yeah, it could have occurred afterwards," Smith answered. "[But] after this type of injury, you can get a honeymoon period. Unlike something like head injury where, once a lethal head injury occurs, you're no longer normal, the literature would suggest that in fact, with blunt abdominal injury, you can get a honeymoon period where an infant appears essentially normal but as the abnormalities continue in their process—be it, you know, leakage of blood or leakage of bile or leakage of enzymes or whatever—then symptoms will certainly kick in.

"My hunch is that [Jenna] probably had some initial symptoms from the injury if it was a single event. She may well have had a period of time when she appeared normal or near normal. Obviously, internally she's not normal but she may have appeared normal. [Or] no, she may not have had this honeymoon period. She may have been injured and never been normal from that point forward, but she could have had a honeymoon period."

And yet Smith said that initially he had suspected JD was responsible for Jenna's injuries because of the grid-like burn on her forehead. "You know, you've got a burn which we know was not there when the mother left the home . . . I can tell you that my personal opinion initially was that the babysitter had to be responsible because whoever caused one mark would have caused presumably all of them."

Thompson had raised the question of sexual assault during his examination of Smith. In response, Smith said there was no physical evidence that Jenna had been sexually abused.

"Now, having said that, let me be very careful here. You need to understand that it is quite possible that someone, you know, who is not a parent, not a caregiver who is looking after her in terms of bathing her, it's quite possible someone touched her inappropriately but I have no marks at autopsy which indicate injury that could be contributed to sexual abuse."

Hauraney returned to this line of questioning during his cross-examination. He noted that the attending doctor and several of the nurses at the hospital in Peterborough made observations that suggested the child may have been sexually abused. Smith, however, remained undeterred.

"Part of what happens, and I've seen it on more than one occasion," he explained, "is that with changes attendant upon death, a person can make observations which, in the living child, are alarming but in the dead child are not. I've had cases sent to me that are, you know, people are absolutely adamant [they] are child abuse and in fact it's normal post-mortem change. But the observations are made by people who don't make those observations in dead children or they're made in difficult conditions as opposed to at the autopsy, where we have lots of light and that's not something that you can necessarily do with the living child."

Smith explained that normal, natural changes the body goes through after death can be misconstrued by untrained or inexperienced observers as signs of sexual abuse. "It's very common for people to say there's anal contusion or there's been anal interference, but it's by people who are not familiar with the anus post-mortem," he said.

The mysterious hair seen by emergency room staff was also discussed at Brenda's preliminary hearing. Hauraney asked Smith about a note made by the attending doctor, Dale Friesen, in his report, about "a curly hair around the vulva area." He asked Smith, "Would you expect this young girl to have a curly hair on her vulva?"

"No. No, I assume that's some pick up. That's something which has landed there."

Hairs sometimes fall off paramedics or emergency staff and onto the patient during resuscitation efforts. But Hauraney pointed out to Smith that Friesen didn't think this hair was a contaminant. "I understand in speaking with him he was satisfied it was consistent with a dark pubic hair?"

"You know something I don't know," Smith replied.

"But does that . . . does that raise alarm bells?"

"Yes, sure."

"And I take it then, as far as you know, the police didn't bring any pubic hair to you for examination?"

"No."

"And did they advise you that there may have been a pubic hair found?"

"I can't. I can't remember."

What Hauraney didn't know at the time was that Smith *had* found a hair in Jenna's pubic area during the autopsy. What's more, Smith had brought it with him to the preliminary hearing, tucked into a sealed envelope. That hair was *in his pocket* at the very moment he was denying its existence on the stand.

The question of why Smith would take a potentially crucial piece of evidence to the preliminary hearing but not mention it to anyone became one of the central questions swirling around the pathologist when the scope of his incompetence and misconduct started to surface.

Smith also testified that he didn't do a rape kit exam on Jenna. At least, he couldn't remember doing one.

"Did you take any swabs?" Hauraney asked him.

"You know, I was wondering if I did," Smith answered. "I don't have any record of it, and so without that I don't know if I did a rape kit or not."

"Would that have at least satisfied you in some regard whether or not there may or may not have been some interference with the vagina?"

"The rape kit certainly doesn't rule it out. You know, if you have evidence, then yes, you can say there's interference but the lack of evidence doesn't mean there's been no interference."

At the end of the preliminary hearing, Brenda was ordered to stand trial on the charge of second-degree murder.

The ruling was not unexpected, and Brenda's legal team believed it was still a winnable case. Jenna's babysitter, JD, remained a viable suspect; Hauraney just needed to find medical experts who would challenge Smith's opinion on the timing of Jenna's fatal injuries. He spoke to several experts in Hamilton: Chitra Rao, a forensic pathologist at McMaster University; Dr. K. C. Finkel, who worked in the Department of Pediatrics at the university's Faculty of Health Sciences; Dr. Peter Fitzgerald, a pediatric surgeon at McMaster Children's Hospital. All of them disputed Smith's opinion on the timing of Jenna's injuries, suggesting it was much more likely they occurred within hours of the child's death.

Peter Fitzgerald suggested Hauraney speak with Sigmund Ein, a colleague of Smith's at the Hospital for Sick Children. Ein was widely considered the top pediatric surgeon in the country. Fitzgerald believed his opinion would carry a lot of weight.

On November 3, 1998, less than two weeks after Brenda's preliminary hearing, Hauraney spoke with the surgeon.

Dr. Ein declined to speak to me directly, citing medical, legal and privacy concerns, but his notes of the conversation he had with Hauraney were filed at the Goudge Inquiry. Based on the two handwritten pages, it appears Hauraney did most of the talking, explaining the case history, Jenna's extensive injuries and her behaviour throughout the day before she died. He pointed out that JD began babysitting Jenna late in the day, and she was dead by 1 a.m. Hauraney made the case that the child must have been beaten by the babysitter that evening, less than six hours before she died. Ein's notes state the lawyer also said Dr. Fitzgerald was of the same opinion, and claimed that Smith was too.

Ein agreed. However, his notes also refer to Brenda having beaten Jenna the night before she died. The notes don't explicitly state who voiced that opinion, but Ein hadn't yet reviewed the case; he was relying on the information Hauraney was relaying to him.

The two-pronged theory that would structure Hauraney's defence was beginning to take root: Jenna's fatal injuries occurred after Brenda had given her to JD to babysit, but the child had been previously beaten by her mother as well.

Hauraney agreed to send Ein the autopsy report and other material related to the case so the surgeon could review it all himself. On November 26, 1998, he wrote in his notes: "I read most of the document Mr. Haraney [sic] sent me and altho' she was beaten by mom the nite before she died, the next day she was up and about all over the city. If she had suffered a perf bowel (the nite before) she may not have died, but she would at best be bedridden with a sore belly, legs drawn-up & vomiting. She suffered her fatal injuries on the evening of her death!"

In Smith's autopsy report, Ein found further evidence of the timing of the fatal injuries: a quarter to a third of the child's blood had accumulated in her abdomen, and there was no evidence of inflammation of the peritoneum (the thin layer of tissue that covers the inside of the abdomen and most of its organs). A stomach injury as severe as the one Jenna had suffered would undoubtedly cause such inflammation, but it wouldn't be instantaneous. The absence of peritoneal inflammation told Ein "that the injuries she suffered were that evening, not 24 hours" before her death.

Hauraney's focus was firmly on the murder charge and Brenda's upcoming trial. He now had a highly credible medical expert who would forcefully challenge Smith on the timing of the fatal injuries. And yet in those same notes, Ein asserts as fact Brenda's beating of Jenna the night before the day Jenna died, an assertion that would become an increasingly serious issue as Brenda's case proceeded.

Ein also noted that he needed to discuss the case with Smith directly. Smith wouldn't be hard to find; they both worked at the Hospital for Sick Children. He contacted Smith the following week. And he was apparently very persuasive, because after discussing the case with Ein, Smith came to agree with him: the blood pooling in Jenna's abdomen, along with the lack of inflammation, showed that her fatal injury must have happened on the evening of her death.

Despite having testified at the preliminary hearing only six weeks earlier that Jenna's fatal injuries occurred twenty-four to twenty-eight hours before she died, Smith was now ready to say the injuries occurred within hours of her death—while she was in the care of JD.

Hauraney met with Ein on December 10. Ein again went over his medical opinion and recounted his meeting with Smith. His recollection hadn't changed. He still said Dr. Smith agreed with him.

Hauraney struggled to control his excitement. But he still needed to hear that from Smith himself. Within days, he had the pathologist on the phone. Was his understanding correct? Did Dr. Smith now agree that Jenna's fatal injuries occurred within hours of her death?

Smith said he did. He now felt there were two assaults on the child: Jenna's fatal abdominal injuries occurred within hours of her death, but the child had also suffered injuries to her liver and ribs that happened earlier than that.

Hauraney asked if he would put his new opinion in writing.

Smith said he would.

As Hauraney waited for Smith's new written statement, the pathologist was wavering. On January 7, 1999, Smith wrote to Jim Cairns, the province's deputy chief coroner and his supervisor at the Coroner's Office. "I am not entirely certain as to why [defence counsel] wants a letter from me, after spending a day on the witness stand at the preliminary hearing. Should I agree to his request?"

It's not known how Cairns responded, but Smith never did write a letter for Hauraney.

Ein did, however. His letter arrived later that month. He wrote: "I have reviewed the police report that you sent to me in November 1998, and I have discussed the autopsy of this case in detail with Dr. Charles Smith. I believe the fatal injuries Jenna suffered occurred on the night of her death."

Hauraney was ecstatic, but he knew he still needed Smith's agreement in writing, and he was starting to doubt that he would ever get it. He decided to change tactics. He asked Ein to host a meeting with the key players to discuss of timing of Jenna's injuries. It took months to arrange, but Smith did agree to attend. On April 23, 1999, at the Hospital for Sick Children, in Toronto, the two doctors met with Hauraney, Crown Attorney Brian Gilkinson, and the two investigating officers, Detective Constable Lemay and Sergeant McNevan. Gilkinson asked Ein when he thought Jenna's fatal injuries occurred.

He said it was impossible to pin down the exact times and reactions for all of her 111 injuries. But Ein said he was "99.9% certain from the autopsy findings that the injuries came > 5 pm," according to his notes of the meeting.

Gilkinson methodically worked through the painfully long list of the child's injuries and wondered if any of the tumbles she'd taken earlier that evening—a fall on the fence as the babysitter lifted her out of the back-yard, her fall on the slide—could account for any of them. He asked if the internal bleeding or the perforated bowel could have occurred earlier, and if the onset of symptoms might have been delayed.

According to Lemay's police report of the meeting, Ein said that he had difficulty believing Jenna would have been able to play at the park given the extent and severity of her injuries. He said she would be in immediate distress. She would have been "relatively immobilized" from the time of the injury. Blood in her stomach would have caused irritation. "The child would not be the same," Ein said, according to Lemay's notes. He said if she was struck with one blow, it was of "great significance," causing more severe injuries than the child would have suffered from falling on a picnic table or sliding on ice. She would have shown pain within two to three hours of the fatal assault.

But Ein also said he thought some of Jenna's injuries were older. "It's pretty obvious she was a . . . battered child," he wrote in his own notes.

The Crown's case against Brenda was beginning to crumble, and Hauraney worked hard to continue its disintegration. Less than two weeks later, he again wrote to Gilkinson, reminding him that Ein's opinion was not his alone, that three other specialists he'd spoken to concurred. "I was advised by each and every one of these individuals that this child would not have gotten out of bed after trauma was administered either accidentally or on purpose. The indication is that the child would be lethargic, would have suffered pain immediately, would not have wanted to eat and, at some point or other would have commenced vomiting. The explanation given by the three experts comes to the same conclusion as Dr. Ein and, as I understand Dr. Smith's discussion, he is in agreement with this."

Gilkinson, however, wanted another opinion.

At the time of the preliminary hearing, Brenda was almost three months pregnant. Although she hadn't told anyone except her parents, Justine, her lawyer Jim Hauraney and Children's Aid, she was starting to show, and reporters were suspicious. Brenda denied she was pregnant, but the *Peterborough Examiner* ran with the speculation. The pregnancy wasn't planned. The father was Steven Baxter, an old friend. (This is not his real name.) Because of the murder charge, Brenda had already lost custody of Justine, and she knew Children's Aid would take this child as well. But it didn't matter. She was having the baby.

"My theory was God wouldn't give me anything that I couldn't handle. So I decided on my own I was keeping him," she would tell me years later. "I was keeping him no matter what."

Brenda didn't know what to expect. She prayed that she'd be allowed to have the child in peace and then take him home with her. Laird Meneley, her family lawyer, had already written to Children's Aid requesting that the agency not apprehend the child. He informed them that the Crown was to meet with Ein and Smith the week before Brenda's due date, April 30, and there was an increasing likelihood that the murder charge would be withdrawn. Meneley was frank with Brenda; he wasn't sure how much sway the letter would hold while the murder charge was still in place.

Toward the end of April, Hauraney told Brenda that Smith had also changed his opinion. Brenda couldn't believe it. If Smith changed his opinion, the Crown had nothing tying her to Jenna's murder—other than her since recanted statement to police. Still, Hauraney could not say for certain whether the charge would be dropped.

Brenda hated Peterborough Civic Hospital. To her, the place reeked of death. The thought of giving birth there made her skin crawl. Not that she had any choice. Her bail conditions barred her from leaving the county of Peterborough, and the Civic was the only hospital in the county. Brenda was scheduled to be induced, so a home birth was out of the question.

Steven Baxter was going to be there for the birth as well. By then, he and Brenda were on the outs, but Brenda was happy to have the baby's father present.

Alex Baxter was born on Saturday, May 1, 1999. (This is not his real name. Brenda's son is not allowed to be identified by name by court order.) Steven gave Alex his first bottle. The newborn looked so happy tucked in protectively against his father's chest.

Brenda didn't see her son again until the next day, and then only in the nursery. She wasn't allowed to take him out of that room. And they weren't allowed to be alone together. Still, in the nursery, under someone else's watchful eye, she could at least hold her baby, bathe him, change him, feed him. In that moment, it was enough.

TWO

ON MONDAY MORNING, May 3, John Van Dorsser, Brenda's new family doctor, told her she was good to go home but that Alex needed another day in the hospital. The infant was jaundiced, and the doctor wanted to keep an eye on him. Brenda asked if she could take Alex home on Tuesday. The doctor was shocked. She would not, he told her, be able to take her baby anywhere. The order to apprehend Alex had been approved the day of his birth. Van Dorsser was trying to avoid having Alex placed in care, but the next Family Court date wasn't until May 5, Wednesday, and the longest he could keep the baby in hospital was Tuesday.

Laird Meneley had been Brenda's family lawyer for years, since the first time she called Children's Aid, so she was keeping him up to date on the criminal investigation, especially as Dr. Smith's opinion on the timing of Jenna's fatal injuries started to shift.

On April 30, Brenda submitted her first affidavit, signed in the hospital while she was getting ready to give birth to Alex. In it, she outlined the five medical opinions (from Ein, Rao, Fitzgerald and Finkel, plus Smith's own revised opinion) she knew of that stated Jenna had suffered her fatal injuries on the night she died.

On May 4, when Alex was only a few days old, Meneley went to the hospital to get Brenda's statement ahead of her first custody hearing the next day. Brenda wrote in an affidavit, "I am informed by Mr. Hauraney and do verily believe that Jenna had a compression fracture of one rib and this occurred sometime in the 48 hours prior to her death. This fracture was caused by compression and could have been caused by a fall, a strong hug, rough play, from CPR, or from intentional injury inflicted by the person or persons who caused Jenna's death. There were many people in the company of Jenna in the 48 hours before her death. I did not intentionally cause any harm to Jenna." That same day, Alex was taken from the hospital to a foster home in Lindsay, Ontario, outside of Brenda's bail parameters. It was impossible for her to see her newborn son unless CAS brought him back to Peterborough.

"Surely there was a foster home inside Peterborough that could have taken him," Brenda would say years later. "Surely to God! But apparently not."

The indignity was short lived. The judge at her court hearing on May 5 ordered that Alex be returned to Brenda's care, with one large caveat: she was required to have a nurse with her twenty-four hours a day. Children's Aid and Brenda's parents, with whom she was living, would pay the cost. The arrangement was good only until the next court date, which was two days away.

The Kawartha Haliburton Children's Aid Society was working behind the scenes to do what it thought necessary to protect Brenda's children, but it needed help from police to determine the potential danger to Justine if she were returned to her mother's care and if Brenda were allowed to keep her newborn.

In the months leading up to Alex's birth, Brenda and Meneley repeatedly told CAS that the medical evidence against her was crumbling and that she expected the murder charge against her to be dropped. But police and the Crown told the agency they were still bullish on proceeding.

On April 28, a couple of days before Alex was born, a Children's Aid case worker, Sylvia Sullivan, met with Crown Attorney Brian Gilkinson. According to Sullivan's notes from the meeting, Gilkinson told her he would not be dropping the murder charge at Brenda's next court appearance. He told her that Brenda "is definitely a child abuser but whether she is a child killer needs to be determined." On May 6, almost a week after Alex's birth, Sullivan met with Lemay to discuss the case. The detective had previously been reluctant to disclose the Crown brief on the case, but during this meeting he did share police interviews, the autopsy photographs and Brenda's statement to police the day she was arrested. Ahead of Brenda's May 7 hearing, Sylvia Sullivan swore an affidavit that purported to lay out the police's criminal case against Brenda.

In building their case, though, the police excluded key pieces of evidence: there was no mention of the pubic hair seen on Jenna's genital area by the emergency doctor at the hospital; there was no mention that the diaper Jenna was wearing the night she died was lost by police; there was no mention that the towel JD used to clean up Jenna's vomit on the night she died was not seized by police; there was no mention that JD's shirt, which Jenna had vomited on, was not seized either.

And there was no mention of the latest developments in the case: neither Dr. Ein's opinion that Jenna's fatal injuries occurred on the evening of her death while she was in JD's care, nor Dr. Smith's stunning reversal of his own opinion.

Almost two years earlier, Mr. Justice Alan Ingram of the Ontario Court of Justice Family Court had ordered the Peterborough police to share with Children's Aid their full investigation into Jenna's death. But Brenda increasingly feared that the police never did share or that they did, but Children's Aid was manipulating the evidence to strengthen its custody case against her.

"I thought the reason for Judge Ingram's order of July 30, 1997 was to ensure that the Family Court was fully and appropriately informed about the progress and evidence in the criminal investigation," Brenda wrote in a second affidavit on May 7. "I do not feel that this purpose had been accomplished."

On May 7, the court ordered Alex into the custody of his father, and allowed Brenda daily twelve-hour visitation rights. She had been annoyed about the intrusive round-the-clock nurse, but at least Alex had been at home with her. This was even worse.

Alex was almost a week old, and Brenda had yet to spend a minute alone with him. Justine had been in foster care since the day of Brenda's arrest, almost twenty months earlier. After two years, Children's Aid said it was going to apply for a Crown wardship order for Justine that would revoke all of Brenda's parental rights. Her criminal trial wouldn't take place until the following year. By then, Justine could be put up for adoption, lost to Brenda forever.

Jennifer Brown, another CAS case worker, spoke to Smith on the telephone. She told him that Brenda was fighting in court for custody of her new child. "Well, I guess I'll be doing his autopsy too," Smith replied.

He mentioned to Brown Jenna's small size at the time of her death. "It really makes me worry that she may have been a failure-to-thrive child," suggesting that she had been malnourished and otherwise not properly cared for by her mother.

Brown made that call in May, after Alex was born. Smith had already met with Dr. Ein by then, agreeing with his assessment that the timing of Jenna's fatal injuries meant Brenda could not have been responsible. But he failed to mention that to Brown.

In the days after Brenda gave birth, Crown Brian Gilkinson was looking for one more opinion on the case. He took his questions directly to Smith's peers. On May 10, he met with Dr. Bonita Porter, the deputy chief coroner for inquests at the Chief Coroner's Office. She was also the acting chair of the Pediatric Death Review Committee. Gilkinson explained the difficulties he was having in determining the crucial issue of timing in Jenna's death. Porter offered to review the case.

She examined the coroner's report, Smith's autopsy report and a transcript of his testimony at the preliminary hearing. Later that month, Porter issued her report. "The time between the injury sustained by Jenna and her death had to be less than six hours. There may be different opinions from pathologists, given differing experiences with paediatric trauma cases, as to how much less but I think all have agreed that certainly not more than six hours."

On May 28, 1999, two days after receiving Porter's report, Crown Attorney Brian Gilkinson met with the lead investigator on the case, Dan Lemay. He told the officer he would be withdrawing the murder charge against Brenda Waudby.

But throughout May, CAS continued its Crown wardship application for Brenda's newborn. After Brenda's May 7 Family Court hearing, Laird

Meneley began to suspect the delays in her case were a combination of intransigence on the part of police and wilful blindness on the part of Children's Aid. On May 31, he examined Sylvia Sullivan under oath.

"The police have been very reluctant to give me any information whatsoever," Sullivan told him.

Meneley asked her, "You have a court order still effective, that entitles you to all information in the police files?"

"Yes."

"Have you made any inquiries, anything, to the police since April 30?"

"Myself, no."

"Has anyone else?

"The two people that have been assigned to go to the police to make all inquiries of the police have been Linda Mitchelson and then later, Jennifer Brown."

"Have those two persons only asked questions that benefit your protection application, or do they ask for all the evidence?"

"I was not present at the time when they went over there, so I do not know."

Indeed, it became increasingly clear during the questioning that Children's Aid workers weren't asking the most important questions, and therefore didn't have the most relevant, up-to-date information in the case.

"You've had the order since July 1997 for the production of the police records," Meneley pointed out. "Is that correct?"

"That's correct."

"And you received this affidavit [from Brenda] on April 30," he continued, referring to the one that included the five medical opinions agreeing that Jenna's fatal injuries had occurred within hours of her death. "Is there any indication that anyone asked the Crown attorney or the police about these medical reports?"

"Not to my recollection."

"Are you aware, and it's indicated in my client's affidavit, that the Crown attorney wishes to obtain a sixth medical opinion, independent of the Hospital for Sick Children?" This sixth report was from Bonita Porter, a deputy coroner at the provincial Coroner's Office—the same office that hired Smith to conduct Jenna's original autopsy.

"Prior to reading this affidavit, no," Sullivan admitted.

"Do you know that he since obtained that opinion?"

"No."

"You don't know that the sixth opinion, obtained independently of the Hospital for Sick Children, confirms the other five opinions?"

"No."

"Will you undertake to actually ask someone about those things?" he asked.

In the end, the CAS lawyer, Robert Lightbody, asked Meneley if Brenda would supply the information. "Mr. Meneley, if you're prepared to provide us with a list of the doctors, the names of the doctors and the dates," Lightbody asked.

"I don't have an order for production of the police file," Meneley replied.

"You seem to have certain information . . . I'm asking you to identify that information."

"If you include me on your order, I'll go and get it. Most definitely," Meneley answered. "If you'll consent to my being added onto that order of July '97, it will definitely come out. However, you at the current time have that order and you have an obligation to produce the whole story, not just the part of the story that the Society wants to hear. I'm asking you to phone [the police and Crown attorney] about these medical opinions. Because they indicate that Ms. Waudby was not responsible."

"Okay. I'm asking you to identify [the doctors]," Lightbody said. "I understand that this information is available to Ms. Waudby through her criminal counsel. She could get that information and through you put it to us and we'd be pleased to consider it."

"It's the Society's duty to investigate," Meneley responded. "Are you telling me that the Society, with information such as this, is declining to investigate properly?"

"I'm not declining anything," Lightbody responded. "I'm asking you to identify what you wish us to investigate."

"There have been medical opinions rendered about the death of Jenna Mellor," Meneley said. "How much more clearly do you need it spelled out? Do you need it clearer than that? I mean, I can't make it any clearer than that. There are five medical opinions that indicate Ms. Waudby was not there when the death of Jenna Mellor was caused by injury. And I'm saying as a Society, you have an obligation and you've got an order from the court to get this information that you've known about since April 30. Now, will you undertake to go and get it?"

After more back and forth, the agency finally said that it would.

Around the time of Meneley's exchange with Lightbody, Jim Hauraney called Brenda into a meeting at his office. Brenda's parents, Robert and Gladys, and her sister, Colleen Ward (who happened to be Hauraney's accountant), went with her. Hauraney told them that the Crown was prepared to withdraw the murder charge. But there was a catch.

The Crown wanted Brenda to face some kind of charge. The state still believed she was guilty of something, if not murder, then child abuse. They wanted her to plead guilty to either assault causing bodily harm or a child abuse charge under the Child and Family Services Act. But a plea bargain of some sort was what it would take to make the murder charge go away. Without the plea, the Crown would proceed to trial on the murder charge.

Brenda protested that all the medical evidence pointed at JD, but Hauraney reminded her that the police had her confession: she had admitted to hitting Jenna, even if those blows were not fatal. Hauraney suggested she talk to Laird Meneley, who would be able to advise her on which plea would work better for her in the Family Court proceedings. Hauraney said the child abuse charge was the less serious of the two. It wasn't a Criminal Code offence, and so Brenda wouldn't go to jail. Colleen didn't understand why Brenda had to plead guilty to anything. If Colleen had seen Brenda's confession, Hauraney said, she would have a better understanding of why. He again told Brenda to talk to Meneley about the implications of each option for Family Court.

Brenda took a deep breath. She could make the murder charge go away. She could unburden her parents. She could get Justine and Alex back.

She would just have to plead guilty to something she didn't do.

That is Brenda's version of the meeting. And Colleen's. (Colleen signed an affidavit on September 23, 1999, swearing that her recollection of the meeting was truthful.)

But Hauraney has a different recollection. He denies he told Brenda she had to plead to a lesser offence before the Crown would withdraw the murder charge. He believed the Crown was going to drop the charge regardless. Yes, the Crown was also pushing for a plea to a lesser charge, but it was not a quid pro quo, and Hauraney said he never said it was. Brenda was welcome to fight a child abuse or assault charge if either was ever laid.

Hauraney said he was okay with Brenda pleading guilty to either of those. While the blows she'd confessed to police didn't account for Jenna's fatal injuries, Brenda had admitted to hitting her child. Furthermore, medical evidence pointed to older rib injuries. And it wasn't just Smith's evidence. Other medical experts reached the same conclusion, including Sigmund Ein, who had just helped Hauraney knock down the murder charge.

On the phone, Laird Meneley asked Brenda how her meeting with Hauraney had gone. She explained that the Crown would be dropping the murder charge but she would have to plead guilty to a lesser offence.

Meneley wasn't surprised. The Crown had a lot invested in Brenda's prosecution. It wasn't going to let her walk away scot-free. He did advise her to stay away from the assault charge. If she pleaded guilty to that, she'd never get her children back. Like Hauraney, he told her the child abuse charge was not as serious—it wasn't a Criminal Code offence.

Plead guilty to abusing her child—something she didn't do—or take her chances on the murder charge. But while Brenda awaited trial, Children's Aid might put Justine up for adoption. She couldn't afford to wait for her day in court. Even if she won, she'd still lose: Justine would be gone.

Brenda Waudby's choice was not unique. Plea bargains are common in the judicial system. Of the twenty cases the Goudge Inquiry examined, eight involved plea bargains.

It was finally going to be over. Brenda fidgeted in her chair in the small courtroom in downtown Peterborough. She'd spent too much time in this building over the past two and a half years.

Brenda stared at Crown Attorney Brian Gilkinson as he addressed the court. "Ms. Waudby is prepared, based on evidence obtained of old injuries during the investigation of more serious offences, to enter a plea to abusing her child pursuant to Section 79 of the Child and Family Services Act."

"Could I ask a question?" inquired Judge Thomas C. Whetung. "So, the matters here today do not relate to the matters before the other [criminal] court?"

"Absolutely not," Gilkinson replied. "Absolutely not." He went on, "The point of the matter is that the Crown will be withdrawing those more serious charges. If further evidence comes forward with respect to those more serious charges, it would be the Crown's position to relay them, whether it is with respect to Ms. Waudby or perhaps to take further action against other individuals, depending upon what further investigations may reveal."

The spectre of a murder charge would remain.

The court clerk read out the charge: that between January 2 and 18, 1997, Brenda Lee Waudby knowingly inflicted abuse on her child Jenna Mellor.

The dates didn't make sense to Brenda. She did spank Jenna, and accidentally dropped her on her crib's guard rail, but that was on the night before she died, which was four days *after* January 18. And even if the Crown was basing the charge on her now recanted confession, that alleged beating happened the night before as well. But she told herself it wouldn't matter. She would be getting her kids back.

"How do you plead, guilty or not guilty?" the clerk asked.

"Guilty."

—

The rest of the court appearance floated by. Brenda had a hard time focusing. Gilkinson read the agreed statement of facts into the court record, explaining that the investigation into Jenna's death had involved several experts who found signs of pre-existing injuries to the child. "In particular," he said, "post-mortem examination revealed old rib/head injuries that would have occurred during the time frame."

Hauraney assured Brenda that the Crown was talking about injuries to the head *of* the ribs—where the ribs adjoin the spine—and not separate injuries to the head *and* the ribs.

Hauraney and Gilkinson made a joint submission recommending a sentence of one year's probation, with the stipulation that Brenda comply with any direction given by the probation officer, in conjunction with Children's Aid, for the care and management of her children if and when she had other children under her care.

The judge accepted the submission. "Ms. Waudby, there will be a probation order for you to sign today before you leave and, after you sign that, you are free to leave. Thank you."

Four days later, Brian Gilkinson withdrew the second-degree murder charge against Brenda Waudby. But even with that out of the way—for now—Brenda quickly realized that she would still have to fight Children's Aid for custody of Justine. And Children's Aid immediately began using her guilty plea against her.

Ken Munks, a CAS case worker, claimed in an affidavit that Brenda had confessed to "swinging her arms and striking the child on the torso an uncertain number of times." The reference to Jenna's torso is significant because Dr. Smith and all the other medical experts agreed that the child died from blunt force trauma to her abdomen—the implication being that Brenda had confessed to striking the child in a way that accorded with her cause of death.

However, Brenda had never confessed to hitting Jenna on the torso in either of her statements to police. She responded in an affidavit of her own: "Mr. Munks is trying to exaggerate the nature and content of what was said by me to the police on the night of my arrest for a murder that I did not commit in an attempt to mislead the court."

Despite the efforts of Children's Aid, Justice Ingram returned Justine to Brenda's care on July 21, 1999. CAS's appeal of that ruling was rejected.

Alex was returned to Brenda's care in March 2000. Both children have remained in her care ever since.

THREE

THE POLICE INVESTIGATION into Jenna's death continued. Three days before Brenda pleaded guilty to child abuse, JD agreed to take another polygraph test, this time to be administered by the Ontario Provincial Police. But as with previous efforts, JD was found not to be suitable for the exam. He became agitated and upset when the officer told him they would be unable to conduct the test. He continued to insist that he had done nothing wrong, and only wanted to clear his name.

On July 20, 1999, Det. Const. Dan Lemay arranged for JD to visit Dr. Arnold Rubenstein, a forensic hypnotist in Toronto. However, the doctor was unable to get JD to relax enough to be hypnotized. Rubenstein felt he genuinely wanted to be hypnotized, as the teenager asked him to try doing it without his knowing. JD did go over his recollections of the night Jenna died, and his account was consistent with his earlier statements to police: he said Jenna was a little whiny that evening but no more than usual; he said he still couldn't believe she had died. Other than when Jenna bumped her head on the slide, he said it was a "perfect day."

The doctor did note that the teenager seemed fixated on his hair, constantly fixing it throughout the interview. JD said he put a lot of pressure on himself to be perfect, and worried what people were saying about him because of the investigation. He also admitted that he had a temper and that when he was younger he would throw and break things.

A number of physical items were also sent to the provincial Centre of Forensic Sciences in Toronto for analysis, including Maggie's hair dryer, several baby blankets, the mattress from Jenna's crib and her diaper, and T-shirts and other items of clothing seized from the apartment and hospital.

It's unclear why it took the Peterborough police two and a half years to send this crucial evidence for forensic analysis, but the results didn't move the investigation in any new directions. The items were checked for bodily fluids: two T-shirts had blood on them, but no semen was found. Police also sent more DNA samples to compare with the anonymous letter accusing Brenda, but there were no matches.

Police made further pleas for help from the public, but no useful leads were forthcoming.

Meanwhile, Brenda had become very vocal in the media. She complained that she had been harassed by police and wrongly charged, which had left her daughter's murder unsolved. She launched civil lawsuits against the Peterborough Lakefield police and Dr. Smith.

Despite the public's appetite for resolution, the police investigation was petering out by the fall of 1999. In September, police seized Brenda's file from Dr. Mark Ben-Aron, a Toronto psychiatrist she had spoken to a year after Jenna's death. The file turned up nothing useful to the investigation. That was the last investigative step Lemay would take. By the end of that year, the detective had moved on to other matters. The investigation into Jenna Mellor's death had ground to a halt.

It stayed that way for more than a year and a half. Then, in July 2001, Det. Sgt. Larry Charmley was assigned to review the case from beginning to end. The shifting medical evidence had pushed the investigation off the rails, but police did not lose sight of the crime. A young child had been beaten to death in her own home. Her unsolved murder continued to haunt the community, and it was a stain on the police. Charmley had not been involved in the initial investigation. In fact, though he had been with the Peterborough police for almost fifteen years and had assisted on other homicides, he had never led a murder investigation before getting the call from the police chief.

Charmley soon learned that the original investigators still believed that Brenda was responsible for Jenna's death. JD, the only other suspect, had been co-operative throughout the investigation, and his story remained consistent. The pressure on the teenager had been intense and constant for years, and the police thought he was too young to lie so effectively.

Charmley spent the next several months going over all the documentation, statements, videos and evidence collected during the initial investigation. One of his first meetings, only five days after beginning his review, was with Jim Hauraney. Brenda's criminal lawyer told the detective he was still deeply concerned about the case. He believed there was ample medical evidence suggesting the child had been sexually assaulted, which was never properly investigated. He also pointed out that the ER doctor at the hospital, Dale Friesen, noted seeing a hair in Jenna's vaginal area, but the hair had disappeared before being processed.

Charmley interviewed old witnesses, chased down old leads, developed new ones. He asked the Chief Coroner's Office to hire an independent specialist to review all the medical evidence and help him better understand not only the conflicting reports but also Charles Smith's evolving opinion. He prepared a lengthy list of questions he hoped to get answered, which he gave to Bonita Porter at the Coroner's Office. And he tried to find out whether the mysterious hair Hauraney mentioned had ever existed, and if it did, what happened to it.

Charmley interviewed the emergency room doctor and nurses: they all told him that they remembered seeing a hair in the child's vaginal area. A police officer who'd been present at the hospital recalled seeing a foreign object there as well, although he thought it was likely a thread rather than a hair.

The detective had a still from the autopsy video enhanced, and indeed, there appeared to be a hair sticking out of the child's labia, although he couldn't be sure. He reviewed all the autopsy photos. None of the pictures of the child's pubic area showed a hair or thread. However, one photo of a bruise on her upper leg also happened to capture what looked like a hair sticking out of the labia. Technicians, however, were unable to enhance the image because the hair was on the periphery of the photo.

On October 5, 2001, almost three months into his investigation, Charmley spoke with Charles Smith. He asked the pathologist if he remembered seeing a fibre in the child's vaginal area during the autopsy. Smith said he did, although he said it was more likely a hair. He said he had offered it to the police at the time, but they said it wasn't pertinent, so he kept it himself. Smith added that it was likely a contaminant—a stray hair that fell on Jenna during resuscitation efforts, but he could dig it out of his files if Charmley still wanted it.

The detective said he did.

The detective then spoke with Const. Scott Kirkland, who had attended Jenna's autopsy and who had since retired. Kirkland said he had no recollection of Smith finding anything in the child's genital area. And he seriously doubted he would ever have said it was unimportant. "It was Dr. Smith's autopsy," the officer explained. "He was the one running the show. He told me what was important, and what pictures to take."

As soon as Charmley obtained the hair, he submitted it to the Centre for Forensic Sciences, along with the anonymous letter written in the days after Jenna's death and several handwriting samples for comparison.

While he waited for the results, he continued re-interviewing everyone who had come into contact with Brenda, Jenna or JD in the hours or day before the child's death. Nothing new turned up, although Charmley did speak with JD's mother about a rumour he'd heard that JD didn't have any body hair. Maggie confirmed that her son did have trouble growing body hair and said the teenager's eyebrows had only recently grown in. She said she had taken him to see a doctor about it years before, but she couldn't remember the doctor's name. And she wasn't sure if he would have had pubic hair at the time of Jenna's death.

The forensic analysis of the hair turned up nothing that could move the investigation forward. The hair did not have a root, which was needed for standard nuclear DNA analysis, but the forensic lab was able to determine that it was from the chest or pubic area likely of a Caucasian. A forensic pathologist at the Centre of Forensic Sciences said the hair could still be tested for mitochondrial DNA. That was not as precise as standard DNA testing, and likely would not identify a specific person, but it could narrow it down to specific maternal lineage. The testing would have to be done at a different lab, because the centre didn't do the procedure.

—

By early 2002, the case was again the subject of widespread media coverage in Peterborough and Toronto. In February, word that the missing hair had been recovered was leaked to the press. Both the police and Smith were pilloried for bungling the investigation.

Police decided to have the hair tested for mitochondrial DNA at an FBI lab in Washington, D.C. Comparison hair samples were taken from both Brenda and JD in June. It would be several months before the results would be ready.

Meanwhile, the medical review Charmley had requested was completed later that summer. The Chief Coroner's Office had hired Ken Feldman, a pediatrician with the Children's Hospital and Regional Medical Center, in Seattle, Washington, to complete the review.

Most troubling among Feldman's findings was his opinion that, while abdominal trauma was the most likely cause of death, he couldn't rule out a brain injury as the culprit either. Smith's autopsy and the six reviews had been completed, yet this was the first time anyone had suggested another possible cause of death. Rather than provide clarity, Feldman further muddied the waters of the medical evidence.

Signs continued to point to JD as the more likely culprit, but none of them were definitive, or useful as evidence. In November 2002, Charmley received a copy of a report by the Complaints Committee of the College of Physicians and Surgeons of Ontario, after Brenda launched a formal complaint about Smith's conduct in the case. Two forensic pathologists and a pediatric pathologist, all independent, reviewed Smith's work. The trio of specialists found several deficiencies, but considered Smith's overall approach to be acceptable. However, what was of most interest to Charmley was their opinion on the timing of the fatal injuries.

"The review of these records indicates that the injuries had to be received within two to three hours of her death," the report said. "The clinical history of the child should have enabled [Smith] to refine his conclusion that the injuries had to have occurred within 2-3 hours of death. . . . Clearly the timing of the major injuries all occurred shortly before her death since she would have been unable to play, eat and appear to be normal after receiving such injuries."

It was a strong opinion, echoing the position of the four experts Brenda's lawyer hired years earlier, with the bonus that the committee members were completely independent from the legal case. But when Charmley asked the College for the names of the three independent assessors so he could question them further about their opinions, his request went unanswered. Legal counsel for the College told him police should not view the report as giving an opinion on the timing of the injuries. Further, the detective discovered that although all three assessors were pathologists, they were not clinicians and had not been given the full medical file for their review. In the end, Charmley decided that he couldn't rely on their opinion.

Then, in December, a former girlfriend of JD's came forward, saying she suspected he might be responsible for Jenna's death. The two had dated for about two years after Jenna's death. She said JD had a short fuse, especially when he smoked marijuana, and that he had assaulted her during their relationship. However, she had no evidence to back up her suspicions about JD's involvement in Jenna's death, and conceded that JD always denied having anything to do with it.

The results of the mitochondrial DNA tests came back on May 1, 2003. All the suspect hairs, including Brenda's and JD's, were negative for a match, ruling them both out as the source of the hair. Charmley told Brenda the results, but he didn't tell JD, hoping that it might lead him to slip up or even confess. He didn't.

A school friend of Justine's told police that she knew Brenda was responsible for Jenna's death. Colleen MacDonald claimed that Justine told her she had seen her mother beat Jenna to death with a bat. But given the suggestibility of young children, and the trauma Justine had endured, the detective felt the only way to judge the validity of Justine's claim was to have her hypnotized. Brenda was initially wary, but Charmley persuaded her to allow it after he confided that the police were now focusing their attention on JD.

It was May 7, 2003. Jenna had been dead for almost six and a half years, and it was the first ray of hope Brenda had ever received from police.

Justine was hypnotized the next month. The doctor thought she resisted being fully hypnotized, but Justine believed she went fully under. Although she didn't provide any information about who caused Jenna's death, she did describe the last hours she had with her sister.

Jenna, she said, had been upset when Brenda first left but eventually calmed down. JD's mom made them hotdogs and Kraft Dinner for supper. After they ate, Justine asked if they could play outside. It was freezing and dark already, but JD took the girls into the backyard. Justine wanted to go to the playground in the housing complex behind the house. It had slides and a jungle gym. She climbed over the back fence, then JD passed Jenna over. Justine remembered that Jenna's snowsuit felt puffy as she grabbed her. Then she saw that her little sister's eyes were rolled back in her head, and all she could see was the whites.

Justine yelled, and Jenna snapped out of it, her eyes rolling back into place as Justine lowered her to the ground. Jenna whimpered, but the jungle gym improved her mood. JD left them alone, sitting on a bench nearby as they played. Jenna liked the red twirly slide the best, and it was even faster in the winter cold. Justine tucked Jenna in between her legs so they could ride down together. But Jenna wanted to go on her own. She started pushing herself forward, away from Justine, who was holding her by the hood. Jenna started to whine. Worried she might be choking the fidgeting toddler, Justine let go.

Justine heard a heavy thump. She raced down the slide. Jenna pointed to her head. She had bumped her head on the final turn at the bottom. JD came over to check on her. She wasn't even crying. She seemed fine.

After they got home, Justine went to watch *Dragonheart* with JD's brother, Kevin, who had come back with his mother. But the film had barely started when JD called her into the bathroom. Jenna was sitting on the toilet. The lid was down. JD was standing in front of her, his mother's blow-dryer in his hand, its noise filling the room. The skin on Jenna's forehead was red and blotchy. Justine asked what happened. JD said she was fine, but Jenna looked scared. She wasn't crying, but the red marks on her face looked painful. Still, JD was fourteen. Justine was seven. She listened to her babysitter.

Justine went back to Kevin's room to finish watching the movie. When it was over, they moved into the living room to watch *Independence Day*. Justine sat on the floor, her back propped up against the couch. Jenna came up the stairs with JD. It was after eight, past her bedtime. She was wearing Justine's pyjama top, which looked more like a dress on her tiny frame.

Justine offered to tuck her in, but JD told her not to worry, he could get her down. He led Jenna back downstairs to bed, and Justine went back to watching her movie. That was all she could remember.

Charmley continued to focus his investigation on JD. He told Maggie that the hair found on Jenna was not JD's. Hoping that JD, who was now twenty, would now be able to take a polygraph test, he convinced Maggie that the test would clear her son. But JD was not willing to take it. He said he had been harassed enough already and was done with the police investigation. He said his lawyer advised him not to take a polygraph and that he did not have to talk to police. In early 2004, he moved out on his own, and his family refused to say where he was living. Charmley decided not to pursue the matter any further at that time.

FOUR

MORE THAN TWO and a half years after he had started his review, Det. Sgt. Larry Charmley completed his report in March 2004. The detective believed he had done all he could. He passed his report on to a number of investigators and agencies, including the Crown Attorney's Office and the Chief Coroner's Office (for which Smith no longer worked).

The Coroner's Office ran with his report. Deputy Chief Coroner Jim Cairns asked the office's new forensic pathologist, Dr. Michael Pollanen, to do a complete review of Smith's work on the case. Suddenly, the medical side of Charmley's investigation had new life.

A case conference was held that June at the chief coroner's office to go over Pollanen's findings. Charmley was in attendance, along with other members of the police investigation team, as well as Gilkinson, Pollanen, Cairns, Huyer, Dr. Barry McLellan, the acting Chief Coroner, and Dr. Robert Wood, a forensic odontologist, or dentist, with the Chief Coroner's Office. Pollanen agreed with Smith's findings on the cause of death—the child had died from intra-abdominal hemorrhage, or bleeding, caused by blunt force trauma to the abdomen. He also found evidence that the child had suffered other forms of recent violence, including head and chest injuries, burns and even bites. Pollanen's findings diverged from Smith's original finding on the crucial timing of the injuries, which, he said, were "inflicted within hours of death. The lethal injuries did not occur, for example, many hours or days prior to death."

The signs of bites were of particular interest. Wood assisted Pollanen in assessing a photograph of marks and bruising on the child's right knee, which Wood considered signs of two probable bites, although he couldn't be certain because of the poor quality of the photograph. The markings had not been handled properly at the autopsy, which should have been halted as soon as the marks were discovered so they could be properly photographed. As well, DNA swabs of the area should have been taken.

Yet neither was done. And because it had been seven and a half years since the child died, and the main suspect was a young teenager at the time, a useful comparison would no longer be possible.

Pollanen suggested police get another clinical opinion on how the child's behaviour would have changed as the symptoms of the abuse developed. He said that a separate consultation with a clinical expert in child sexual abuse would be useful as well.

Pollanen's report also examined Jenna's rib injuries, which were the basis of the charge of child abuse Brenda had pleaded guilty to. While he said he couldn't be definitive, he could find no evidence that the rib injuries were older than the child's fatal injuries. However, he did find evidence of one other older injury—a laceration to Jenna's liver, which showed early signs of healing. This injury could have occurred several hours or days before her death, and Pollanen suggested it would have been caused by blunt trauma to the abdomen. The liver injury fit into the twenty-four-hour window in which Brenda had confessed to hitting Jenna, but she had recanted that confession. And the child abuse she pleaded guilty to occurred days to weeks earlier than the child's death.

At the case conference, Charmley was given the names of two pediatric surgeons to review Pollanen's report and the case history. Huyer agreed to do a sexual abuse assessment.

Dr. David Wesson, from the Texas Children's Hospital Clinical Care Center, in Houston, and Dr. Mark Walton, a pediatric surgeon at McMaster University Medical Centre, in Hamilton, did clinical assessments. Both found that Jenna's fatal injuries occurred within hours of her death—just as Dr. Ein had reasoned years earlier. Dr. Wesson put the timing at "within three hours of her death, although there is an outside chance that they occurred as much as six hours before she died." Likewise, Walton thought her fatal injuries happened during the evening of her death: "Trauma resulting in these injuries earlier in the day would have caused notable symptoms of lethargy and abdominal pain and would have been noticed by even a girl of Justine's age."

Wesson also suggested how Jenna's fatal injuries may have occurred: "On two occasions in the last few hours before her death she was held over the edge of a toilet bowl. A force from behind her when she was in such a position," pressing her against the rigid rim of the toilet, could have caused her abdominal injuries.

Walton also noted that callus had not begun to form at the rib fractures, suggesting they happened at about the same time as the fatal injuries. Even then, he still reasoned that they "might have occurred in the days beforehand." He added, "There is little in the history to help us know what events caused the other [rib and liver] injuries that were seen at autopsy."

Dirk Huyer completed his sexual assault assessment in late August. His challenge was separating Jenna's physical injuries, which were numerous, from signs of possible sexual abuse. In the end, he thought sexual abuse was unlikely. "The lack of specific injury to the genitalia of Jenna Mellor does not rule out possible sexual abuse, but indicates that forceful penetrating injury did not occur."

Shortly after Huyer completed his report, Charles Smith's lawyer contacted a lawyer for the Chief Coroner's Office. Smith had heard— mistakenly—that police intended to charge JD with Jenna Mellor's murder based on new evidence of sexual assault from Dirk Huyer, and he forwarded his long-missing notes to the coroner's office to show that Huyer had examined Jenna for signs of sexual abuse at the time of the autopsy. When asked years earlier at Brenda's preliminary hearing if he had taken autopsy notes, Smith said that he didn't think so. It turns out he had just misplaced them.

The notes state that Huyer examined the child's hymen. While Huyer's opinion is not included in the notes, it is implied that he helped Smith reach the conclusion that there were no signs of sexual abuse.

Det. Sgt. Larry Charmley completed a second report reflecting these new reviews and forwarded it to his superiors and the Crown prosecutor, Brian Gilkinson. On February 17, 2005, Gilkinson emailed the detective to say he still didn't have enough to proceed with charges. "It appears the evidence will never be definitive enough to mount a prosecution against anyone absent . . . [someone] entering the station and insisting on giving a full, independently verifiable, voluntary confession," he wrote, adding that while JD and his mother were the logical suspects, "this case is so fraught with evidentiary issues that [reasonable and probable grounds] for anyone's arrest does not appear to exist."

Charmley agreed. Given the investigation's tumultuous history, medical and physical evidence would never be strong enough for a conviction. What police really needed was a confession.

Peterborough police launched a so-called Mr. Big sting, using an undercover officer to befriend JD and induce him to join a criminal organization.

On December 16, 2005, JD met with Mr. Big. His real name was Sgt. Paul Staats, a seventeen-year veteran with the Hamilton Police Service. The meeting took place at Hilton Suites hotel in Markham, north of Toronto. It was set up by "John," another undercover agent who befriended JD and posed as a member of Mr. Big's crew, which JD was being recruited to join. (John was not present at the meeting.)

Staats played the honesty card in the meeting, repeatedly talking about trust and family. "It's all about money, but more importantly it's about honesty and trust," he told a hopeful JD.

The conversation gradually shifted over to the one obstacle to JD's recruitment: the ongoing police investigation into Jenna Mellor's death still swirling around him. "One of the things I cannot have ever is having heat on this organization," Mr. Big warned. But he had a solution. "Number one is: Do you believe that I can fix our problem?"

"Yes. See, the only problem I have is, like, you know, the problem," JD said. "It's that it just won't go away."

"Do you believe that I can make it go away?"

"I hope so. I do believe that."

Mr. Big asked JD what he wanted from life. Money was the answer. "I want to have nice things," he said. "I just, I want it all."

Mr. Big told him he would pay him well, and the young man would be able to have the things he wanted. But before he could bring JD into his crew, he needed to take care of his "problem." And to do that, he needed details. "And I will tell you why," Mr. Big said. "It's because I have to know exactly what happened because I have someone else take the heat over this and if they take the heat over this, they have to know the details."

"See, but ahh, there really could be no one else to take the heat because there was the mom, and who else would it have been?" JD asked.

"I'll ask you again," Mr. Big said. "Do you believe I can make it go away?"

"Oh yes."

"All right. What I'm offering you here is to eliminate your problem."

"That would be great."

"All right. If you feel you cannot be honest with me and lay it all out on the table right here, right now, then you can walk out that door. We never had this conversation. We never met. And all the ties that you have with John will be immediately cut."

"I definitely don't want that."

Mr. Big told JD to tell him what happened. But he warned him that he had done his own investigation and knew many of the details already. He would know if JD wasn't being completely honest with him.

So JD told him what happened. They had had a normal evening, he said. He took Jenna and Justine to the park. Everything was fine. Then the child suddenly got sick in the middle of the night. "She was choking, so I took her to the toilet. I was holding her there. I stood her up a bit. She fell back. It was horrible," he said. "And then the eyes started rolling back in her head. I took her upstairs to my mom and told my mom what was happening and my mom called the ambulance."

That was it. The child died, but it wasn't his fault. With some coaxing from Mr. Big, JD did mention burning Jenna with a hair dryer as he was trying to dry her hair, but he said it was an accident.

The minutes ticked by. Mr. Big kept prodding JD, telling him he'd heard a different version of the events of that night. "I want to tell you something, all right? This is the deal. This is a test right now for you," he said.

"Oh ya, I believe it is."

"You fail the test, you walk out that door."

"Oh ya."

"All ties with me, all ties with John are eliminated. You are on your own."

"Oh, for sure."

"And what I can tell you, what I know is the cops are looking at you real hard."

"Really, ahh."

"And I, listen to me. They are looking at you real hard. And you know what?"

"What?"

"It's just going to be a matter of time when you're on your own that they hook up and take you in for it."

"Ya."

"Now, I want to tell you something right now. All right. I can make that go away but if it happens while you are in the family because you weren't honest with me and you bring heat on me, then we have a big problem."

JD kept denying any responsibility. He mentioned Jenna's internal bleeding and broken ribs, but he said Brenda was to blame. He mentioned the hair, but said it wasn't his. Mr. Big told him he thought the police were looking at the right suspect.

"Really?" JD replied. "Well, I don't like the way you think that. I honestly don't."

"Like I told you. I need to know the details. I make it go away. That's the only reason I need to know. All right. I don't care. I told you. I'm sitting here. I'm not judging you."

But JD kept denying it. He voiced indignation at what Mr. Big was suggesting. He said he had God on his side. But Mr. Big did not let up the pressure. He kept telling JD the police knew what he did, that he would be arrested. "It's just a matter of time," he warned.

"Fuck. That's awful."

"Before they come and handcuff you."

"Really?"

"And put you behind bars. Let me ask you something. Have you ever been behind bars before?"

"Not really, no."

"You ever been to a local jail?"

"Just in the drunk tank a couple times. I was so drunk."

"You go to prison, or a detention centre . . ."

"I'd get killed."

"You'd wish you had this night back."

After about thirty minutes, JD finally cracked.

"Can you help me, sir?"

"Ya, I can."

"Will you please?"

"I will."

"Oh, I don't feel like a man though. I did do that. Will you not see where I come from?"

At first JD said he didn't remember what he'd done. And then he did. "I guess I must have hit her," he said.

"Tell me what happened."

"All's I can say is, I must have got mad. That's it. I don't know why or what happened."

"Where did you hit her?"

"In her stomach."

"How did you hit her?"

"Poking and shit. Poking. I didn't think it was that hard."

"Poking, like what?"

"Poke, poke, poke. Really kinda pissed off, I guess. I don't know, sir, I'm sorry."

"You don't have to be sorry. I tell ya."

"I don't want to go to jail."

Mr. Big explained how he could stop that from happening. He had someone already in prison who was going to take the rap. Another life sentence wouldn't matter to this guy, he explained. Mr. Big was going to look after his family.

But that didn't make sense, and JD knew it. How could someone else have done it? There were only two suspects. How could someone else have been responsible?

JD was suddenly terrified that Mr. Big was a cop. "I don't know what to do," he said. "I'm just so scared about it. I don't know whether you're a policeman or what."

Mr. Big huffed and chuffed, acting indignant at such an insult, then carefully steered JD away from his suspicions and back to his confession. He told him he needed details, precise details, so his fall guy would be convincing when police questioned him.

"Well, ah, I was changing her, and fuckin', I just looked and stuff and I didn't really touch that bad or nothing. For some reason there seemed to be something about sexual assault and stuff, right?"

Mr. Big nodded.

"That's it. I poked her too hard, and I touched her too much or whatever. I should never have did it. That's all I can say."

"Did you, did you stick something up inside her?"

"No. No. Maybe my finger, just around the outside." Three of four times, he said. Just his finger. "I never forced anything right up there or anything."

"Okay, so how could she get a broken, er, get broken ribs?" the undercover asked.

"It must have been the punches, like the pokes." He admitted they were more like punches than pokes. "Not my hardest. Like, I would never hit anybody my hardest. And it wasn't my hardest. It was just a jab. But she was small." Five shots, he said. Five or six punches to the child's rib cage. Hard enough to break her ribs.

He said he was mad because he didn't want to babysit that night. He wanted to go out. So he took it out on the child. "When I first got her after the mom had just left, I was like, fuck. Whack, whack."

Then she bumped her head on the slide, and thinking he would get in trouble for it, he got even more frustrated. Then when he was blow-drying her hair, he accidentally burned her. By now, he was so angry that he punched her in the stomach two or three more times, even harder. And then he punched her in the head.

"You were pissed at that time?" Mr. Big asked.

"Ya, pissed; well, mad because fuckin' she'd hit her head, she had a burn on her head and I was like, 'She looks like shit.' She's fucking not moving or nothing."

He put the two children to bed and two friends came over to visit. They were listening to music when Jenna started coughing. He took her out to the living room. "She couldn't stand up. They were like, 'Oh, what's wrong?' I was like, 'She must be feeling a little sick.' So I took her back to the room." He punched her again several times in the ribs. She kept standing up in the crib, so he hit her again, trying to get her to stay down. Then, JD said, after his friends left, that's when he sexually assaulted her. With his fingers.

"I was younger," he said. "I hadn't did anything yet with anybody. I was. I didn't really know better. I don't know. I guess I should have known better but I didn't know. I was an awful fucking little boy."

But it wasn't the first time. He had sexually assaulted Jenna when he was babysitting her two days earlier. And not just with his fingers. But on the night she died, JD said, he only touched her. "And then, an hour after that she was coughing. I grabbed her, took her to the toilet. She fell back and hit her head. I ran upstairs with her and yelled to Mom something's wrong. And that's what happened."

JD also mentioned that police thought Jenna had rib injuries from an earlier assault before he started babysitting her, but he thought he was probably responsible for those too.

"You think, or you know?" Mr. Big asked.

"I . . . okay, I know." The six times JD punched her, it wasn't full force, he said. But he thought it was hard enough to break ribs.

JD said his parents had never asked him about that night in an accusatory way. He thought his mother might have had some doubts, but she never brought them up. And the police didn't seem all that suspicious of him either. JD said the officers who investigated him initially said the only reason he was a suspect at all was because he was taking anger management classes just before Jenna died. "And they, the police said to me that hadn't I been in there, they'd never would have looked at me. And the only policeman that I guess, well, you say there's a lot of them, but the only one that really ever bothered me was the last one who did it. It was this Larry Charmley guy. And he fucking seemed to hate me."

JD had never told anyone what had happened. He had been the only one there, the only person who was responsible. There was no other version of the truth.

Charmley met with Brian Gilkinson to review the undercover operation and JD's confession. There are laws governing coercive confessions. Confessions made to a person in authority, such as a police officer, must be made voluntarily. There can't be any promises of leniency or threats of punishment that could influence the confession.

Police use Mr. Big stings because confessions to friends, family or crime lords are fair game, even when those people are in fact undercover agents. In JD's confession, coercion had been involved, but it was driven by JD's own desire to have the police investigation end so he could join Mr. Big's crime syndicate. JD said he was motivated by money. He wanted to buy a dirt bike, and working for Mr. Big would earn him the money to do that. The undercover officers never threatened the young man, either explicitly or implicitly. In fact, JD was told early on in the meeting that he could walk away without any consequences. Otherwise, JD would have to be honest and tell Mr. Big everything, but it was purely for his own benefit: to end the police investigation. As Mr. Big operations go, this was a strong one.

Charmley and Gilkinson then met with Cairns and McLellan from the Chief Coroner's Office. Dirk Huyer was also present. The medical experts agreed: JD's confession fit with Jenna's injuries.

Charmley finally had enough to lay charges. On December 28, 2005, JD was arrested and charged with second-degree murder and two counts of sexual assault.

It had been almost nine years since Jenna Mellor's death, and police finally had the answers that had for so long eluded them. Mr. Big stings were controversial, but this particular operation seemed solid. Unlike Brenda's recanted confession, JD's statements to the undercover agent aligned with the child's fatal injuries; he had punched and poked her in the abdomen hard enough to break ribs.

The sexual assault, however, was a problem. That part of JD's confession didn't line up with the prevailing medical opinion. During his consult at the original autopsy and again at his review years later, Dirk Huyer dismissed suggestions that Jenna had been assaulted or raped. Other medical professionals had seen signs of sexual assault, but Huyer said no. Even though JD had confessed, the lack of medical evidence would make proceeding on the two sexual assault charges more difficult.

A year later, Gilkinson negotiated a plea bargain with JD. The Crown dropped the second-degree murder charge in exchange for JD pleading guilty to the lesser charge of manslaughter. The accused, now in his early twenties, was sentenced. Given his age at the time of the crime, he was sentenced as a youth.

The two counts of sexual assault were dropped. Gilkinson told the judge there were "certainly evidentiary issues that the Crown would not be able to surmount with respect to establishing those matters beyond reasonable doubt."

The plea deal and twenty-two-month sentence were particularly troubling for Brenda. It didn't seem harsh enough for the person who killed her daughter. But she was also frustrated because she didn't know what was going on. Brenda knew JD had been charged with sexually assaulting Jenna, and that the charges were then dropped. She didn't know why. And she still didn't know exactly how Jenna had died. JD's confession was not entered into the court record, and neither the police nor the Crown ever shared it with her. And in another cruel twist, the court reporter made a crucial mistake in the transcript of the proceedings.

In summarizing JD's plea, Gilkinson said JD admitted hitting Jenna with "good solid jabs to the stomach" but he believed they "wouldn't have" had enough force to break ribs.

That one word—*wouldn't*—meant the punches JD confessed to did not account for Jenna's broken ribs. JD's confession did not contradict the evidence that underpinned Brenda's conviction for child abuse years earlier.

Except that's not what JD, or Gilkinson, said.

In fact, the babysitter had told Mr. Big that he believed his blows to the child's abdomen were powerful enough that they *would* have broken her ribs. That's what Gilkinson stated in court. Only the court reporter misheard him.

Brenda had met with Gilkinson just before JD's plea, but no one took notes. The purpose of the meeting was to explain why the Crown was accepting JD's plea to manslaughter and why the sexual assault charges were being withdrawn. Gilkinson believed he fully explained the Crown's position, but if he did, Brenda didn't absorb his explanation. Given that Gilkinson was the same Crown who had prosecuted her years earlier, and given the lingering trauma of the case and JD's confession and sudden plea bargain, Brenda had a hard time absorbing the legal intricacies of the case against her daughter's killer. Gilkinson never told her the substance of JD's confession or showed her a transcript, and Brenda never thought to ask.

It would be another five years before Brenda Waudby finally learned the truth.

ATHENA

ONE

FOR ANTHONY KPORWODU, waking up rested was the first sign.

He and his partner, Angela Veno, had a three-month-old daughter and a sixteen-month-old son. The baby had not been sleeping well. She had been irritable, crying almost constantly. But on that Friday morning, March 6, 1998, Anthony opened his eyes to a silent household.

Anthony may have been rested, but his body ached. Angela worked an overnight shift; that plus the volatile sleeping patterns of two young children meant the sleeping arrangements in their crowded two-bedroom apartment in Scarborough were in constant flux. Anthony had spent most of the night dozing on the living room floor; baby Athena was in her car seat nearby; her big brother, Julius, was asleep in his bedroom, while Angela sprawled out on the couch.

The twenty-four-year-old glanced at the clock: it was almost seven thirty. Athena's silence was not unwelcome, but it was unusual. Then, suddenly, his brain processed what his eyes were seeing: staring at Athena's tiny body in the car seat, he realized that her chest wasn't rising. Anthony scrambled across the floor. He put his hand on Athena's forehead. It was cold to the touch. He put his fingers on her lips: cold. He opened her mouth. Her tongue was colourless.

"Wake up! Angela, wake up!" he yelled. "There's something wrong with Athena. She's blue."

Angela looked at the lifeless body of her daughter and started to scream. Anthony reached for the phone and dialled 911.

Anthony Kporwodu and Angela Veno met in the summer of 1995 while studying at the DeVry Institute of Technology, a community college in Toronto. Anthony was in his early twenties, and Angela was in her late teens. He was born in Ghana and had come to Toronto as a seven-year-old with his mother and brother.

Angela Veno was born in Nova Scotia. Her parents moved a lot, so she hopscotched around the province as a child, growing up in several small communities. She married her high school sweetheart right after she graduated from high school in June 1995. The newlyweds ran off to Toronto, but the relationship quickly fell apart. Angela met Anthony that August, and they were living together by December. She gave birth to Julius the next year. Athena was born in 1997, the same year Angela's divorce was finalized.

Anthony studied briefly at York University before completing one semester of a business administration course at DeVry. He then cycled through a variety of jobs: sales rep, assembly line worker, machine operator, window and eavestrough cleaner. His most recent job was as a duct cleaner, but it was intermittent work at best. Angela didn't stick with DeVry either, but she did complete a banking course at another college. She'd had her own assortment of short-term, low-wage jobs: telephone attendant, teller, credit tracing officer.

Athena was born on December 2, 1997. Anthony's duct-cleaning work had mostly dried up over that winter, so money was tight for the family, but he was home to help out with the baby and her big brother. Athena was a good baby; she ate well and slept as much as a newborn does. It was a hectic, tiring time, but Angela and Anthony were happy.

By mid-January, the couple knew one of them had to get back to work. It was Angela who landed a job first. A friend who worked at a massage parlour in downtown Toronto told her it was great money; if Angela needed work, she could probably get her in.

Angela wasn't keen, but what could she do? Their phone had been cut off, they were struggling to keep up with the rent, the transmission in

Anthony's van had just died, and they had two children. It wasn't a hard decision to make. And Anthony was okay with it; he trusted Angela. When she said nothing untoward would happen, that's what he chose to believe.

It was depressing work, and painful for Angela to be away from the children, but it *was* good money: She made $400 her first night. The shifts were overnight—seven till four—and Angela was soon working doubles, even the odd triple. Oftentimes she just slept on the couch at work until her next shift started.

It was not an easy life, but it wasn't all hardship and struggle. Their apartment was in a townhome complex overflowing with kids. It felt like a safe place to raise a family.

The 911 operator explained how to do CPR. Anthony tried to push air into his daughter's lungs, but she wasn't responding.

The paramedics, firefighters and police arrived within minutes. A paramedic opened Athena's mouth, his finger flicking inside to check her airway. He slipped an adult-size face mask over her mouth. As the paramedic squeezed the bag, Athena's chest rose slightly. And then she was gone, whisked out the door on a stretcher to the waiting ambulance for the sprint to the Scarborough Centenary Hospital.

At 8:05 a.m., barely thirty minutes after her father's frantic 911 call, Athena Kporwodu was pronounced dead.

Athena Agnes was born shortly after midnight on December 2, 1997. The doctor was immediately worried about the newborn. Her white blood cell count was high: 34,000. The normal range at birth is 9,000 to 30,000, with a mean of about 18,000. A high white blood cell count can be a sign of infection, and Group B Streptococcus, or GBS, turned up in Angela's vaginal swab. It's a common, easily treated infection for women, but it can be very dangerous, even fatal, if passed from mother to child during birth. The doctor wasn't taking any chances. Athena was given intravenous antibiotics for forty-eight hours, and that did the trick. Her blood cultures came back negative for GBS, and she was cleared to go home after two days.

The child initially did well at home. The young family celebrated their first Christmas as a foursome. But Athena's health had deteriorated by early February. Her appetite dropped off, and what she did eat she quickly spit back up. She had diarrhea. She was irritable, crying lots and sleeping little. Athena would calm when she was picked up, cry when she was put down. Angela and Anthony bought her a swing chair, and it was the only other thing that would settle her.

Angela took her to see their family physician, Dr. Tak Lo, on February 2, 1998. The doctor found nothing too concerning. He said Athena had gastroenteritis, a virus that causes inflammation in the stomach and small intestine. He prescribed Pedialyte for twenty-four hours to replace fluids. At a follow-up visit the next day, Athena already showed signs of improvement: her diarrhea and vomiting had stopped, and she was less irritable. Lo told Angela to feed the child soy milk for a few days, and to bring her back in a couple of weeks for another checkup.

But Angela was back in his office eight days later. Athena was vomiting again and had lost about a quarter of a pound. She was dehydrated but didn't have a fever. Lo chalked it up to the gastroenteritis she was fighting and prescribed more Pedialyte. At a checkup the next day, Athena appeared to be stabilizing: she was still mildly dehydrated but was keeping down the Pedialyte. Her weight was the same. Lo decided they should focus on getting her through the illness first and evaluate the weight loss later.

The Pedialyte helped only for a day or two, and then the vomiting and diarrhea started anew. The child was irritable and cried almost constantly. Sometimes it almost sounded like screeching, which Anthony found worrying. Angela tried to reassure him. But Anthony was exhausted. Everyone was on edge. Athena had looked ill for weeks. Her skin was pallid, almost grey. And she wouldn't stop crying.

And then, in mid-February, she had a seizure. She was in the car seat in the back beside her brother when her whole body stiffened up.

After that, she wouldn't sleep. She wouldn't stop crying. She was not eating well, and she vomited after almost every feeding. Anthony was so worried that he resorted to trying to squeeze a half bottle of water into her mouth, just to get some fluids into her. On March 4, after Anthony gave Athena a bath and tried to feed her, she had another seizure. Her tiny body stiffened as she held her breath and squeezed her eyes shut.

He phoned Angela and described how Athena's eyes were pointing in different directions. Her body stiffened again, then relaxed, as if she was being hit by aftershocks. Angela said she was coming home. They'd take her to the hospital together.

In the end, the couple decided to take Athena back to see Dr. Lo rather than go to the hospital. They didn't want to risk a long wait in the ER, and since Lo had seen her recently, they thought he would be better able to figure out what was wrong. They called a cab. Athena seemed more alert during the drive over to his office.

By the time they saw the doctor, Athena was no longer vomiting and didn't have diarrhea. Lo found no signs of an upper respiratory tract infection. There was no fever, and the seizures had stopped, although Athena did stiffen up for a moment. Anthony described what Athena's seizure had looked like. Lo thought it sounded like breath-holding spells. A child stops breathing, sometimes for up to a full minute, and then passes out or has a seizure. The body may twitch or go rigid. The skin turns red or bluish purple, especially around the lips. The spells are commonly caused by a change in the child's breathing pattern, such as when angry or scared, and less commonly by a slowing of the heart rate, usually in response to pain. They are not considered dangerous.

But breath-holding spells normally occur in children six months to six years old, and are most common in one- to three-year-olds. Athena was three months old.

In any case, Lo was not especially concerned. Athena was not dehydrated. She was alert and awake. He did not order further tests.

Angela went back to work. Anthony managed to get two feeds into Athena, which she didn't vomit back up, but it barely added up to half a bottle. She sucked hard on the bottle and slept.

When she woke, Anthony tried to feed her a small amount of a Pedialyte and baby formula mix. Athena wouldn't latch on the nipple of the bottle, though, so he resorted to squeezing it into her mouth. It took forty minutes to feed her another half a bottle. The feeding and constant crying wore her out, though, and she slept fitfully throughout the day.

Angela and Anthony decided they needed a change of scenery that evening. Everyone was going stir-crazy in the apartment. And besides, they had just picked up their new car that afternoon, a used Pontiac Sunbird. It would be Angela's car; they were spending a small fortune on cabs getting her home from work in the early morning. Buying a car was a big step for the young couple, and dinner out with the kids would be a nice way to mark the occasion.

They went to a Vietnamese restaurant, but were out in half an hour because Athena wouldn't stop crying. So they just drove around the city. The motion of the car soothed both children, and the quiet was a welcome respite for the exhausted parents.

It was eleven thirty when they pulled the car into their apartment complex. Athena stirred as Angela lifted out her car seat, and she was wailing again by the time they were at their door. Anthony hustled everyone inside, anxious the neighbours would call the police because of the noise.

An officer had already visited them. A neighbour had called the police two days earlier, worried about Athena's incessant crying. The visit unnerved Anthony and Angela. They were happy their neighbours were concerned about Athena's crying, but it was hard not to take it personally. Athena was sleeping when the officer knocked on the door. Anthony was worried he might be charged with neglect, but the officer nodded knowingly when he explained that they had a cranky newborn. He left without seeing the child.

Anthony put Julius down to bed while Angela fed Athena. The child devoured a full bottle of formula and still seemed hungry, and the formula was staying down so far, so Angela gave her another. Anthony hopped in the shower while Angela finished up. She was cradling the baby gently, rocking her toward sleep, when she seized again. Angela now understood why Anthony had been so distraught the day before. It was terrifying to watch. The couple reminded themselves of what Dr. Lo had said.

They weren't sure Athena was holding her breath, though. If anything, her breath appeared to quicken, not stop. But they told each other they were just overreacting. There was no need do take her to emergency. They agreed to watch her through the night.

It was almost one thirty before Athena finally fell soundly asleep in her car seat. Anthony kissed her on the forehead and lay down to sleep on the floor beside her.

A pediatrician who viewed Athena's body found the soft spot on the top of her head tense and bulging. That is often a sign of meningitis, a potentially fatal inflammation of the membranes surrounding the brain and spinal cord. Athena's other symptoms—difficulty breathing, diarrhea, vomiting, appetite loss, stiffening and irritability—were non-specific, but were consistent with meningitis. One of the most common causes of meningitis is Group B Streptococcus, which Angela was carrying at the time of Athena's birth. Perhaps the antibiotics Athena had been given as a newborn beat the condition back but didn't eradicate it.

Meningitis can be highly contagious, so Athena's body was quarantined. Dr. Allan Hunt performed the autopsy at Scarborough Centenary later that day. He was an experienced pathologist, specializing in anatomic and general pathology, and had been working in the Toronto area for thirteen years. He had gone to England to obtain his two forensic pathology certifications because no forensic certification existed in Canada at the time.

Hunt knew he would have to be careful. Two police officers and the coroner, Dr. Ross Bennett, were present for the autopsy.

Hunt began by ordering X-rays. No abnormalities were detected, but it was hard to be sure because of the poor quality of the images. He then turned to the body itself. The child's abdomen was distended. An endotracheal tube was still in her mouth, but its lower end was in the esophagus instead of the trachea. One of the paramedics had inserted it incorrectly, blowing air into her stomach rather than her lungs.

There were no scars on the body, but Hunt did see several areas of discoloration on her chest and abdomen. She had a small scratch on the base of her nose. There were also several discoloured areas on her back. They looked like they could be Mongolian spots, bluish-grey birthmarks that are sometimes mistaken for bruises. But the marks on her chest and abdomen definitely looked like bruises. They could have been caused during resuscitation efforts or they could be signs of abuse. She also had a red mark on the back of her head.

And the bruising appeared to be getting worse. In his post-mortem report Hunt wrote, "Over time the discoloured areas of skin on the head and torso indicative of possible bruising are becoming more obvious."

Hunt did a cisternal puncture at the base of the child's skull. If the cerebrospinal fluid he collected contained granulocytes, a type of white blood cell, that would signal that the child had bacterial meningitis. Spinal fluid is usually clear; what Hunt withdrew was deep, dark red, which could be a sign of infection or bleeding in the brain (or be caused by a botched puncture). Tests on the cerebrospinal fluid ruled out meningitis. That left bleeding in the brain as a potential cause for the bulging soft spot—a sign of trauma.

Hunt cut into the body.

As he began the internal exam, he found more signs that troubled him. There was bleeding in the soft tissue around the rib cage. Some of the bleeding lined up with the possible bruising he had seen on her skin; other spots had no obvious cause. There were signs of fibrosis on the left side, suggesting an earlier soft-tissue injury. He palpated several of her ribs and found signs of healing fractures. The surface of her liver was depressed and had a whitish colour, also suggesting an older injury.

Hunt had seen enough. His findings pointed to possible child abuse, most likely shaken baby syndrome. He immediately stopped the examination. The stakes were high—Athena's injuries could lead to criminal charges—and pediatric pathology was not his area of expertise. A pathologist from the Ontario Pediatric Forensic Pathology Unit would be better suited to complete the autopsy.

TWO

DET. SGT. MATT Crone and Det. Larry Linton of the Metro Toronto Police Force arranged to meet Anthony and Angela at the police station for questioning. The couple had gone home after the trauma of the morning, but were waiting at the police station when the two officers arrived.

"We're very sorry for your loss," Crone said, taking first the mother's hand, then the father's. "Thanks for coming in. We take these matters very seriously, and we're looking to answer questions not only for us and our investigation, but for you as well."

The detectives explained that they needed to ask them each some questions separately. They led Angela into the interview room first.

She explained her personal history, how she and Anthony had met, Athena's birth and her recent poor health.

"Okay, now I have to ask you this and before I ask, I have to tell you that the tape is on and whatever you say is being recorded," Crone said.

Angela said she understood.

"Did you ever lose your temper with Athena at all?" the detective asked.

"Never with my daughter. Never with my son."

"Okay. You never shook them or hit them?"

"No, if they're crying to the point where we start to feel agitated, we'll put them in their room and either go on the balcony, living room, just sit down and breathe. Because it's better to let them cry in their crib than to hurt them."

Crone's questions shifted to Angela's impression of Anthony.

"Do you ever know Anthony to hit or . . ."

"Oh, Tony, no. I couldn't even imagine. He's the one who taught me how to take care of kids." Angela said her parents didn't teach her anything about being a mother.

"He basically taught me everything."

286 - JOHN CHIPMAN

"So he's a good father?" Crone asked.

"Very good father. He's amazing. Amazing."

Angela said they had left Athena with a babysitter only twice: once with a friend named Karen Black when Athena was about a month old, and once with a friend's younger sister, a sixteen-year-old named Melissa Sarmiento. After both occasions, Athena had seemed fine. Neither baby-sitter raised any concerns, other than Athena cried a lot.

As the questioning continued, Angela recalled two incidents involving Athena's brother, but they sounded innocuous: Julius had once kicked Athena's car seat while they were driving. She was jostled a bit, but they didn't see any marks or injuries on her afterwards. Another time, Julius scratched his sister's face, leaving a small mark near her eye. That was it, until this morning.

"Anthony was telling me that . . . after he [did] CPR, he noticed like a bruise on her chest. So he thought maybe he was giving her CPR, that he was pushing too hard."

Crone asked her why she went back to work so soon after Athena's birth. Angela was blunt: they needed the money. Anthony had been working as a duct cleaner but his shifts had dried up, so she picked up the slack.

The interview ended shortly afterwards. The two detectives led Angela out to the waiting room and brought Anthony in. He described Athena as a good baby, saying she had even slept through the night occasionally, until about a month earlier, when she had stopped eating and started vomiting. And crying. A lot. It got so bad, he said, the neighbours had called the police earlier that week.

After the parents left, Linton called the coroner. He wanted to know if a crime had been committed. Dr. Bennett said he couldn't say until the autopsy was completed because some of Dr. Hunt's findings suggested non-accidental injuries. He said it could be shaken baby syndrome, but it was too early to say for sure. The coroner said Charles Smith at the Hospital for Sick Children was taking over the autopsy, which would be completed the next day.

Linton and Crone discussed how they were going to proceed. They would need to wait for the autopsy results before they could determine if there were grounds to search the couple's apartment. In the meantime, though, they needed to maintain the integrity of a potential crime scene. The family was staying with a friend that night, but the detectives decided to keep the officer guarding the scene there overnight, just to make sure no one entered.

Crone arrived at the apartment just after eight that night. The constable at the door said he'd had a lot of curious people around, but no one who had any information. An insurance man from London Life had come by. He'd just left his name, Robert Schindelheim.

Athena's body was sent to Toronto's Hospital for Sick Children, where Dr. Charles Smith would finish the autopsy. Matt Crone and Larry Linton met with the pathologist beforehand to discuss the case. Dr. Hunt joined them as well.

After looking at new X-rays, Smith told the detectives there didn't appear to be any head injuries. But the ribs were another story. He pointed out small lines on several X-rays, indications of healing fractures on the ribs.

The damage was plain to see. To Linton, the ribs almost looked misaligned. Crone asked if they could be resuscitation injuries. Smith said the fractures were more than two weeks old, and they were in the wrong place. He said there appeared to be about fifteen rib fractures. And one of the child's toes, the first metatarsal, was broken on her left foot. And there could be a fracture in her left knee, but he would need to examine more closely to be sure.

Smith said some of the fractures were consistent with shaken baby syndrome. "In the absence of another explanation, these injuries are non-accidental."

The second autopsy began at 11:35. With five police officers on hand, along with Dr. Hunt and Smith's assistant, it was crowded.

Smith rhymed off a laundry list of injuries to the police as he worked: bruising on the upper buttocks and at various points on the back; small round bruises on the right side of her chest; dark reddish marks on the right ribs under the skin; small bruises to the skin over the left rib cage; an abrasion at the elbow on the left arm; evidence of an older bleed on the inner skull; a laceration in the liver; other signs of healing in the tissue that pointed to older injuries. But the most damning evidence was the ribs. Smith noted so many fractures that Linton had to make a chart in his notebook to keep them all straight. There were twenty-one confirmed fractures, plus signs of another eleven possible ones. They were literally everywhere: front and back and both sides. Every single rib was fractured, most of them in more than one place. Some were hairline fractures; some were breaks all the way through.

Smith's conclusion: Athena died from multiple non-accidental traumatic injuries. Crone asked if he could say when her fatal injuries occurred. Smith said he could not. Crone pushed him for a ballpark estimate. Smith said the rib fractures all occurred within the last month of her life, but he couldn't be any more precise than that.

Matt Crone had been a police officer for more than twenty years, an investigator for twelve. He'd worked dozens of cases, including several involving children. And yet he still found it hard to accept what Smith was telling him. Not hard to believe; just hard to accept.

"It's hard to get your head around the fact that someone would wilfully kill something as inoffensive and precious as a child," the detective recalled years later. "Your mindset when you are investigating is 'Someone tell me this was an accident. Someone tell me there was some unfortunate thing that happened that can explain all this.' Because I really don't want to charge somebody with this. As a human being, I'm really having a tough time believing someone could do this intentionally."

Crone had crossed paths with Charles Smith before, but this was going to be the first time the detective had worked with him while leading a homicide investigation. Smith struck him as reasonable during the autopsy. He didn't overreach on what he knew. It would have been helpful to their investigation if Smith could have dated the child's injuries more accurately, but Crone respected the pathologist for being prudent. The detective knew how difficult child deaths can be to crack. Often, injuries don't add up. "One of the really, really difficult problems with investigating child death," he recalled, "is causation, where you can have a number of injuries that are all survivable but the child will die."

Smith was certain Athena's rib fractures had been caused by trauma. But rib fractures aren't fatal on their own. Could the liver laceration have killed her? Or could that have been caused during CPR? Crone said, "There wasn't one of those injuries in Athena that had it occurred in an adult would have been life-threatening, yet this child died. So that's always the larger issue."

The pathologist had once told the detective, "If you ever want to get away with a murder, kill a child." Smith said he was certain Athena Kporwodu had died a violent death from multiple non-accidental traumatic injuries. So the case would come down to timing: When did Athena suffer her fatal injuries, and who had access to her at that time? The detectives would have to consider the babysitters, but the child had barely left her parents' care during her brief life. The parents were the obvious suspects. But could both of them be responsible? If it was hard to imagine one person responsible for such a disturbing crime, the detective found it even harder to believe that two people could be involved.

Anthony and Angela went back to the police station that afternoon. Their daughter had been dead for little more than twenty-four hours. The day before, they had been grieving parents. Now they were prime suspects. The detectives questioned Angela first.

She asked what the results of the autopsy were as they led her into the interview room. Crone told her the post-mortem examination found that Athena died of non-accidental injuries. He said criminal charges might be laid related to her death.

Angela started sobbing. She said there must have been some mistake. Crone assured her there wasn't. Athena's injuries were severe. She had suffered a large number of rib fractures.

Angela said the rib fractures didn't make sense. She asked the detective if the pathologist considered brittle bone disease. She had seen a show about it on television.

Crone said the pathologist found no congenital reason or disease that would account for her death.

Angela was distraught, and it took several minutes for her to calm down enough to take an oath and begin answering questions. Once she finally composed herself, she walked the detectives through the three short months of her daughter's life.

Crone asked her how she ended up working at a massage parlour.

"We were having money problems and for me to go back to the bank, the pay wasn't very good so my friend was talking to me about working in a massage parlour and I, we thought about it, we talked about it for a week or so and then decided to try," Angela explained.

"Okay and how did Anthony feel about you working in a massage parlour?"

"At the time, we needed the money very badly so to him, it was fine. He trusted me totally, so he wasn't any problem. There hasn't been any problem."

Angela detailed Athena's medical history. She recalled two eye infections that required trips to the doctor's office, and the antibiotics she required at birth; there was the vomiting, the diarrhea, the trouble eating, the seizures. And the crying. It was almost constant during the last month of her life.

"This constant crying, did it cause you or Anthony aggravation?" Crone asked.

"No," Angela replied, then added, "Like any parent, it does [a] little bit, of course."

"Were you losing sleep because of it?"

"A little, yeah."

The detective asked if she and Anthony argued much. Angela said she could only remember two times since Athena was born. Both times it was about their money problems.

"When you came back from the hospital [Friday morning after Athena died], did you have a fight?" Crone asked.

"No. We were just basically silent. In shock. I just," Angela paused, struggling to find the words. "There was no argument. We were just scared."

"Why were you scared?"

"Because my little girl, because . . ." Angela started to cry. "My whole pregnancy I just wanted a, I just wanted [a] girl so badly." Her sobs overwhelmed her words, making her almost impossible to understand. "I know when I gave birth to her, I was like going crazy. I [could] jump off the bed, I was so happy." She sniffed back her runny nose. "I just grabbed her from the doctor. I was so ecstatic I had a girl. From the time I was a little girl, I've always wanted a daughter." Sobs twisted her words into unintelligible sounds for a moment, and then they came back to her. "She's gone."

Next, Anthony was brought in for questioning. "How did she die?" he asked almost immediately.

Crone told him they didn't have the cause of death yet, but that Athena had suffered serious non-accidental injuries. He said they would like to record the interview. Anthony said he was fine with that. Another officer came in to read him his cautions and take his oath.

Crone again had Anthony walk the detectives through the three months of Athena's life. He asked him about his recent struggles to get work, and Angela's decision to start working at a massage parlour.

"Do you know how she came to work there?" Crone asked.

"It was out of desperation pretty much because we reached, at one point, where the money was running out and I had to keep up with the bills." He said the phone was cut off; they had back bills on their vehicle; and rent was coming due. "So we figured that something had to be done in order for money [to] be coming in." Angela started looking for work, and that's when a friend mentioned the massage parlour. She said the money was great. "[Angela] figured okay, once she gets a little bit better, or heals a little bit more, then she might pursue it."

"What specifically does she do?"

"Ah, basically, it's like um, um, massage. She um, she, people come in and she gives them massage and, ah, and she gets paid for it."

The detective moved off the topic for a minute, asking Anthony about Athena's health again and the two babysitters they had used. "Okay, now,

Angela started working in January. How did you feel about her working in a massage parlour?" Crone then asked, shifting gears again.

"I don't mind actually. We were talking about it and she found it hard to make the decision, but I just figured, I just said, well, there's not much we could do." But Anthony stressed that he left the decision up to Angela. "I wasn't overly, y'know . . . uncomfortable with it or anything like that."

"But would you agree with me that there's generally a negative connotation associated with massage parlours?" Crone asked.

Anthony said that generally there was, but it wasn't an issue for him. "The thing is that I trust Angela. I've known her for a while. I trust her wholeheartedly so I didn't for one minute even believe that she . . . anything would be done other than, ah, just what she worked at," he explained. And the money was good. Anthony said Angela made $1,000 a week.

The conversation shifted back to Athena's health. Specifically, her crying.

"Was there ever a period of time in the three months that you were concerned about the amount of crying that Athena was doing?" Crone asked.

"We were. Ah, a little bit, because even though . . . it wasn't that different, that much off of what Julius was. It wasn't the amount of crying, it was . . . the extremity." Anthony said she wasn't crying so much as she was screeching. He wondered why. "Angela usually said that it's because she's a girl . . . yeah, well, that's the truth. But it wasn't anything that I thought to be abnormal."

Crone asked him about the police officer who came to the apartment on Tuesday. Neighbours had complained about a crying baby.

"Don't you think that was strange that someone called?" the detective asked.

Anthony said he and Angela did find it odd. Athena was crying the night before and in the morning while he prepared her bottle. But that wasn't unusual. "She cried all the time. Why would they think that anything was wrong?" He said her crying jags were like clockwork, every three to four hours when she was hungry. There was nothing out of the ordinary about Monday night or Tuesday morning.

"Well, if I were to tell you that three separate people phoned the police and reported her crying all night, would that surprise you?" Crone asked.

"Three separate people?"

"Um-hum." Crone said the neighbours said the baby was crying non-stop all through the night. Anthony said that wasn't true.

The detective asked how she was during the day on Tuesday. Normal, Anthony replied; she cried a lot. But he worked extra hard to soothe her. He didn't want a neighbour calling the police again.

"I was worried that, someone might . . . get worried that either the child was being neglected or the child was being abused or anything like that, so I tried to keep her as quiet as I could by holding her as much as I could."

Crone asked Anthony about Athena's condition on Wednesday, when she seized up after he gave her a bath. "I tried to look into her eyes 'cause she had her eyes closed. When I opened her eyes, the one eye, the one pupil [was] looking one way and the other one looked like it was just like focusing on nothing." Anthony said he panicked and called Angela. He told her something was wrong with Athena and she had to come home. He was going to take her back to the doctor.

"This is something pretty unusual," Crone noted.

"Yeah, that was unusual."

"You were nervous and scared?"

"Yeah," Anthony admitted.

"You didn't think of calling an ambulance?"

Anthony said no. He and Angela had seen a report on the news a few days earlier about people waiting three or four hours at the hospital. They thought the family doctor was a better plan. "Who would know her condition [better] than the doctor we had [been] seeing?"

By the time they got her to the doctor's office, Athena's symptoms had receded. She was fine. Dr. Lo didn't think she had had a seizure. He said it was breath-holding syndrome.

At the end of the interview, Crone asked Anthony for his permission to search the apartment. "You're well within your rights to refuse, and one of the things I have to tell you [is] that if we were to find evidence in there that you were guilty of an offence relating to this, and I told you this could be as serious as murder . . . That may be used against you in evidence," Crone warned.

"Well, I'm not worried about that 'cause I know that I didn't do anything and pretty sure that Angela didn't do anything." Anthony said he was fine with police searching the apartment.

Crone reached to turn off the recorder, but Anthony had a question of his own.

"Would you be able to tell me, like, how or what she sustained or something," he asked.

Crone said he didn't know yet because the medical experts were still completing their examinations, and those were expected in two or three weeks. "But I can tell you that she sustained some very serious injuries."

"From what? I mean, from a beating or somethin'?" Anthony asked.

Crone said he couldn't tell him.

The detectives took Anthony back to the waiting room, where Angela was sitting with Julius. Reality was setting in for the parents. Athena was gone, and they were murder suspects. Linton slipped out as his partner explained what would happen next in the investigation. Angela watched Linton go. She knew what was coming. She asked Crone if they were calling Children's Aid.

Crone nodded. "Due to the nature of the injuries to Athena, CAS will be involved. Someone will be coming by shortly to talk to you. They may want to examine Julius."

Angela begged the detectives not to let them take him. Anthony asked if Julius could stay with family. He had an aunt and uncle who could look after him. The detective said that was a possibility, but it would be up to Children's Aid.

It was a thirty-minute wait. Finally, the door opened. Detective Linton stepped in with another man, who introduced himself as Brian Prousky. He said he worked with Children's Aid and he was taking custody of Julius. Angela and Anthony told him about Anthony's aunt and uncle.

Prousky said the child could stay with them temporarily. After that, he would be placed in foster care.

"For how long?" Angela asked.

Prousky said he wasn't sure. "The initial apprehension will be for a few days, maybe a week. You can go to court to ask for custody back."

"While the police are investigating us?" Angela asked.

"The two matters are separate, but how the police investigation proceeds will assist the court in determining custody."

On March 6, 1998, Anthony Kporwodu and Angela Veno lost their three-month-old daughter. The next day, they lost their son.

THREE

NEITHER ANGELA NOR Anthony was allowed to see Julius for a week after his removal. After that, visits were kept to twice a week and only under strict supervision. Angela and Anthony ping-ponged between outrage and despair. They suddenly had no say in decisions about Julius's health or education. And Angela couldn't see any effort being made to help him understand why he had been taken away from his parents.

Julius's behaviour started to change almost immediately. The good-natured toddler became erratic and aggressive. Angela found bruises on his head during one visit. She was told he had slipped on a concrete step and bumped his head. A doctor examined him. He was soon moved to another foster home.

Police continued their investigation. Detective Sergeant Crone canvassed neighbours. He spoke with a twenty-one-year-old woman named Christine Oakley who had been living in the townhome complex for four months. She said that during the past week she had heard a baby crying in the couple's apartment all the time. At night, the crying was loud enough to wake her up. Oakley said she was sure something was wrong. When Crone asked her to explain, she said it was just a lot of noise from their apartment. Lots of banging around, like someone was shifting furniture around. And she also heard people arguing during the day. A man and a woman yelling. Crone asked if she heard anything Friday morning. Oakley said she didn't. It was quiet when she left for work. No arguing. No crying baby.

It was useful information. But Oakley called Crone back three days later and backtracked on most of it. Much of what she had told him, she said, came from someone babysitting for her at the time. Oakley did hear a baby crying Monday or Tuesday night, but she slept off and on so she couldn't say the baby was crying all night. She never heard the baby scream, and she didn't hear anything on Thursday night, the night before Athena died. And in the week since she hadn't heard Angela and Anthony fighting at all.

Crone and Linton tracked down Anthony and Angela's two babysitters. Melissa Sarmiento said she looked after Athena only once, on February 10. Angela and Anthony dropped her off for a few hours that evening. Melissa's brother and parents were home with her at the time. She said Anthony warned her that Athena had a bit of a cold and would likely cry a lot, but Melissa said the baby wasn't too bad.

Karen Black had met Angela at a telemarketing firm where they both worked, but it wasn't until Karen got laid off that they became friends. Karen also said she babysat Athena only once, a couple of months earlier. She went to Angela's apartment; both children were already asleep when she arrived. As for Angela and Anthony's relationship, she said she didn't know them well enough to have an opinion. Karen said Angela did mention that they were having financial problems.

Dr. Lo, the family physician, told Crone they seemed like reasonable parents. He'd also cared for Julius and had never seen signs of abuse. They stayed up to date with the children's vaccinations. He said he had seen Athena a fair bit recently. She was sick over the last month of her life: vomiting, diarrhea, crying spells, then a breath-holding spell. The doctor examined the child during each visit but said he didn't find any signs of serious illness or infection. He told the detectives that when he saw Athena in February, she had the flu. When he saw her the last time, two days before she died, Lo said he was a little concerned about her weight. She had only put on two ounces in two to three weeks. He explained that one to two pounds a month would be normal for a child Athena's age. Anthony and Angela had scheduled another visit on Friday, the day she died.

The detectives asked if the doctor saw anything during his examinations that suggested Athena was being harmed in any way. Lo said he saw no signs of abuse. "They appeared to be caring parents."

Detective Linton called Anthony and Angela the following Tuesday. Athena had been dead for four days. He wanted to find out if they would take a polygraph test. Angela was crying when she answered the phone. She passed it to Anthony.

He asked why no one had told them when they could pick up Athena's remains. Linton said that wasn't a police matter. The funeral home makes the necessary arrangements. But the detective offered to find out when the body would be ready to be released if Anthony and Angela had any problems.

Anthony also said he and Angela had been speaking with Children's Aid officials, who said they were both suspects in Athena's death. And that she had died of shaken baby syndrome.

Linton told him the cause of death had not been determined, and police wouldn't know what it was until the pathologist finished his final autopsy report. All he could say for now was that the pathologist believed Athena had suffered multiple traumatic injuries that were non-accidental in nature. And as for suspects, he said police were not looking at any one person in particular. He and Angela were as suspicious as anyone else who had been in contact with Athena.

Linton then asked Anthony about taking the polygraph test. Anthony said that it sounded fine, but he needed to run it by his lawyer. The detective asked Anthony to get back to him as soon as he could.

The ultimate question in any homicide investigation is: Who did it? But an even more fundamental question needs to be asked first: Did a crime actually occur?

Answering that question is much more difficult in pediatric homicides than in adult cases. Michael Pollanen, Ontario's chief forensic pathologist, described the difficulties at the Goudge Inquiry. As an example, Pollanen used an infant who dies in her sleep. She has no external signs of injury. She has no medical history of life-threatening illness. There are no witnesses. There is no circumstantial evidence. And there is no physical evidence of a crime at the scene. The first and only evidence of a homicide is found by the pathologist.

That reality adds even more weight to the autopsy findings. It's why independent review is so important. Mistakes in an autopsy will be amplified because there is no other evidence to consider. So when Anthony

Kporwodu contacted James J. Grosberg about representing him should criminal charges be laid, the lawyer's first piece of advice was to get a second autopsy. Otherwise, there was a good chance the entire case would come down to Hunt's and Smith's opinions.

But Dr. Smith had not completed his autopsy report. Further testing was needed to determine the exact cause of death. And a second autopsy would be costly, an expense that Anthony and Angela could ill afford. They still had to pay for Athena's funeral. So they decided to wait until Smith's autopsy report was done before deciding. They still hoped his report would show they had nothing to do with Athena's death.

The couple had already signed a contract with Highland Crematorium and Ogden Funeral Home, but after speaking with Grosberg, Anthony told both businesses not to cremate Athena's body without their consent. He also told police and the coroner that he and Angela might be ordering a second autopsy.

Coroner Ross Bennett warned Anthony it would be a costly procedure, and would likely have to be done in the United States. A day earlier, Bennett had issued a certificate to the funeral home saying there was "no reason for further examination of the body." He did not revoke that certificate after speaking with Anthony. He also never told Anthony that the coroner's office could, if asked, preserve Athena's body until the couple decided about a second autopsy.

Two weeks after the memorial service, the funeral home told Angela that Athena's body needed to be transferred to the crematorium. She immediately called the crematorium and reminded them not to cremate Athena without her and Anthony's consent. The crematorium official said they could not hold the body forever, but agreed to contact her before doing anything.

That was on April 1, 1998. Angela and Anthony did not speak to anyone at the crematorium again until June 7, when someone called asking them to pick up Athena's ashes.

She had been cremated a week earlier.

Athena's remains were her parents' responsibility at the time of her cremation. The coroner did not order her cremation, nor could he. But Dr. Bennett did not revoke his certificate, which contradicted the family's wishes. He did not reiterate Anthony's wishes about retaining the body with the funeral home or the crematorium. And he did not tell Anthony or Angela that the Chief Coroner's Office could hold Athena's body until they decided whether to do a second autopsy.

The Ontario Court of Appeal would eventually rule that it was not Dr. Bennett's responsibility to do any of those things. He did not have to do anything more than he did.

But he could have.

Anthony took the polygraph test, which he failed miserably. He scored 99 per cent for deception. But it was far from a smoking gun. Polygraph results are inadmissible in Canadian courts. (Angela had declined to take the test.)

The detectives weren't overly concerned. Anthony's results supported the theory they were starting to formulate: if Smith's autopsy report showed Athena's death was indeed a murder, then her father most likely killed her. They were starting to think of Angela as more of a potential witness than a suspect. Anthony was Athena's primary caregiver. When Angela did care for her, Anthony was also around, especially in the last month of her life when her health deteriorated. And Crone doubted the couple were conspiring to abuse the child together. They appeared to be caring, responsible parents. There was no evidence that Julius had been abused. The detective didn't think he was dealing with manipulative psychopaths. If someone did beat Athena, as Smith was suggesting, it seemed most likely that it happened in a moment of exhaustion or frustration. Probably a shaken baby case.

What police really needed was the pathologist's final report. His opinion would drive their entire investigation. Linton first called Smith to inquire about his progress on March 23, less than three weeks after the child's death. Smith said he hadn't dissected the child's brain yet, but expected to get to it later that week. He told Linton he expected to have his final post-mortem results ready for police in three to five weeks.

The wait for that final report, however, stretched on through the spring, summer and fall of 1998. It was frustrating, and not just for the detectives. With the possibility of a second autopsy now off the table, even more was riding on Smith's findings for Anthony and Angela.

At the time, pressure was growing on the Pediatric Forensic Pathology Unit to speed up completion of its autopsy reports. Although widely respected, Smith had developed a reputation among doctors, police officers and Crown attorneys for lengthy delays in completing his work. Dr. David Chiasson, then Ontario's chief forensic pathologist, was pushing to have 90 per cent of autopsy reports finalized within ninety days of the autopsy. There was pressure from outside as well. The commission investigating the wrongful conviction of Guy Paul Morin, whose conviction for first-degree murder was overturned on the basis of DNA evidence, tabled its report the same month Athena died, and one of its recommendations emphasized the importance of timely forensic services. In most cases, toxicology reports can be completed within sixty days, allowing another month for a pathologist to consider the test results and complete the autopsy report.

Chiasson pushed his initiative in a meeting with Smith in 1998; Dr. Laurence Becker, the chief of Paediatric Laboratory Medicine at the Hospital for Sick Children; Dr. Jim Cairns, Ontario's deputy chief coroner; and Dr. William Lucas, a regional coroner in Toronto, were also present. While the initiative's merits were endorsed at the meeting, Chiasson testified at the Goudge Inquiry that it never took hold.

Everyone in the room knew that Chiasson was setting an ambitious goal. Three months might be reasonable for straightforward autopsies, but complicated cases could easily take six or even nine months to complete. In Athena's case, one that Smith would later describe as one of the most complex of his career, he had to consult three other specialists at the Hospital for Sick Children: a radiologist for a skeletal survey, another radiologist for a CT scan of the rib cage and a pediatric specialist to analyze the brain.

On top of that, the provincial Centre of Forensic Sciences ran numerous toxicology tests on Athena's blood, liver and stomach contents, and those test results weren't finalized until September, six and a half months after Smith had made his initial post-mortem examination. Despite knowing Chiasson was trying to speed up autopsy reports, at no point did Smith ask the centre to expedite its work in Athena's case. Meanwhile, Smith received all three reports from the specialists he'd consulted at SickKids by the end of April (although one wasn't signed until July).

In a 2003 ruling, Superior Court Justice Brian Trafford noted that Smith could have taken another month to consider the specialists' findings to determine a cause of death and completed his autopsy report by the end of May. It wouldn't contain the toxicology results, but at least the preliminary report would have been completed within Chiasson's goal of ninety days.

Anthony and Angela were waiting to see Dr. Smith's autopsy report before deciding if they needed a second autopsy. The three specialists' reports were in Smith's hands by April 29, exactly one month before Athena Kporwodu's body was mistakenly cremated.

FOUR

IN THE SUMMER of 1998, Angela told a social worker with Children's Aid that she was pregnant. The woman's advice: get an abortion, because there was little chance the agency would let her keep the child. The worker also told her that if police cleared Angela and Anthony in Athena's death before the baby was born, then Children's Aid would probably drop its custody application for the new child, and for Julius as well.

Anthony started calling the coroner's office and the Hospital for Sick Children. In an affidavit, Angela said he spoke to William Lucas, a regional coroner in Toronto, and Dr. Smith. Neither would tell him when Smith's report would be finished. Angela and Anthony would soon have to decide whether to continue with the pregnancy. Then their lawyer told Angela that they their names had been listed on the province's Child Abuse Register. They could only be removed if they were cleared of any wrongdoing in Athena's death.

They were suspected child killers, registered child abusers who had already been forced to give up their son. They thought about finding a nearby relative to take the baby, but who? They had failed to find someone in the family to look after Julius. They considered adoption, but under the circumstances, it seemed unbearable.

So they decided on an abortion.

Angela spiralled into a morass of depression and anger, frustration and loss. She sought medical help, but no amount of drugs or therapy could touch her grief. In the eyes of the police, in the eyes of the child welfare workers, all of this pain and suffering was of her own doing: she was a mother unfit to raise her own son, a mother unable to protect her newborn daughter, a mother who may have had a hand in her newborn's unexplained death.

Twelve days after leaving the abortion clinic, Angela received the call she had been waiting for: Smith's autopsy report was finally done.

Detective Linton asked Angela and Anthony to come down to the police station to discuss the results.

Police had actually received the autopsy report seven weeks earlier. It reinforced Smith's initial findings—multiple traumatic injuries to the head, ribs and liver—but it didn't advance the detectives' understanding of what had happened.

Linton spoke to Smith on October 27 after receiving his final report. The pathologist told him he couldn't put a precise time frame on the fractures. He estimated they were one to two weeks old, but not a month. There is no literature in this area, Smith explained. He was dating the fractures based on his autopsy experience. Kids heal faster than adults, he explained, but there is no research on three-month-olds.

He did say that the injuries occurred during more than one assault. The rib fractures were likely weeks old, but her liver injury was acute.

Smith added that the child also suffered an acute head injury, and there could be older head injuries too.

Linton asked if any of the injuries could have been caused by CPR. The pathologist said the head injuries were definitely not resuscitative. The liver injury could have been caused by a fist or compression. It was hours old, not days. The detective noted that the parents had taken her to the doctor, who didn't report any signs of abuse. Would there be signs from these injuries? he asked. Smith said not necessarily. The family doctor could have missed them.

Linton asked about bruising. The pathologist said some bruising may not appear from trauma. He thought the child's death could have been caused by shaking, but it wasn't a classic shaken baby case.

Investigators needed more evidence, which is why they waited to discuss the final autopsy results with Athena's parents. They would bring the couple down to the police station, and meanwhile a surveillance team would install listening devices in their apartment. The police hoped to capture some incriminating evidence when the suspects discussed the autopsy afterwards on their own. Linton had gone to court to get permission for the surveillance. The only problem now was figuring out where Anthony and Angela were living.

Linton had received word that a sheriff's office eviction order was posted on the door of their apartment. The surveillance affidavit was put off until police figured out their new address.

Linton received a voicemail from Anthony that he was able to track back to the Idlewood Inn, a rundown motel in Scarborough, in Toronto's east end. When the detective called back, Angela said they probably wouldn't be staying there for long. The detectives decided to wait it out until the couple settled at a more permanent address. A week later, Linton got another message from Anthony. They had moved into the Gateway Inn, another Scarborough motel, and would be staying there until at least the end of the year. The two detectives went back to court and received authorization to surreptitiously record in Angela and Anthony's residence.

Detectives Crone and Linton arrived at the motel shortly after 7 p.m. The ride down to the police station was sombre.

Angela and Anthony had heard much of what the police were telling them now, months before, in their first conversation after the autopsy: Dr. Smith's findings showed that Athena had suffered multiple traumatic injuries to the head, liver and ribs. The toxicology tests, which had caused so much of the delay, had come back negative, ruling out drugs or poison as a cause of death.

The conversation ended, and Anthony and Angela were walked back out to the cruiser for the drive back to the Gateway Inn. In the ninety minutes they were gone, the police installed listening devices in their motel room. They set up a listening post in a nearby room and another one down the road.

That first night, Angela and Anthony were as steadfast on their own as they had always been with police: the autopsy report must be wrong; how could Athena have those injuries?

For the next thirty days, police continued to monitor the couple's conversations. They talked about Bill Clinton's impeachment. They talked a lot about Julius and finding a way to keep him in the care of family members if they couldn't care for him themselves. At one point, Anthony called Linton to ask about further DNA testing to see if that might explain the injuries. The detective said it might be possible, but it would take months.

Police released a press release on December 21. Angela and Anthony called friends and family to tell them they had not done anything to hurt their child.

And then, the next day, Angela called Linton. She was sobbing, and her words were barely intelligible. She told him that she thought she now knew the truth. And she was terrified Anthony was going to kill himself.

Linton asked if she wanted to talk in person.

There was silence on the phone. And then the answer the detective was hoping for: yes.

Angela was going over to a friend's place. The detective said he would meet her there later that evening.

Linton couldn't reach Matt Crone, the lead investigator on the case, so he asked another detective to accompany him for the interview.

Angela led the two detectives into the kitchen, where they sat down at a small table. The friend, Karen Black, stayed in the living room.

She told Linton she and Anthony had been watching the news and saw a report about Athena's death. The reporter went to their old apartment, talked to one of their former neighbours. The woman said she heard noises coming from their apartment. It wasn't just crying. The woman said she was scared to go back to her own apartment.

Angela said she looked at Anthony, who said, "'You think I did it, don't you?' And I started to cry." Angela was sobbing again, recounting the scene. She said she realized that she did have a little doubt, and she didn't want anyone to think she would put anyone before her children.

Angela said Anthony told her that if she thought he did something to Athena, he would leave. But it was Angela who ended up going. As she was leaving, she saw him write something down on a piece of paper. And then it hit her. He was going to kill himself.

Linton asked her if Anthony had hurt himself. Angela wasn't sure, but she didn't think so. He had gone to stay with a friend.

"Even if I have the littlest doubt," she said, "I don't want to be with him."

Linton asked her if he could record their interview. All the other interviews had been recorded and it would be odd if this one wasn't, he explained. She agreed. But no sooner had Linton finished recording the introduction when there was a knock at the door.

It was Anthony. He wanted to speak to Angela in private.

Linton clicked off the tape recorder. Angela and Anthony were together less than ten minutes, just enough time for Linton to have a cigarette. They came back down to the living room, and Anthony asked for the White Pages. Karen said she didn't have one.

Angela returned to the kitchen and sat down again.

Linton asked her if she wanted to continue speaking to him. She said she didn't want to speak on tape without talking to a lawyer first.

Linton tried to salvage the evening. He explained that it didn't matter whether she spoke to him on tape or not; he could simply take notes if that made her more comfortable. He summarized the evidence of the case so far: the autopsy findings, the financial stresses they were under, the timing of Athena's injuries.

But Angela wouldn't budge. She said she never saw any bruises. They took her to the doctor, who didn't see any either. How was that possible? she wondered.

Linton said the pathologist who did the autopsy believed Athena's injuries could have been missed by their family doctor.

Angela shook her head. The interview was over.

It was the closest police would get to an admission or confession from either Angela or Anthony. Linton asked the monitors to continue listening in on the motel room through the night, in case the couple talked about their meeting with police and revealed something incriminating.

But the surveillance team didn't get anything useful. The couple returned to the motel that night, picked up some things and left. They returned around four in the morning, but the recording was hampered by a scheduled system shutdown. The team scrambled in an attempt to record them, but the tape's sound quality was so poor, it was useless.

The couple spoke with a lawyer the next day and returned to their long-held position: Dr. Smith must have missed an underlying medical condition at autopsy that explained Athena's death.

The surveillance continued for almost a month, wrapping up in the middle of January. The team lost track of the couple for a couple of days at the end of December, when they moved out of the Gateway. They eventually found them at a nearby motel, but it took another week to get a tap on their new phone.

Detective Linton and another officer were waiting for her one day in early January when she showed up for work at the massage parlour. They spoke outside. Linton said he was worried about how their conversation had ended at her friend's house. It looked like Anthony may have threatened her. Angela said he hadn't. He'd just reassured her that he had done nothing wrong.

The detective told her about another neighbour who had come forward, saying she had also heard Athena crying. The news didn't sway her.

"Well," Linton said, "if Anthony didn't do it, then it must have been you, Angela, and I don't believe that." He asked her to think about all the information the police had about Athena's death. Angela said she would. They made awkward small talk about Christmas, and then Linton asked about Julius, who was still in foster care. The detective pointed out that he was a healthy little boy. There was no indication he was ever harmed. "I feel bad that he has to be separated from you right now," he said. He told Angela to call him anytime she wanted to talk.

The surveillance turned up nothing more of use. Crone wasn't surprised. He knew it was unlikely that Anthony was simply going to admit to killing the child, to Angela or anyone else. If they were lucky, Anthony might try to explain or rationalize her death in a way that would point to his culpability. But he didn't.

It was time to review the case with the Crown. It looked like everything would rest on Smith's autopsy report. But was that enough to warrant an arrest? The first person the detectives approached was Assistant Crown Attorney Margaret Creal. After reviewing all the material, Creal told them the case looked like a difficult one for the Crown. She wasn't sure there was a reasonable chance of conviction.

On March 1, 1999, almost a year after Athena's death, the detectives arranged a meeting with Smith, Chiasson and another assistant Crown attorney, Anthony Loparco, to review the investigation. Smith said he believed Athena's head injury was several days old. He said the bruising was also days old and evolving.

But the parents had taken her to their family doctor two days before she died, and he hadn't noticed any bruising on the child at all.

Smith said the laceration to Athena's liver was caused by a compressive force, as if someone or something had squeezed her lower chest or stomach area. "It could be from a blow, from a fist hitting her in the abdomen," he explained. "We also see this kind of injury in car accidents, from the seatbelt pressing against a person forcefully. But that's obviously not an issue in this case." The pathologist said the liver injury occurred separately from the injuries to the head and ribs.

At the end of the meeting, Loparco offered no opinion on how to proceed.

Then, nine days later, another development. Dr. Bill Lucas, the regional coroner responsible for the case, called Crone: London Life Insurance was requesting a copy of the autopsy report. Angela was making a claim as a beneficiary on a life insurance policy she and Anthony had taken out in Athena's name.

Looking back through the case file, Crone noticed that the insurance agent had shown up at their apartment the day Athena died. Had he found the missing link in the case: a motive for the child's death?

The detective was less enthused after running it down. A life insurance policy can also be used as a savings fund. A portion of the premiums would go toward insurance coverage; the rest would grow as a cash investment within the policy, which the holder could withdraw later in life. Life insurance plans are often sold to parents as an education savings fund. The insurance agent, Robert Schindelheim, was a customer at the massage parlour where Angela worked. He had sold a similar plan to one of Angela's coworkers. Less than two weeks before Athena died, Angela and Anthony had purchased plans for the whole family. Schindelheim had shown up at their apartment the day Athena died only because they still had paperwork to complete. Athena's plan was worth $15,865. Crone found it coincidental, but not quite a smoking gun given the circumstances of the purchase and the relatively small payout.

Eight weeks later, the two detectives took the case further up the chain to Crown Attorney John McMahon—and finally had a breakthrough. After reviewing the evidence, McMahon told them he thought it would be appropriate to charge Anthony Kporwodu with manslaughter in the death of his daughter.

On May 3, 1999, almost fourteen months after Athena's death, her father turned himself in to police. He was released the next day, after a $15,000 surety bond was posted by a family friend.

Assistant Crown Attorney Rita Zaied was assigned to prosecute the case. That July, she asked the investigating detectives to set up a meeting with Smith. They met on July 20.

Zaied asked the pathologist when the lacerated liver occurred. Smith said he believed it happened within twelve hours of her death.

Crone couldn't believe his ears. He had already gone over the timing issues with Smith. During the autopsy, the pathologist told him he couldn't date any of the injuries. Now, apparently, he could.

Smith's timing of the liver injury brought Angela Veno into the crime. Both parents had told police they were home for the full twenty-four hours before Athena's death, which meant Angela was also home when the liver injury occurred.

With one sentence, Smith had expanded the entire scope of the case.

"Well, that's it. She's in," Zaied said.

She pointed out that according to Smith's report, Athena was beaten on multiple occasions. Her parents may not have intended to kill her, but they knew, or should have known, that she could die from the repeated beatings. The charge for both parents, she said, should therefore be upgraded from manslaughter to second-degree murder.

Smith's opinion on the timing of the liver laceration caught Crone off guard, but it wasn't actually new. In his autopsy report he called the laceration "acute." He called it the same thing in a telephone conversation with Linton the day he completed the report. But the significance of that one word eluded the detectives until this meeting, nine months later. In medical terminology, acute can mean of rapid onset or short term—that is, an acute injury would have occurred shortly before death. Smith never specifically spelled out the significance of the timing; it was only mentioned in passing during an overview of the findings. And while it is in his report, it was a single word buried in fifteen pages of highly technical medical jargon.

This time, when Smith uttered that one word a lukewarm case suddenly became red hot. It had taken meetings with three Crown prosecutors for the detectives to feel confident in laying a manslaughter charge against Anthony. Now they were being told to charge both parents with second-degree murder.

Crone understood the Crown's reasoning. Even if Anthony was the one who did the beatings, Angela, being present during the twenty-four hours before Athena's death, would have to have known about them.

But he still felt uncomfortable with the direction Zaied was pushing the case. The picture she was painting of Angela and Anthony wasn't the same picture he'd painted for himself during sixteen months of investigation. Yes, he could picture a scenario in which Anthony shook Athena violently, or hit her out of exhaustion or frustration. But what the Crown was now describing required a level of intentional callousness that he simply did not see.

Crone left the meeting without voicing his concerns, but he couldn't shake his growing unease. How had they gone more than sixteen months into their investigation and only now be dealing with the timing of the liver laceration? Smith's eccentricities were well known among police, coroners and Crowns. He spent his career dissecting dead children, so eccentricities were to be expected. But recently Crone had started to hear rumblings of something much more troubling. The pathologist was chronically disorganized and often late finishing his reports. The detective had seen it firsthand.

Crone was a member of the Ontario Homicide Investigators Association, and he'd bumped into a detective with the Sudbury police, Robert Keetch, at a recent meeting. Idle conversation turned to cases, including the Kporwodu file. Keetch was shocked to hear that Toronto police were still working with Dr. Smith. He said the pathologist had botched one of their investigations. A toddler in Sudbury named Nicholas Gagnon had died in his mother's care. Smith said the medical evidence pointed to a homicide, but the Crown advised police to not lay charges against the child's mother because of concerns about the quality of Smith's autopsy report.

Crone didn't think Smith's assessment of Athena's injuries was wrong, exactly. Pictures were taken during the autopsy, and other qualified specialists had assisted in examining the body. The detective wasn't worried about the strength of the evidence.

Crone's concern was that Smith was inconsistent. He clearly remembered Smith telling him during the autopsy that he couldn't date the liver laceration. And now he said he could. To the detective, it sounded like the pathologist was contradicting his own initial opinion.

During a phone call on October 27, Smith did tell Crone's partner, Larry Linton, that he believed Athena's liver laceration was acute—the information was in his autopsy report as well. But the pathologist never explained to Crone that this was a new opinion, or that it was evidence of multiple assaults.

Now Crone was being asked to upgrade the charges to second-degree murder on the pathologist's words—words he was starting to distrust. If Smith changed his opinion yet again, Crone would be left with charges he could no longer support. The whole case could collapse.

His solution: get Smith to put his opinion in writing. If the pathologist felt the liver laceration was less than twelve hours old, then he'd have to say so in an addendum to his autopsy report. The detective wouldn't charge Anthony or Angela with second-degree murder until he had that opinion in writing.

Crone asked Smith for a written statement within days of the July meeting. The pathologist grumbled but said he would provide one. But no statement arrived. Three months later, the detective asked again.

"Fine," the pathologist replied. "I'll finish it tonight."

A week passed. The detective paged Smith at the hospital. He left him a message asking him to call. Both attempts went unanswered. A month later, the detective tried again. And again, Smith said the statement would be ready the next day. And again it wasn't.

By late November 1999, almost twenty-one months since Athena's death and seven months since Anthony's manslaughter charge was laid, the detectives needed to get the case moving or the delays could start to become an issue. Under the Charter of Rights and Freedoms, defendants have a right to have their charges heard in a timely manner. If a judge rules that delays in bringing a case to trial are unreasonable, under the Charter, the charges can be thrown out. Even murder charges.

The Crown was livid that the upgraded charges had yet to be laid. On November 30, Zaied called Crone to say that she'd spoken with her boss and that he agreed: they had grounds to charge both parents with second-degree murder. The message was clear: stop stalling and lay the damn charges.

Frustrated, the detective decided he could wait no longer. For months, Smith had been promising to complete the addendum but had yet to produce it. Crone felt duty bound to move forward with the murder charges. On December 6, he called Anthony's lawyer, James J. Grosberg. The same day, on Grosberg's recommendation, Angela hired her own lawyer, John Rosen.

Rosen is a big player in the world of Canadian criminal defence lawyers. He defended convicted murderer and rapist Paul Bernardo, but that was only one of many high-profile cases he'd handled over more than twenty-five years in the business.

Rosen told Angela that she was going to have to turn herself in. He made arrangements for her to surrender.

FIVE

DETECTIVE SERGEANT CRONE was being pressured to lay charges based on Dr. Smith's opinion, an opinion the pathologist had yet to put down in writing. And only a month earlier, the CBC program *the fifth estate* had aired a documentary, "Diagnosis: Murder," examining Smith's shoddy work in several cases, including those of Lianne Gagnon and Sam MacIntosh (who went unnamed in the report).

Crone was also familiar with the Brenda Waudby case in Peterborough; his wife had worked with Maja Schlegel, the undercover officer on the case. The legal and judicial communities were abuzz over the accusations against Smith, which reinforced rumours that had been circulating for years. Taken together—Smith's flip-flop in Athena's case, plus the questions swirling around several of his other cases—the signs were too much to ignore. Crone decided he could not upgrade the charges until Smith put his opinion in writing.

He called Crown Attorney John McMahon to voice his concerns. He called Assistant Crown Rita Zaied. The detective convinced them both. And then he called John Rosen and James J. Grosberg to tell them there would be no murder charges until Smith produced his written statement.

Another six weeks passed and there was still no addendum. On February 1, 2000, Crone put his request in writing. The situation was escalating, and now he wanted a paper trail. The detective explained to Smith that the delay had ground the case to a halt, and that it had compromised the police and Crown's disclosure requirements. The case the Crown was building would turn on what Smith said about the timing of the liver laceration. But the detective couldn't disclose this information to the Crown because he didn't have it in writing.

"Despite my many phone calls and your assurances," he wrote to Smith, "I have not yet received the additional information requested. I fully appreciate how full your schedule is, but the situation is now critical and I must formally request, in the strongest possible terms, that the additional information I have requested be forwarded to me as soon as possible."

No response.

Zaied wrote a similar request weeks later.

No response.

On March 6, 2000, on the second anniversary of Athena Kporwodu's death, Anthony appeared in court for the fifteenth time. Most of the court dates so far had been largely inconsequential while the Crown and police waited for Smith's written addendum. Zaied's frustration was palpable in court as she explained to the judge the efforts to obtain it.

"We've written letters, I've called, the police have called numerous times. Understandably, counsel is anxious to get on with this and so is the Crown. I am considering taking the unusual step, Your Honour, of sub-poenaing the doctor to come to Court to get some explanation as to when we're going to get this other report . . . Without [it], we're sort of stuck."

The Crown's threat was unprecedented, but even that didn't prompt Smith to write his addendum. So, on April 3, Crone followed through, subpoenaing Smith to appear in court the next week.

That finally did the trick. Smith's addendum arrived on Crone's desk the next day.

His letter outlined Athena's injuries, stating that she had suffered head injuries on at least two occasions; one was acute, less than a day old, and the second was weeks old. He said the child's fractured ribs may have resulted from a single assault or repeated beatings. She had acute injuries to her chest wall and lungs that were less than a day old. The liver laceration was also acute, less than twelve hours old. Smith believed the child was beaten on at least two occasions and possibly more, one of which was within a day of her death.

It was a single page, 265 words long. It had taken Smith 260 days to produce it.

But, finally, it was written confirmation of what Smith had told Crone and Zaied the previous July: the child's injuries showed a pattern of repeated abuse, including a beating that occurred within a day of her death, when she was in the care of both parents.

It is worth noting that most of this information was already in Smith's post-mortem report. The addendum did summarize his opinions on the timing of Athena's various injuries more clearly and concisely than in his final report. But the timing of the liver laceration, which is what prompted Crone's request for a written addendum in the first place, was listed as acute in the original report. If the purpose of the addendum was to establish Athena had suffered multiple injuries on multiple occasions, including at least one acute injury while she was under the care of both parents, the autopsy report already did that.

When I asked the detective about this, years later, he said that what he'd wanted from Smith was his methodology. "If you say to me, 'How can you tell an old rib fracture from a new rib fracture?' well, [a pathologist] can give you that answer. I can give you that answer; I know what that means," he told me. "But if you are going to tell me that the liver laceration is acute, I want you to tell me why you know that it's acute or why it happened in the last twelve hours of her life. I need to know why."

Given Smith's growing reputation for being unreliable, the detective wanted a solid footing for the case. Yet Smith's addendum did not address his methodology. It did not explain how he came to his conclusions.

Nevertheless, police and the Crown proceeded with the upgraded charges.

(Years later, Dr. Smith would complain to Detective Linton that, in his view, an autopsy report should include only an opinion on the *cause* of death. Smith felt Crone's request for written confirmation of his opinions on the timing of Athena's injuries was inappropriate. He even considered seeking legal counsel before responding to the request. This was the first time he'd ever voiced such concerns. In fact, he testified at the preliminary hearing that he understood one of his duties as a pediatric pathologist was to determine, whenever possible, the timing of the fatal injuries to establish a suspect's exclusive opportunity.)

With the addendum finally in hand, the case started moving again. In May 2000, Angela and Anthony were charged with second-degree murder. The previous four months had been devastating for the couple. Worried Julius would become a Crown ward, lost to them forever before the case was even heard, Anthony and Angela signed over custody to Anthony's parents. They were happy he was being raised by family, but there was one large caveat: Anthony's parents lived in Ghana. Julius had flown to his new home in early April. Angela and Anthony had expected to be charged with murder in December, but then they heard nothing more. They were left on tenterhooks, wondering if the charges were ever coming.

Angela and Anthony surrendered to police on May 15, 2000. They were released on bail later that day. Their preliminary hearing was set to start in January 2001.

Cindy Wasser was John Rosen's law partner at the time, and her eyes lit up when he told her that they were taking a case in which Charles Smith would play a prominent role. Wasser had a history with Smith. She had faced him in a trial more than a decade earlier and had been so disturbed by what she witnessed that she had been hoping ever since to get another crack at him.

Julie Bowers's murder trial was a media sensation at the time. Her eleven-month-old son, Dustin, had disappeared on January 14, 1988, in Kincardine, Ontario. Bowers told police that Dustin was snatched from his car seat when she left him unattended for a minute to run into the bank. A tragic case, to be sure, but what caught the media's attention was the manner in which the boy's body was found the next day. Bowers told police that she had a dream about her son the night after he disappeared. She then joined their search and led them to his body, which was found in a patch of dense bush outside town.

To investigators, it looked like a clear-cut case. There was no abduction; Bowers had killed her son. Overcome with guilt, she then led police to his body. How else could she have known where it was?

Julie Bowers was charged with second-degree murder. Fresh out of law school, Cindy Wasser was junior counsel on the case under Jack Pinkofsky, a leading criminal defence lawyer at the time. Another fast-rising lawyer, James Lockyer, was also on the defence team.

Despite the damning circumstances surrounding the discovery of Dustin's body, Wasser was convinced the child *had* been abducted and Julie Bowers was innocent. The case against Bowers hinged on the time of death. She told police that Dustin disappeared from her car at 1 p.m. If the time of death was before that, it would be evidence of her guilt. If it was after that, it would support her story of an abduction.

Smith did the autopsy, and his estimate of the time of Dustin's death was a moving target. He initially suggested Dustin was placed in the snow at 5:30 p.m., more than four hours after the reported abduction. But according to media reports of the trial, by the time Smith took the stand he'd changed his opinion, concluding that Dustin could have been abandoned in the snow as early as 8 a.m., five hours before Bowers said he was taken. Smith said the child died of hypothermia.

Pinkofsky brought in an expert witness who had a very different opinion. Janice Ophoven, a pediatric forensic pathologist in Minnesota, was troubled by her interactions with Dr. Smith from the earliest stages of the trial. She requested that he send her the slides he took during Dustin's autopsy so she could do her own review, but there were inordinate delays. Then, when he finally sent them, they were the wrong ones: they belonged to an elderly patient with Alzheimer's.

At the time, Cindy Wasser and the rest of Bowers's legal team dismissed the mistake as a sign of Smith's disorganization and unprofessionalism. But Ophoven was deeply disturbed. She said there were strict protocols governing the handling of autopsy specimens to prevent just this type of error. (Media reports suggested the mix-up occurred because Smith kept some of the specimens at his home.) The mistake had put Ophoven on high alert.

When Ophoven arrived in Toronto for the trial, Wasser picked her up at the airport and they went out to dinner. Wasser recalled years later, "She sits down and she says, 'I did not want to do this on the phone but here's what I've discovered: Dustin was likely still alive when he was found and could have been resuscitated. The tissue slides show that he actually died of suffocation in the rubber body bag.'"

Wasser remembers all the air being sucked out of the room as those words sunk in: Dustin was likely alive when he was found, he could have been saved, but the coroner had inadvertently killed him. It was almost beyond comprehension.

And it fell to Wasser to tell Bowers about Ophoven's suspicion. She remembers the long trek over to Bowers's hotel. Julie's husband had come down to Toronto to be with her for the trial. The lawyer told them there was compelling evidence that someone else was responsible for Dustin's death. It should have been good news, but then came the kicker: they believed that that someone else was the coroner.

In court, Dr. Ophoven explained that death by hypothermia is a slow process. Vital signs can disappear before a person actually dies. "Re-establishing a normal temperature, re-warming and resuscitation before deciding absence of life is the case, is important and in my opinion must be done," she testified.

According to media reports, court was told the coroner pronounced Dustin dead at the scene after failing to detect vital signs. The child's body was moved to the side of the road while the death investigation continued. But Ophoven testified that Dustin should have been rushed to hospital immediately; she suspected he was, in fact, still alive. She said the only sign of freezing she found in his organs was slight freezing in his voice box. The only sign of frostbite was on his left foot. Skin and testicles show the first signs of freezing. Dustin's testicles appeared normal. Ophoven testified the child was likely left in the snow between 10 p.m. and midnight the night before he was found. Her expert opinion was that he died on the side of the road, or worse, he suffocated in the rubber body bag used to transport his body to Toronto for autopsy.

Wasser said the death investigation team would have been less experienced in a rural area of the province like Kincardine, and Smith would have been its most experienced member. She believes Smith should have known hypothermia resuscitation protocols and shared them with the local coroner.

Ophoven had previously explained to the defence team that at autopsy she took the internal body temperature with a thermometer, inserted anally, and then made calculations based on what the person was wearing and the temperature outside at the time the body was found to determine how long the body had been left out in the cold. Ophoven said the process was standard practice for pathologists. But Wasser said when the defence asked Smith about it on the stand, he testified that the Hospital for Sick Children didn't have any of those thermometers, so he had used a different method to calculate how long Dustin had been left in the cold.

Wasser found it odd that SickKids, a world-class hospital, would not have one of these thermometers on hand, so during a break she and a colleague walked over to the hospital to double-check. She recalled, "We went up to this particular wing and spoke to some nurses, and asked, 'Do you have these kinds of thermometers? We need one.' And she said, 'Oh, we've got boxes of them in the supply room. How many do you need?'" Wasser then asked the nurse if the hospital had always had these thermometers. The nurse nodded.

"At that moment, I stood there and thought, 'Wow, this forensic pathologist who is like a god has perjured himself.' I had never experienced that as a young lawyer, but it's the stuff that you watch in movies."

Wasser asked the nurse to come to the courthouse to testify. They brought a box of thermometers. Smith was called back to the stand.

"You could see the jurors' faces, the disgust, when Jack confronted him. He was so unconcerned about it," she recalled. "As he got off the stand and walked past the jury, it looked to me like they were actually going to hurl spit at him. That was the look on their faces."

Julie Bowers's legal team was also able to challenge the significance of her dream. An expert witness testified that the details of her dream—that Dustin was outside in the snow—could easily be understood. He said it was perfectly reasonable for Bowers to dream about her son lying out in the snow. He had just gone missing; it was the middle of January. Her defence team argued that it was her desperation and doggedness—and a lot of luck—that led her to find him.

The jury agreed and came back with a verdict of not guilty.

After the trial, Cindy Wasser waited for the other shoe to drop. Given how Smith's opinion on when the child was dumped in the snow kept changing, given how Pinkofsky eviscerated him on the stand and, most troubling, given that Smith did not know the proper resuscitation protocols in child hypothermia cases, Wasser thought there were going to be consequences.

Smith's incompetence was plain to see. If winning was the Crown's objective, he didn't help. If justice was the objective, he was on the wrong side of that as well. And if Dustin's survival had really been in the cards, as Ophoven believed, the failings of Dr. Smith, the coroner and the rest of the emergency response team on the scene cost them the chance to save him.

But there were no consequences.

The young lawyer watched helplessly from the sidelines as Smith continued his professional ascent. But she vowed that if she ever got another chance to face him in court, she would make the most of it.

A decade later, her second chance arrived.

Cindy Wasser's partner John Rosen was lead counsel for Angela Veno. Anthony Kporwodu replaced his old counsel, James J. Grosberg, with a more experienced criminal lawyer, Delmar Doucette. Wasser says she was keen to challenge Smith on the strength of his medical opinions, but Rosen thought this wasn't the right case to challenge him directly. The evidence was incontrovertible. With Athena's head injuries and thirty-plus rib fractures, it seemed obvious that someone had beaten the child. The question was who. The defence strategy for both Angela and Anthony would be to point suspicion at one of the babysitters.

Doucette's theory was that the child had been severely beaten on a single occasion sometime in the weeks leading up to her death, and that had caused all her rib fractures and her head injuries. At trial, he was going to argue that Athena's acute injuries—specifically, the laceration to her liver—were accidentally caused during CPR by Anthony or the paramedics.

Anthony and Angela didn't agree with their own defence counsels. They didn't think either of their babysitters was any more capable of hurting Athena than they were. Both parents pushed their lawyers to challenge the Crown's case on the medical evidence itself. They believed there had to be an underlying medical reason for Athena's death. Wasser was keen to try, but she said Rosen steered her away.

"I kept saying to John, 'No, I want to pursue Smith. I want to pursue Smith,' and he kept telling me to stop it, that it was an emotional issue and I had to back down. He spoke to the other counsel, who tried to have nice warm, soft talks with me about backing down."

The couple's preliminary hearing began on January 15, 2001, almost three years after Athena died.

A week into the hearing, another bombshell involving Smith landed. The headline in the *Toronto Sun* screamed, "'Justice' Done as Woman Freed." The accompanying story explained the Crown's decision to stay a second-degree murder charge against a Toronto woman, Maureen Laidley, in the death of her boyfriend's four-year-old son, Tyrell Salmon. And Charles Smith was at the centre of that case as well.

Tyrell died on January 23, 1998, only six weeks before Athena. Laidley told investigators the boy had been jumping on a couch and fell, hitting his head on a marble table or tile floor before he died. But Smith, who conducted the autopsy, concluded that Laidley's explanation could not explain the child's death.

In preparation for the trial, Laidley's lawyer, John Struthers, contacted three forensic pathologists who contradicted Smith's evidence, arguing that Laidley's explanation of an accidental fall could indeed explain Tyrell's death. The Crown also consulted with a colleague of Smith's at the Hospital for Sick Children, neurosurgeon Robin Humphreys, who could not say whether Tyrell's head injury was accidental or non-accidental. Given the conflicting medical opinions, Crown prosecutor Frank Armstrong decided there was no longer a reasonable prospect of a conviction and withdrew the murder charge.

Smith's already tarnished reputation took an even harder blow just three days later.

On January 25, Crown counsel withdrew a second-degree murder charge against Louise Reynolds for killing her daughter, Sharon Reynolds, in Kingston, Ontario. The seven-year-old had been reported missing on June 12, 1997. Officers with the Kingston police found the child's body in the basement of her home. It looked as though she had been savagely attacked, with dozens of penetrating wounds to her partially clad body. A large piece of her scalp was ripped off and flung nearby. Officers noted a strong smell of animal urine and feces in the basement, but the only dog present in the house at the time was a small family dog.

Smith performed a post-mortem exam in Toronto. At the time, he had little experience with penetrating wounds, having seen only one or two stab-wound cases and one or two others involving dog bites. He did the autopsy anyway, and concluded that Sharon had died of blood loss caused by multiple stab wounds.

A day or two later, though, police learned that the small family dog hadn't been the only animal in the house that day. A neighbour's pit bull was also there. According to the Goudge Inquiry, police learned that the pit bull had a red substance on its chest and paws when its owner picked it up on the night of Sharon's death. There was blood on the dog's collar, and its feces may have had blond hairs in it for days afterwards. The dog was euthanized two months later because of an unrelated nipping incident.

After discovering the pit bull's presence in the home, a police officer raised concerns about some of the markings on Sharon's back. Smith told the officer definitively that a domestic or wild animal did not cause the marks. Nine days later, Louise Reynolds was charged with second-degree murder. The police's theory was that she had killed her daughter in a fit of rage over Sharon's head lice. Reynolds was held in custody without bail while she awaited her trial.

Reynolds maintained her innocence. The defence's position was that Sharon died in a vicious attack by the pit bull; her wounds were dog bites, not stab wounds. The Crown countered by hiring a forensic odontologist to study her wounds. Robert Wood reviewed photographs from Smith's autopsy and concluded that, "without equivocation," Sharon's injuries were not dog bites. The Crown now had two expert opinions supporting its theory that Louise Reynolds stabbed her daughter to death.

It took Smith nine months to complete his autopsy. As in Athena's case, police had to issue a subpoena to get him to appear in court to produce the report. In it, he maintained his earlier position that Sharon suffered multiple stab wounds.

Undeterred, Reynolds's lawyer hired his own forensic odontologist. Robert Dorion reviewed the same autopsy photographs and prepared a report that directly contradicted Smith and Wood. Dorion believed the child was bitten at least twenty times, and the marks were caused by a powerful animal, most likely a dog.

Smith testified at Reynolds's preliminary hearing, which ran for fifteen days over seven months starting in April 1998, the month after Athena died. Wood did not testify. According to the Goudge Inquiry, Smith was unequivocal in his testimony: Sharon suffered multiple stab wounds; a pair of scissors was the likely weapon. When asked about the possibility that a dog may have been responsible, Smith responded dismissively, "As absurd as it is to think that a polar bear attacked Sharon, so is it equally absurd that it's a dog wound." On November 19, the judge committed Louise Reynolds to stand trial for second-degree murder. At this point, she had been in custody for seventeen months.

Three months later, Dr. James Young and Dr. Jim Cairns, the top two officials at the provincial Coroner's Office, attended a meeting of the American Academy of Forensic Sciences, where they learned that Dr. Dorion was not the only respected expert questioning the Crown's position in the Reynolds case. Another forensic odontologist, Lowell Levine, and two forensic pathologists, Michael Baden and Rex Ferris, also disagreed with Smith's opinions. They warned Young and Cairns that a miscarriage of justice might be unfolding in Kingston.

Cairns met with Smith, Wood and David Chiasson, the province's chief forensic pathologist. Smith and Wood maintained their position that a dog was not responsible for Sharon's wounds, but the group decided to disinter the body and conduct a second autopsy to be sure.

Sharon's body was exhumed in June 1999. Smith and Wood were joined by Dorion and Ferris, both of whom were retained by the defence. Upon completing the autopsy, Wood and Smith both revised their opinions. A dog had attacked Sharon, they now said, but it was still possible that some of the injuries—particularly some marks on Sharon's skull and neck— were caused by a weapon.

The defence experts disagreed, arguing that all of the child's injuries were bite marks caused by a dog. Ferris, in particular, criticized Smith's methodology and conclusions.

Still faced with opposing expert opinions, the Coroner's Office hired another expert to review the two autopsies and all the accompanying reports. They settled on Steven Symes, a forensic anthropologist from the University of Tennessee who was an authority on saw and knife marks. Symes concluded that most of Sharon's injuries were suffered during a dog attack. He did note that there were marks on the child's skull that appeared to be unrelated; he thought their likely cause was a scalpel or sharp knife.

By December 2000, even Jim Cairns—one of Smith's staunchest sup- porters—was skeptical of Smith's opinion in the case. The next month, Crown Attorney Ed Bradley spoke to Smith again. For the first time, Smith acknowledged that he could not dispute the evidence offered by the other experts, although he still believed that at least some of Sharon's injuries were not caused by a dog attack.

On January 25, 2001—in the midst of Anthony Kporwodu and Angela Veno's preliminary hearing—Bradley announced that he was withdrawing the second-degree murder charge against Louise Reynolds, concluding that the Crown no longer had proof that Sharon's death was caused by stab wounds.

Reynolds had spent twenty-two months behind bars awaiting trial. Her surviving daughter had been seized by Children's Aid and placed for adoption.

Within the course of one week, Crown attorneys had withdrawn charges in two murder cases that heavily relied on Smith's medical opinions. Other forensic pathologists provided compelling evidence that he might have been, or was, wrong. The media reported that Smith's professional conduct was under "heavy assault."

James Young, the province's chief coroner, worried that all the media scrutiny was bad not just for Smith's reputation but for the Chief Coroner's Office as well. Smith had become a lightning rod for scrutiny, and Young decided that both Smith and the Chief Coroner's Office would be better off if he temporarily stopped working on coroner's cases. It was the first time anyone had considered taking any such action. For Young, the issue was not Smith's competence or the quality of his work. He still had confidence in both. Rather, he felt the move would help maintain the reputation of the Coroner's Office. He reasoned that the added scrutiny Smith was facing would impede his ability to work on coroner's cases anyway. David Chiasson, the province's chief forensic pathologist at the time, did have some concerns about Smith's competency and welcomed the decision to remove him from coroner's cases.

Young and Cairns told Smith of their decision. They gave him the option to resign voluntarily. On January 25, 2001—the same day the charges against Louise Reynolds were withdrawn—Smith wrote a letter to Young requesting he be removed from performing forensic autopsies and requesting an external review of his work.

Young agreed, but didn't publicize the decision. He would later tell the Goudge Inquiry that he considered it an internal matter. Issuing a press release would damage Smith's reputation and make it more difficult to rehire him. Within days, however, reporters were asking Young if the embattled pathologist was still doing autopsies for the provincial Coroner's Office. At this point, Young announced his decision—explaining it had come after a request from Smith himself. The province's top coroner added that an independent external review of Smith's work would be conducted before he would be allowed to return.

At a meeting on January 26, senior officials discussed an extensive independent review of Smith's work. All that was decided then was that any review should include Smith's role in the Sharon Reynolds case. Calls were made to pathologists outside Canada to gauge their interest in and availability for a review. (Locating and organizing the relevant files related to Smith's work was a problem. Officials found information on all the autopsies Smith had done on coroner's warrants going back fifteen years, but the details were scarce. The files didn't indicate which cases went to trial. They contained no records of his consultations.)

On January 31, John McMahon, the director of Crown attorneys for the Toronto region, met with Cairns and Chiasson to discuss the controversy regarding Smith. McMahon expressed concern about Smith's reliability and the effect his involvement could have on current homicide prosecutions. It was agreed that all Smith's active criminal cases would be reviewed by the Chief Coroner's Office to ensure that his opinions were medically sound. Cases in which his opinions were sound but might reasonably be disputed at trial by qualified medical experts would be referred to an independent expert for further review. McMahon advised that reviews be conducted by an outside pathologist not connected to the provincial Chief Coroner's Office to ensure they were independent.

McMahon left the meeting with the understanding that a thorough review of Dr. Smith's work was under way. Crown attorneys and police worked on pulling the files together. Three months later, McMahon's office sent to Cairns a list of nineteen potential cases for review. McMahon believed a review of all or at least some of those cases would be undertaken. He assumed the Coroner's Office review would be wide in scope and would examine possible wrongful convictions.

However, James Young believed the purpose of the review was to determine whether Smith should be allowed to resume doing coroner's autopsies. According to the Goudge Inquiry, Young did not consider a review by the Chief Coroner's Office to be either in the public interest or a tool to determine whether Smith had contributed to any miscarriages of justice. Senior officials at the Coroner's Office weren't even on the same page about the scope of a review. Young and Cairns thought it should extend only to cases that were still before the courts. Chiasson thought it should encompass all active and completed criminal cases. The review was in disarray before it even began.

Within three weeks of his decision to conduct the review, Young changed his mind. On February 8, 2001, Louise Reynolds launched a $7 million lawsuit against the police and several medical officials, including Smith. As Young would later testify at the Goudge Inquiry, his decision not to reinstate Smith until the Reynolds lawsuit was resolved negated the need for any review, since the only purpose of that review was to determine whether Smith could return to work for the Chief Coroner's Office. Senior officials at the Coroner's Office determined that a review of Smith's role in the Reynolds case was no longer necessary, since it would be reviewed extensively in the context of the civil lawsuit.

Young did not explain to anyone his rationale for stopping the review. He did not tell John McMahon at the Crown Attorney's Office, or anyone else. And he didn't publicly acknowledge the decision until months later.

Meanwhile, the defence teams for Angela and Anthony, along with several police forces, were left with the impression that the Chief Coroner's Office was conducting an extensive review of Dr. Smith's work.

SIX

CROWN PROSECUTOR RITA Zaied realized that Smith's involvement in the case against Angela Veno and Anthony Kporwodu was becoming a liability. She didn't doubt his conclusions—Athena's injuries spoke for themselves—but it would be infinitely easier for the defence to raise doubts about them with all this controversy swirling around Smith's work on other cases. She also knew the clock was ticking. It had been almost three years since Athena died, almost two since the manslaughter charge was first laid against Anthony, and they weren't yet through the preliminary hearing for their joint trial. A Charter challenge was beginning to look like a real possibility.

Section 11(b) of the Canadian Charter of Rights and Freedoms guards against unreasonable delays for a defendant awaiting trial. Zaied didn't think such a challenge would be successful, but it was another arrow in the defence's quiver. She decided she would finish all the non-medical testimony, then ask the court for a recess. That way she could bring in another forensic pathologist to review Athena's autopsy materials to make sure the Crown was on solid ground. Hopefully, it wouldn't take more than a couple of months. The preliminary hearing was adjourned in early February 2001.

With help from the Chief Coroner's Office, Zaied settled on Patricia McFeeley, a forensic pathologist with the University of New Mexico Health Sciences Center, to review Smith's work in Athena's case.

The defence teams didn't want any more delays. They knew the Crown's case would be easier to knock down if it was supported only by Smith's opinion. So if another pathologist was being brought in, the question was for what purpose. The defence asked the court whether the Crown was using McFeeley to shore up Smith's opinion? Or was McFeeley going to do a truly independent review and come to her own conclusions?

The Crown assured Justice Brian Trafford that the court would be getting the latter.

While McFeeley completed her review, pressure continued to mount for a more formal, public investigation into Smith's involvement in a number of cases. In April 2001, counsel for William Mullins-Johnson twice asked the Chief Coroner's Office to review the work Smith had done investigating the death of Valin Johnson, Mullins-Johnson's four-year-old niece. Smith had testified at the trial that Valin was sexually assaulted at or around the time of death. Although other pathologists agreed that Valin had been sexually assaulted, Smith was the only expert who found signs that she was being sexually assaulted when she died. But Smith did not do the autopsy on Valin's body; he completed a consultation report. And because the Chief Coroner's Office had no way to keep track of consultations, it had no record of Smith's involvement in the case. It did not respond to counsel's request at the time, nor did it conduct any review of the case. Mullins-Johnson would remain in prison for another four years, and it would be six years before his conviction was overturned as a miscarriage of justice.

James Lockyer, a prominent defence lawyer, also wrote to James Young in April 2001, arguing for the necessity of a thorough review of Smith's past cases. Young didn't act on this letter either. He testified at the Goudge Inquiry that he didn't see Lockyer's letter as a request for a broad review, saying that Lockyer, who regularly appeared before the media, would have publicly demanded a review if that's what he wanted. However, the Goudge report noted, "It is difficult to see how Lockyer's letter could have been clearer."

Young's decision to suspend Smith from all coroner's autopsies created a staffing crisis at the Hospital for Sick Children. Ninety per cent of the autopsies Smith did were non-criminal in nature. So Chiasson, in consultation with senior officials at the Chief Coroner's Office, arranged to undertake a quality control review of Smith's non-criminal work, to determine whether he could be reinstated on such cases. They hired Blair Carpenter, a pathologist at the Children's Hospital of Eastern Ontario, in Ottawa, to conduct an internal review of six recent cases. Based on

Carpenter's review, Smith was quietly allowed to resume doing non-criminal autopsies in June 2001.

Angela's and Anthony's defence teams tried to get their hands on the results of the review McMahon believed he had ordered back in January—a review that had never in fact happened. On July 16, Rosen asked the Crown for disclosure. Doucette made a similar request on July 30. He sent another letter on November 2, the day before the preliminary hearing was to resume. Rita Zaied, the Crown, fought disclosure, arguing that which reviews and how much of them should be disclosed was an issue for the judge at trial, not the preliminary hearing. The judge agreed, pushing back disclosure for at least another ten months.

Zaied had hoped to have McFeeley's report in hand by June and so wrap up the preliminary hearing that summer. The court even reserved a week in July. However, McFeeley didn't submit her final three-page report until September. She had reviewed the autopsy reports, including several supplementary reports examining X-rays, a CT scan and the central nervous system. She reviewed ninety-eight autopsy photographs and ninety slides that accompanied the doctors' autopsy reports. Her conclusion: the child suffered a multitude of blunt, traumatic injuries.

The rib fractures were the most obvious. They were older, happening days, weeks, even a month or two before her death. Because of the different stages of healing she saw, McFeeley thought the rib fractures could have occurred on more than one occasion, but determining when and precisely how many times was impossible. She did think that the number of fractures, in addition to their locations and the lack of an adequate explanation (such as a car accident), suggested that they were non-accidental.

She also found evidence of older and acute head injuries. The acute head injury, she believed, was likely the cause of death. The liver laceration could have been non-accidental, or it could have been caused during resuscitation efforts.

"As a whole," McFeeley wrote, "Dr. Smith's autopsy report is complete and extensive."

The preliminary hearing resumed in November and ran for another six weeks.

During this second phase of the hearing, Jim Cairns testified that a number of Smith's autopsies had been selected randomly and sent out for independent review. He said that six cases were reviewed by Dr. Blair Carpenter, of the Children's Hospital of Eastern Ontario, and a further seventeen criminal cases were reviewed by himself, David Chiasson and Barry McLellan at the Chief Coroner's Office. He said ten of those seventeen cases were also externally reviewed at the request of either Crown counsel or defence. All the independent reviews, he said, were completed, except for the review of Smith's work in Sharon Reynolds's case, which was stopped pending the resolution of the lawsuit her mother had launched. Cairns also testified that the three doctors reported their findings to the chief coroner, James Young, in June 2001 and told him that Smith was competent to do pediatric autopsies.

At the Goudge Inquiry, seven years later, Cairns admitted that his testimony at the preliminary hearing and trial suggested the internal review was more thorough and rigorous than it really had been. He conceded that his evidence was confusing and misleading. The defence teams were led to believe the Chief Coroner's Office had done a rigorous, scientific review, which it hadn't. The Goudge report also found that the chart of the seventeen cases Cairns had submitted was incomplete—a fact Cairns knew, since he had received the larger nineteen-case list from the Crown's office a year and a half earlier. Zaied also knew of the longer nineteen-case list, and had not informed the court of its existence. Furthermore, the seventeen-case list was inaccurate about the level of agreement other experts had with Smith's conclusions. The inquiry found the chart would lead a reasonable person to conclude that the Chief Coroner's Office had conducted both an internal and an external review, and that the reviewers agreed with Smith in most cases.

Justice Goudge said none of that was true.

In all, the preliminary hearing took eleven months to complete.

On January 17, 2002, Anthony Kporwodu and Angela Veno were ordered to stand trial for second-degree murder. At the couple's next court appearance, the following month, Rita Zaied upgraded the charges to first-degree murder. The justification for the elevated charge appears to be the life insurance policy Anthony and Angela had taken out on Athena in the weeks before her death. Zaied planned to argue at trial that the $15,585 payout provided a motive for the parents to kill their child.

Det. Sgt. Matt Crone thought that was a stretch. "It was just a bullshit, stupid thing," he told me years later. "The amount of the payoff to me was pretty insignificant. I mean, it would have barely buried the kid. It wasn't a lot of money and I just couldn't get my head around it as a reasonable motive."

The small payout wasn't the detective's only issue. There was also the policy itself. It was sold to the couple more as an education savings tool rather than a straight-ahead insurance plan. And then there was how they came to buy it. Angela and Anthony didn't seek out the insurance company; the sales rep approached Angela at the massage parlour, where he was a customer.

Pre-trial motions began on September 23, 2002—four and a half years after Athena's death and almost three and a half years after the manslaughter charge was laid against Anthony. The Crown had taken steps to bolster its case by contracting two more medical experts to review the case. Dirk Huyer did an overview of all the medical findings and testimony. Robin Humphreys, a neurosurgeon at SickKids, also looked at the case, reviewing Smith's autopsy report, the autopsy photographs, the ambulance records, Hunt's autopsy report, hospital records and Dr. Lo's testimony at the preliminary hearing. Humphreys determined that a prior injury could have resulted in a series of seizures that led to Athena's death.

But the court would have legal arguments to sort out before it could hear the medical evidence. Lawyers for the two defendants filed an application for a stay of proceedings under the Charter of Rights and Freedoms, specifically sections 7—the right to life, liberty and the security of the person—and 11(b)—the right to be tried within a reasonable time. What constituted a "reasonable time" would be up to the judge to decide, but the defence teams had been trying to get all review material related to Smith for twenty-two months. The two teams filed an application for all files related to any reviews relating to Smith done by the Chief Coroner's Office and the College of Physicians and Surgeons of Ontario. The lawyers sent subpoenas to both offices requesting the records.

Rita Zaied filed a motion objecting to the two subpoenas. Denise Dwyer, the lawyer for the Chief Coroner's Office, joined it. (Richard Macklin, lawyer for the College, did not.)

Justice Trafford ruled that he would hear the defence's application.

The Crown immediately sought an adjournment of the trial to file an appeal of that decision to the Supreme Court of Canada. The adjournment was denied.

Justice Trafford ordered the Crown to serve notice to all third parties with privacy interests in the records—mainly the parents and direct relatives of the children at the centre of any cases being reviewed.

The defence teams argued that the seventeen reviews should be released in their entirety. Initially, the list didn't even include the names of the deceased children. The Crown and the Coroner's Office argued that the full files couldn't be released, citing the privacy rights of the families involved in those cases. The defence won the argument. The Coroner's Office was ordered to give all seventeen files to the Crown to be disclosed to the defence. However, the Coroner's Office continued to fight the order, seeking a stay of proceedings. The Crown supported the application.

"I appreciate that you and Ms. Zaied do not have much respect for the way that I have conducted this trial. It is fundamentally apparent to me," Justice Trafford told Denise Dwyer in court. "Everything I do is contested by you and Ms. Zaied retrospectively. It is not unusual for either of you to get up and comment on what you perceive to be the correctness of what I am doing here. It is my obligation to do this trial to the best of my ability. This is what I am doing now. That is what I have done throughout the course of this trial. I have told you that I am not criticizing you personally for the way this is unfolding. I am asking you to do exactly what I said, to achieve the greatest measure of efficiency so I can ensure the fairness of this trial. Will you do it?"

"You ordered me, sir. I'll do it," Dwyer replied.

Two weeks later, Justice Trafford dismissed the application to stay proceedings, and the Coroner's Office was again ordered to hand over the seventeen case files for disclosure.

Tensions were reaching a breaking point. Justice Trafford had come down hard on Zaied and Dwyer for their lack of professionalism. He found they had engaged in duplicitous conduct and acted in bad faith. His ruling would have repercussions on the case in the weeks to come. Given the judge's thorough dressing-down of Rita Zaied, the Crown decided that she could no longer effectively represent the state in the case. The Chief Coroner's Office likewise removed Denise Dwyer.

By the time proceedings resumed in January 2003, new lawyers had been brought in for the Crown and the Chief Coroner's Office. Julie Battersby took over for the Crown—and immediately asked for an adjournment so she could familiarize herself with the case. The case did not resume again until April. (In the meantime, Justice Trafford was assigned another murder trial.) Neither Battersby nor anyone else from the Crown's office suggested that Justice Trafford had shown bias in his ruling and his criticisms of Zaied. No one asked the judge to recuse himself.

Meanwhile, the defence continued its efforts to have the murder charges against Angela and Anthony thrown out on Charter grounds, and on June 23, 2003, they won. Justice Trafford entered a stay of proceedings against both defendants under the Charter of Rights and Freedoms, effectively halting all legal proceedings in the case (outside of the Crown's right to appeal). The judge ruled that the delays in bringing the charges to trial had infringed upon Angela's and Anthony's rights to life, liberty and security of the person, and their right to be tried within a reasonable time.

Justice Trafford was critical of both Zaied and Dwyer for contributing to the delay. "They were unduly confrontational," he wrote in his ruling, "with the result being that these applications have taken much more time to complete than they should have in this case."

In calculating the total length of the delay, the judge started the clock at Athena's death on March 6, 1998, rather than when Anthony was charged with manslaughter fourteen months later. This is unusual, but Trafford went with the date of death because he ruled that police and the coroner breached their duties by allowing Athena's body to be cremated.

The judge further ruled that Detectives Crone and Linton should have charged both defendants with second-degree murder on March 7, 1998— the day after Athena died—when Dr. Smith first told them she had suffered multiple traumatic injuries. That way, the defendants could have had a second autopsy completed before Athena's body was mistakenly cremated on May 29. The defence had argued that police and the coroner "knew the defendants, on the advice of counsel, wanted to have a second autopsy if Dr. Smith's opinion tended to incriminate either or both of them, and they failed to take steps necessary to preserve her body." The judge agreed, noting that Ross Bennett, the coroner, had signed a coroner's certificate stating there was no need to hold Athena's body for further examination, even though her parents had clearly said they would like the body held for a possible second autopsy.

"The failure of Dr. Bennett to revoke the certificate, the failure of Dr. Bennett to offer the facilities of OCCO"—the Chief Coroner's Office— "to secure Athena's body pending the decision on the second autopsy, the failure of Dr. Smith to release a timely report, a report that was necessary to the decision by the defendants' lawyer, and the failure of Det. Linton to advise the defendants of the availability of these public facilities amounted to unacceptable negligence in all the circumstances of the case."

Trafford also took issue with Charles Smith's contribution to the delay. "If Dr. Smith had applied himself with the diligence expected of people in his position, the post-mortem released on October 27, 1998, would have included his opinion on the timing of the fatal injuries." Furthermore, Trafford could find no reason why it had taken Smith nine months to complete his amendment, ruling that a month should have been more than sufficient.

Trafford was very troubled by the review of Smith's work. He said that, as the regional director of Crown operations, John McMahon should have requested or required a written report from the Chief Coroner's Office when its review was completed. Similarly, the Coroner's Office informal review—carried out by Cairns, McLellan and Chiasson—should have been much more formal in nature. "They had a duty to preserve the evidence collected during the review and to properly record all other material aspects of the review, such as the meetings concerning the scope of the review and the selection of the experts to do the review," Trafford wrote, adding that the informality of the review was surprising given how important it was to both the Crown and the Coroner's Office.

Rita Zaied, the Crown attorney, did not escape the judge's criticism either. He found that it was "unreasonable, at best," when she became "confrontational" and otherwise resisted the defence teams' efforts to obtain the file related to the review of Smith's work. The judge said there were ways to allow for disclosure and still protect the privacy rights of the families involved in the review: their names could have been stripped out. Zaied, he wrote, also could have interviewed senior Coroner's Office officials at the preliminary hearing, thus clarifying the scope of the review at a much earlier stage. That would also have revealed that Young had terminated the formal review. The judge said Zaied could have asked the detectives to consider using a search warrant to seize the review materials from the Coroner's Office. Zaied did none of these things. Trafford found her conduct "oppressive" and "contrary to her obligations as a Minister of Justice and an officer of the Court in this case."

Deputy Chief Coroner Jim Cairns, too, was criticized. The judge found his testimony misleading, although he did not find it intentionally so. Cairns had testified that Dr. Blair Carpenter's review of six of Smith's non-criminal autopsies was part of the independent review—yet it was not. Similarly, Cairns had testified that the independent review of Smith's work was completed, except for the review of the Reynolds case—yet it was not. And he had testified that James Young was told that Smith was competent to do all autopsies, including criminal cases—yet he was not. Smith was never reinstated to criminal autopsies. Justice Trafford ruled that the errors in Cairns's testimony had a profound impact on the case. If the defence teams had a better understanding of the scope of the review conducted by the Coroner's Office, they would not have needed to make such wide, all-encompassing requests for all the related files.

"While there is a societal interest in a trial on the merits, there is also a societal interest in a speedy trial that is fair and just," Trafford wrote in his ruling. "The defendants, who are presumed to be innocent, have been denied an opportunity of demonstrating their innocence for an unconscionable period of time, 70 months." The judge listed several ways the delays had added to the defendants' suffering: they had lost custody of Julius, they had been unable to preserve Athena's body for a second autopsy, Angela had had an abortion, they had postponed their marriage plans, they had stress-related health problems and they were unable to properly grieve Athena's death.

And with that, the trial of Anthony Kporwodu and Angela Veno was over.

Justice Trafford's decision was almost unprecedented and it sent ripples through the criminal justice system. First-degree murder charges are rarely thrown out. The Crown quickly appealed. The Ontario Court of Appeal recognized the stakes. "The prospect of freeing someone on a charge of first-degree murder without a trial on its merits is almost unthinkable," the court wrote in its judgment.

In the appeal court's decision, Justice Trafford faced some serious criticism of his own. The court disagreed with much of the individual criticisms he had made in his ruling, finding that in some instances they were overstated, if not undeserved. "His findings of misconduct against the original Assistant Crown Attorney [Rita Zaied] and counsel for the Coroner's Office [Denise Dwyer] were inappropriate and most unfortunate. They made it impossible for either counsel to remain on the record."

It found the defence's request for files involving Dr. Smith was overly broad and bordered on a fishing expedition. Zaied and Dwyer, it said, took a reasonable position in resisting the defence's efforts to receive the seventeen review cases. "Positions that are reasonably held and legitimately advanced may, in the end, prove unsuccessful; that, however, does not make them oppressive," the Court of Appeal wrote.

The court also took issue with how Justice Trafford calculated the length of the delay, ruling that the clock should have started when Anthony and Angela were jointly charged, not when Athena died. Trafford had included the lengthy pre-charge period in his calculation because Athena's body was mistakenly cremated. The Court of Appeal noted that the child's body was not in the possession of the police or coroner Ross Bennett at the time it was cremated. Rather, it was under the control of her parents and the crematorium. "While it is true that Dr. Bennett could have reasserted control over the body, on the facts of this case, he was not obliged to do so," the appeal court found. Neither parent ever asked the coroner or the police for help in preserving the body. They had hired a lawyer by this point. The appeal court ruled that the coroner and police were justified in relying on defence counsel to advise Anthony and Angela to seek their assistance in preserving the body if that's what they wanted. "The crematorium had instruction from the respondents not to cremate Athena unless the respondents ordered otherwise. Why the crematorium chose to ignore those instructions is unknown," the Court of Appeal wrote, noting that neither Bennett nor anyone from the crematorium was ever called to testify.

Justice Trafford had also ruled that Smith was negligent in failing to produce an interim autopsy report pending the results of toxicology screening, saying that had the pathologist completed an interim report, Anthony and Angela may have been able to get a second autopsy completed before Athena's body was cremated. The Court of Appeal found the trial judge's reasoning "untenable." It noted that Smith did not know Athena's parents were considering a second autopsy, and neither Anthony nor Angela called him about his autopsy report before Athena's body was cremated. While the pathologist would have been acting competently in completing an interim report, he had no duty to do so.

Likewise, the appeal court disagreed with Trafford's assessment that Zaied and Dwyer had deliberately misled the court by asking for more time to disclose the seventeen review files to the defence. Justice Trafford found that request was, in part, a ploy aimed at gaining more time to appeal his order. In his decision dismissing the Coroner's Office's stay application, Trafford ruled that the two lawyers failed to be "completely candid with the court" and had not acted with the "utmost faith" expected of them. It was because of that ruling that both lawyers were removed from the case, as Trafford's findings of misconduct had "impugned their professional integrity." But the Court of Appeal ruled that his findings were unsupported by the evidence. Therefore, the delay caused by the change in counsel was caused by the court's decision, not by a decision by the Crown or the Coroner's Office.

However, despite all those criticisms, the Court of Appeal supported Justice Trafford's core ruling: that Anthony Kporwodu and Angela Veno faced inferred and actual prejudice because of the Crown's failure to bring them to trial within a reasonable time.

In appealing Justice Trafford's decision, the Crown argued that he had not given enough weight to society's interest in seeing the couple tried, considering the charges were first-degree murder. Trafford ruled that the seriousness of the charge should be considered, but not on its own. If a delay is found to be unreasonable, a defendant's Charter rights have been violated regardless of the charge he or she is facing. The Court of Appeal agreed. "The period of delay for each respondent far exceeds the guidelines suggested by the Supreme Court of Canada. The delay is, on any definition, excessive," the court concluded. "Despite the seriousness of the charges, the delay was unreasonable and a stay is warranted. The appeal is accordingly dismissed."

The court proceedings were over, this time for good. Anthony Kporwodu and Angela Veno would never again be prosecuted for the death of their daughter, Athena.

PART 2

THE INQUIRY

NICHOLAS

THE COURT OF Appeal decision in the case of Anthony Kporwodu and Angela Veno came down in April 2005, more than seven years after their daughter Athena's death. By then, Charles Smith's reputation was mud. Instances of his questionable conduct continued to surface. Justifiable concerns about wrongful convictions started to take root.

Barry McLellan was by then the province's chief coroner. (James Young had retired the year before.) On June 7, 2005, he announced an audit of suspicious child death investigations involving Smith going back to 1991 (plus the McIntosh case from 1998). The review of Smith's cases was needed "to maintain public confidence that is very important to this office," McLellan said at the time. Two Ontario and five international pathologists conducted the review of forty-five cases.

The findings—released on April 17, 2007—were devastating. McLellan said the reviewers took serious issue with Smith's opinions in twenty of the cases. Thirteen of those had resulted in convictions. (In a fourteenth case, the court found the accused not criminally responsible for the child's death by reason of a mental disorder.)

Within a week, Attorney General Michael Bryant announced a public inquiry. Its purpose was threefold: to review how pediatric forensic pathology was practised and overseen in Ontario during the two decades of Smith's career, to investigate whether systemic failures contributed to the mistakes Smith made, and to determine why the provincial Chief Coroner's Office had been unable to catch those mistakes. The Inquiry into Pediatric Forensic Pathology in Ontario, led by Mr. Justice Stephen Goudge, would not answer questions about individual cases. Commission counsel would introduce evidence only if it related to the systemic review.

The inquiry would not determine whether wrongful convictions or mis-carriages of justice had occurred, or whether professional discipline against Smith or others was warranted. It would focus on how Smith and others investigated the children's deaths, not on the criminal investigations into their parents or caregivers. Civil or criminal liability would be left to the courts to decide.

Public hearings began in November that year. Fourteen groups or individuals were declared parties with standing, several of them includ-ing parents or caregivers: among them were Lianne Thibeault, Brenda Waudby, Angela Veno, Anthony Kporwodu and Tammy Marquardt. Forty-seven witnesses were called to testify over three months of hear-ings. Among those were Dirk Huyer, who as a member of the Suspected Child Abuse and Neglect team at SickKids had worked closely with Smith; James Young, the former chief coroner; and Jim Cairns, his deputy chief coroner.

And on a cold, blustery day in late January 2008, the disgraced pathol-ogist himself took the stand.

Tall and thin, with a full head of white hair and wire-rimmed glasses, Smith wore a tailored dark suit and a dark tie. His testimony began with an apology. Lianne Gagnon, there to hear it, wasn't sure what she was expecting, or how she would react. Technically, Smith had already said sorry for his mistakes. At the beginning of the inquiry, one of his lawyers read a written apology into the record. Now, before the questioning began, one of his lawyers, Jane Langford, asked if there was anything he wished to say to the commission.

"Thank you. Yes, if I may," Smith started, his voice barely a whisper. Lianne had to lean in to make out the words. "I would like to confirm and restate the apology that was read on my behalf at the beginning of these public hearings. Through the review of the Office of the Chief Coroner and subsequently through the information which has come out in these public hearings, I have come to appreciate mistakes that I made and I am sorry for them. I also recognize that, at times, my conduct was not professional, and I deeply regret that. I do recognize that many people have questions for me, and I will answer and provide testimony as best as I can to clarify these questions. I do accept full responsibility for my work, for my opinions and for my action. Thank you."

The commissioners quickly moved on to examining Smith's résumé and his role in the twenty contested cases. Smith returned to Nicholas Gagnon just before lunch, explaining his mistakes in detail. He admitted that his focus had been too narrow. He was told the child had bumped his head on the underside of a table, but he hadn't believed that was a reasonable explanation for the child's death and became fixated on finding another, non-accidental cause.

"I believe I concentrated on the head injury component as opposed to stepped back and looked at the whole case, and recognized how limiting or tenuous was the actual evidence for the head injury," Smith told the inquiry.

"Do you have anything you wish to say today about Nicholas's case?" Langford asked.

"Yes. Unlike perhaps some of the other cases, I well recognize that in Nicholas's case, I am solely responsible for all of the difficulties that Nicholas' family has suffered."

After a decade of pain, years of police investigations and Family Court hearings, months of slinking around in the dead of night just to be a mother, the truth was finally out. In front of a judge and lawyers, reporters and victims, Smith finally said the words.

"I do apologize to his family, to his grandparents, and especially to his mother."

Lianne cried. Her father did his best to console her.

Maurice Gagnon had spent two years fighting to clear his daughter's name and preserve her right to parent. He spent the next four trying to hold someone responsible for having made that fight necessary in the first place.

On February 19, 1999, Maurice had launched his first formal complaint about Smith, to the Coroner's Council (a provincial body that investigated complaints about coroners) and the Chief Coroner's Office. It was exhaustively researched and nearly an inch thick. He made similar complaints to the College of Physicians and Surgeons of Ontario in November 1999 and again in March and May of 2001.

He complained to the solicitor general of Ontario about Jim Cairns's role in the investigation, arguing that the deputy chief coroner relied too heavily on Smith's opinions and let his quest to eradicate child abuse impair his objectivity. He complained about the Children's Aid Society's investigation both to the minister of community and social services and to the Child and Family Services Review Board. He filed complaints with the auditor general of Ontario and with the provincial ombudsman. Despite letter after letter, complaint after complaint, nothing happened.

"Our family," he wrote to Clare Lewis, the Ontario Ombudsman, "has been victimized by the negligent, reckless and irresponsible actions of the Chief Coroner's Office in the investigation of the death of my grandson. We have exhausted every known avenue in our attempt to have this matter investigated. Our complaints against the perpetrators of this gross injustice have been summarily dismissed, ignored and, I suspect, not even read . . . As long as pathologists and coroners, operating under the protection of the Chief Coroner, know that they are totally and absolutely immune from personal accountability, they will continue to perform with impunity, producing sloppy and reckless results that will unjustly devastate innocent families."

In early 1999, Lianne's lawyer, Berk Keaney, heard that CBC's *the fifth estate* was in Sudbury working on a separate story, so he quietly approached one of the producers. "Diagnosis: Murder" aired in November 1999 and detailed Lianne's ordeal and the Timmins case. In it, Chief Coroner James Young appeared to downplay concerns about Dr. Smith, but for the first time, someone was publicly questioning the pathologist's work.

The Goudge Inquiry returned to the Timmins case as well, and in particular to Justice Dunn's strong criticisms of Smith in his acquittal of the defendant. In his ruling, Dunn questioned Smith's competence and professionalism, and the judge's words had fuelled Maurice Gagnon's determination to challenge Smith's work on his grandson's case. Smith would later claim to James Young, Jim Cairns and an investigator with the College of Physicians and Surgeons that during the course of the trial the judge had privately admitted to him that he thought the defendant was guilty. In 2001, in an unpublished interview with Jane O'Hara of *Maclean's* magazine, Smith said: "I walked onto the airplane and was stunned when I found myself sitting next to this man, who immediately began discussing the case with me. I'm in the middle of my testimony, and I felt extremely uncomfortable discussing the case with him, and he said that it's fine . . . And that was the first occasion in which he told me that [the defendant] was guilty as sin." Smith added that he found the situation "extremely, extremely unusual" and "absolutely bizarre."

That's because he had made it all up.

At the Goudge Inquiry, Smith finally admitted that he had lied about Justice Dunn's comments. At no time during the trial did the judge discuss evidence with him, suggest he believed the defendant guilty or comment on the credibility of the testimony of Smith and the other SickKids specialists. Smith said he misinterpreted some "complimentary comments" Justice Dunn made during two chance encounters. "I heard what I wanted to hear as opposed to what he actually said," Smith told the Goudge Inquiry.

In an affidavit to the inquiry, Justice Dunn stated that while he did bump into Smith on a flight and at a conference, their conversations were little more than cordial greetings.

Justice Goudge rejected Smith's explanation. "He should have spoken candidly about the criticisms made against him. His failure to do that, and his resort to fabricating statements purportedly made by a provincial court judge about a case, were inexcusable.

"This sorry episode offers a very unflattering insight into Dr. Smith's integrity."

ATHENA
···

ONE

ANTHONY KPORWODU AND Angela Veno did not receive an apology from Smith at the inquiry. Athena's case did come up during his first day of testimony, but in a different context.

Smith's lawyer Jane Langford asked him, "Dr. Smith, you do realize that in one case, the Athena case, your delays contributed to the stay of criminal charges against two individuals?"

"I'm aware of that, yes."

"How do you feel about that today?"

"I'm—I'm deeply contrite."

Smith wasn't apologizing to Athena's parents. He was apologizing to the criminal justice system. For many observers, the bungled trial of Anthony Kporwodu and Angela Veno represented a different kind of injustice. Athena's was *not* among the twenty cases in which the reviewers found problems with Smith's findings. Everyone thought that this time he got the pathology right. Even the defence believed the child was beaten on at least one occasion. Police believed Athena had been killed. Prosecutors believed the same. World-renowned pathologists agreed. Even Angela's and Anthony's defence lawyers believed she had been killed—just not by their clients. And yet her death would never be prosecuted. Smith's delays had contributed to an otherwise solid case being thrown out.

One of Smith's primary goals as a pathologist was to make sure that no child's killing went unpunished. But in a bitter twist, it was his own failings that guaranteed the exact opposite for Athena Kporwodu.

Det. Sgt. Matt Crone became uncomfortable as the delays in Athena's case mounted. The reason he'd waited to lay charges of second-degree murder against Anthony and Angela wasn't that he doubted Smith's medical findings. Rather, he didn't trust Smith to stick to his medical opinion. "It didn't make me feel good. I don't lay the whole delay on Charles Smith. It was my decision," he told me years later. "I'm the guy who dug in his heels. I am the guy that essentially caused a good part of that delay."

Crone did have some misgivings about the prosecution. Rita Zaied struck him as overzealous. Murder charges felt like a reach; Crone believed manslaughter charges made sense. He could see how Anthony, exhausted or frustrated, might have taken it out on Athena. The detective had seen lots of people snap over the years. But otherwise, Anthony and Angela seemed like good parents. Struggling, perhaps, forced to make some difficult choices, but generally raising their children as best they could.

When I began researching this book, I was convinced that someone had got away with killing Athena Kporwodu. Everyone I spoke with told me as much. Even Angela's and Anthony's defence lawyers were going to argue that the child's acute injuries were accidentally caused by Anthony or the paramedics during CPR. They were planning to hang the older injuries on one of the babysitters. They thought police had not properly investigated either of them.

Yet Athena had been outside her parents' care only on two fairly brief occasions, and each time she was happy and healthy afterwards. Police interviewed both babysitters and apparently didn't consider them suspects. Even Angela and Anthony said they didn't think either was responsible. They argued instead that an underlying medical condition must explain Athena's injuries and death.

Cindy Wasser, the junior counsel on Angela's defence team, was the only person I spoke with who was not convinced that the medical foundation of the case was rock solid. And it was just her hunch; she didn't have any evidence or expert's opinion to refute Smith. But after seeing his troubling work up close in the Julie Bowers case a decade earlier, she couldn't bring herself to believe that he got it right this time, even if all the reviews supported him.

Yet Smith's medical opinion about Athena's injuries appeared sound. And it wasn't just his opinion either. Smith's work on the case had been reviewed repeatedly by world-class pathologists, first during the run-up to the trial and again during the Goudge Inquiry. Everyone came to the same conclusion: he had got it right—someone had beaten Athena to death. The only question was who. That's the reason I wanted to explore this case.

In November 2013, I attended a conference and gala hosted by the Association in Defence of the Wrongly Convicted, or AIDWYC (now Innocence Canada). The influential Canadian group was celebrating twenty years of legal work and advocacy. Several of the cases involving Smith had already ended up with AIDWYC.

At one particular session, a panel of doctors and lawyers was talking about the controversies surrounding shaken baby syndrome. Shaken baby syndrome had been a factor in some of Smith's cases, but none that I was focusing on for this book. So I was listening, but not closely. And then Heather Kirkwood began speaking.

Kirkwood is a retired defence lawyer in Seattle who now does pro bono work on cases she suspects may be wrongful convictions, many of them involving shaken baby syndrome.

One of her most memorable cases involved Julie Baumer, who had been looking after her six-week-old nephew in October 2003, when the child became lethargic and fussy and refused to eat. She took him to the hospital, where a CT scan revealed a skull fracture and heavy bleeding in the brain. Julie was charged with first-degree child abuse. Medical experts for the prosecution testified that the child had suffered either blunt force trauma or a violent shaking. Julie's defence counsel did not call any medical evidence to rebut the testimony. Julie was sentenced to ten to fifteen years in prison. Kirkwood took on her appeal in conjunction with the Michigan Innocence Project. A judge overturned the conviction in 2009 on the grounds of ineffective defence counsel. At Julie's second trial, Kirkwood and her legal team called six expert witnesses who testified that the baby had been suffering from cerebral venous sinus thrombosis, a difficult condition to diagnose that some specialists believe can mimic child abuse. The jury acquitted Baumer of all charges.

The Baumer case demonstrated that fractures do not always add up to abuse. But that case involved a single skull fracture caused by a birth injury that was exacerbated by nutritional deficiencies. Kirkwood then stumbled onto another subset of medical conditions that often mimic child abuse.

That morning at the AIDWYC conference in Toronto, Kirkwood crammed an hour-long lecture on shaken baby syndrome into her twenty-minute slot on a three-person panel. She was zipping through an accompanying slide show, and much of what she was saying was highly technical.

"We have the same problems on bones," she said. "I see fractures, and I can't explain the fractures. With rib fractures . . . my questions on these fractures are why don't these fractures hurt? Why don't they swell, why don't they bruise, why don't they bleed? Why don't they act like other fractures? Maybe," she said, "because they aren't fractures."

Fractures that aren't fractures. Suddenly she had my full attention.

Kirkwood started running through some of the cases she had worked on. "The Pereiras—twenty-one fractures. They went through a criminal trial two weeks ago. Vitamin D, rickets. The level of vitamin D was undetectable, but there were the twenty-one fractures, and these were pictures taken during the period the child's bones were being fractured every day." A series of family snapshots flashed up on the overhead projector, pictures of a baby girl, grinning at the camera from the arms of her doting mother and father. "She was happy. People saw her every day. When you have a case like this, it doesn't matter if you have twenty-one or a hundred fractures. Those ain't fractures."

Kirkwood explained that the case changed her mind on fractures. "I used to say I don't take fracture cases. Now, if there's more than five fractures, you can almost guarantee it's metabolic bone disease."

In that moment, my whole perspective on Athena's case shifted. Her multiple rib fractures weren't irrefutable proof that she'd been beaten. There was a possible explanation for them that didn't involve intentional trauma. And if you take the rib fractures out of the equation, the rest of her injuries aren't as damning. It was entirely plausible that the liver laceration was caused during resuscitation efforts; that was what the defence was going to argue at trial. And the brain injury—I didn't know what to make of the brain injury, but could it be it wasn't caused by trauma? Anthony and Angela had repeatedly taken Athena to see the doctor during the last month of her life. Was it possible that she was simply sick? I needed to do some research.

IT TURNS OUT that a multitude of metabolic bone and blood diseases can cause or mimic rib fractures. Some can be mistaken for signs of child abuse. Rickets, a preventable bone disease of early childhood caused by vitamin D deficiency, can lead to soft and weakened bones, fractures, and bone and muscle pain. Children with naturally dark skin, those who don't get enough sunlight and those with diets low in vitamin D and calcium are most at risk. Athena had dark skin and may have had low vitamin D and calcium levels, given her struggles to keep her formula down. During one visit, Dr. Lo recommended Angela feed her soy milk to supplement her diet.

There are also rare genetic forms of the disease. Rickets was previously considered rare in the developed world, but studies have shown that its incidence is much higher than previously thought, and the disease has been found in otherwise healthy young adults, children and infants. In one famous case, parents in London, England, were charged with murder after their four-month-old was found with severe head injuries and multiple fractures throughout his body. Yet they were acquitted after more than sixty prosecution and defence medical experts failed to agree on the cause of death. During the autopsy, a pediatric pathologist discovered the child had congenital rickets, which had gone undiagnosed by two hospitals while he was alive.

Osteogenesis imperfecta, or OI, also called brittle bone disease, is another rare genetic disorder that causes broken bones and fractures and whose symptoms are sometimes mistaken for child abuse. Several still rarer types of OI were only recently discovered—years after Athena Kporwodu's case—and their causes and characteristics are still not well understood. With OI, ordinary activities such as lifting the child, diaper changing or burping can lead to injuries, including rib and spinal fractures, yet there may be no obvious sign of the injuries, other than crying. Bruising may appear with little or no apparent cause. X-rays may reveal old, undetected fractures at

various stages of healing. Some cases of OI are caused by spontaneous muta-
tion, so there may be no history of it in the family, or if there is, a parent
could have mild OI that goes undiagnosed. Likewise, children may not
exhibit the hallmark features of OI, such as bone deformity, brittle teeth or
a blue or tinted colour in the white of the eyes.

Various other genetic conditions popped up in my research that often
featured frequent fractures among their symptoms. Yet I wasn't convinced
any of them were a factor in Athena's death. I could accept that Smith
missed the signs. Some forms of OI were not even known when she died,
in 1998. But I just couldn't believe that world-class pathologists, including
Christopher Milroy, the forensic pathologist who reviewed Athena's case
for the Goudge Inquiry, had missed them too. Milroy, then the chief
forensic pathologist with the Forensic Science Service in the U.K. and a
professor of forensic pathology at the University of Sheffield, had been
specifically tasked with looking for mistakes Smith could have made.

Still, it didn't take much research online to find a wealth of information
about these conditions. If a journalist without any medical training knew
enough to consider these conditions, surely diligent pathologists would
know enough to do the same and rule them out.

I wanted to talk to Heather Kirkwood. She had spent the past fifteen
years looking at wrongful conviction cases, many involving faulty medical
opinions. I was curious whether she would think Athena's case worth
investigating, and I thought I might ask her to connect me with a pathologist and radiologist to review the case with fresh eyes. I also wanted to
talk to Angela and Anthony, but wasn't having much luck tracking them
down. After the court and appeal decisions, they had basically disappeared.
Neither had any online presence, and old phone numbers had been discon-
nected. But I wanted to track them down, for two reasons. I wanted to
speak with them about the case itself, of course, but I was also hoping they
would help me gather all existing slides, specimen blocks and X-rays from
Athena's autopsy. (Privacy legislation prohibited me from doing that
directly.) I wanted to have a new pathologist review the case, and I would
need those original materials.

Kirkwood and I spoke in late September 2014, not long after I sent her Smith's autopsy report and the follow-up reports from the various reviews. She peppered me with near-incomprehensible medical jargon, assuming I was well schooled in medical terminology, but her message was clear: in her preliminary opinion, Athena Kporwodu did not die from trauma.

So what did she die from? I asked. Kirkwood couldn't say. The injuries didn't look right, but she couldn't say exactly why. She didn't think the child had OI or rickets. There were a lot of rib fractures, but the telltale signs of either condition were not mentioned in Smith's autopsy report. Still, the injuries didn't add up. Kirkwood said the brain injury didn't appear to be severe; there was very little swelling. There was a lot of small-scale bleeding in a lot of different places, apparently occurring after Athena died, which was strange. And she believed the liver laceration could also have occurred after Athena died, during the frantic efforts to revive her.

"The child was sick in the last month of her life," Kirkwood said to me. "Maybe that was it. Sometimes sick children die."

Kirkwood's guess was that the child more likely had a blood disease than a bone disease. "What about a family history?" she asked. "There's no indication in Smith's autopsy report that he looked into that."

"What do you mean?" I asked.

"Well, were there any other dead babies in the mom or dad's families? Maybe they have a history of children dying. That could point to a genetic condition that's being passed down from one generation to the next."

It suddenly hit me. In my search for Angela and Anthony, I'd stumbled across an obituary for Angela's father, Albert Veno. It listed all his siblings and children, and I'd hoped one of them might be able to connect me with Angela. The obituary noted that Albert was predeceased by his older sister, Kathleen, and three brothers who died in infancy.

I'd read the obit repeatedly, making note of Angela's eight siblings and the cities where they lived in hopes of tracking them down. But I'd skimmed right over Albert's dead brothers, blind to the significance of their deaths. I found their names in another obituary, this one for Kathleen.

Albert Veno had three siblings who lived into adulthood. Two of them were still alive. Dan was eighty-one years old when I spoke to him in the fall of 2014. He told me the infants Alfred, Frederick and Joseph were his parents' first three children, and they had all died before any of the surviving children were born. His older sister, Kathleen, was born in 1932, which meant the three brothers were likely born in the late 1920s or early '30s. Dan said he was "99 per cent sure" that all three had died during childbirth.

I also tracked down Rosaleen Smith, the baby of the family. She said her parents didn't talk much about the three brothers who died, but she remembered one story her mother told her when she was a young girl. Two of the boys were twins—Rosaleen wasn't sure which two—and when her mother was still pregnant with them, she was struck by lightning. She was cooking in front of their old porcelain stove when it happened. Rosaleen said it must have come down the stove's chimney, through the stove and struck her. Her mother survived, but the babies were stillborn.

It was an unbelievable story—and impossible to corroborate—but if true, it ruled out any genetic or metabolic cause of death for these two boys that might be linked to Athena's case.

But the most troubling thing about Angela's long-dead infant uncles was that I was the first person who had ever called to inquire about them. Charles Smith never looked into Athena's family history. But neither had anyone else—no detectives called, no coroners, no defence lawyers, none of the pathologists who reviewed the case at trial or for the Goudge Inquiry. Dan, Rosaleen and Betty Veno, Angela's mother, all said I was the first person to ask these questions.

What that meant was that no one had thought to investigate Athena's family history to look for genetic conditions that might have explained her death. (When asked if he ever considered Athena's family history, Angela's lawyer John Rosen said the defence's position—had the Charter challenge failed and the case proceeded—was that the key issue was the timing of the injuries, not if there was a non-accidental explanation for them.)[2]

I'd been trying for more than a year to find Angela and Anthony. Her lawyers had all lost touch with her years before. None of the relatives I tracked down had spoken to her in years, and no one had a phone number for her. I did, though, find Julius Kporwodu, on Facebook. He was a teenager now, and he lived in Milton, outside Toronto. I wondered if he'd moved back from Ghana to live with one or both of his parents. I was uncomfortable trying to contact Angela and Anthony through their son, but I was running out of options. I sent a message to him on Facebook, but it went unanswered. His uncle Adrian was Facebook friends with Julius, so I asked his wife to have Adrian relay a message to him. When that also went unanswered, I tried Julius one more time directly. Within days, Angela called.

The conversation didn't start well. She said she wished I'd contacted them directly, rather than going through their son. I apologized and explained that I'd been trying for months to track down her and Anthony, without any success. I explained why it was so important that I speak with her.

She was still very hesitant. She said Athena's death and the criminal investigation that followed had been a very difficult time in their lives and they were reluctant to go back there. They had finally moved on and didn't want their names out in public.

I was buoyed that Angela had called me back, and I hoped that I could get her to talk to me more. But even if I couldn't, I knew there were a couple of crucial answers I needed to get from this conversation in case I didn't have another chance.

"What happened to Anthony?" I asked. "Are you still in touch?"

She said he was sitting beside her.

"So you stayed together?"

Angela said they got married years ago, after the trial ended.

"I can understand your reluctance to talk about all of this. You don't know me or what I'm trying to do with this book," I said. She agreed. She said they would have to decide if they could trust me.

"Let's just put that aside for a while," I said. "What I really need right now is your help. I'd like to hire a pathologist and radiologist to review Athena's death one more time." I explained what I had learned about metabolic bone conditions that mimic child abuse. "I don't know if you're aware of this, but your father had three brothers who died in infancy. And it doesn't appear that anyone investigated whether those deaths might be linked somehow to what killed Athena."

Angela said she was well aware of the infant deaths of her father's three older brothers. And there was more. She said she had an aunt who also lost a child. She didn't think he was much older than Athena.

"An aunt on your father's side?"

She said her name was Rosaleen Smith, her father's younger sister.

Some detective I was! I had already spoken to Rosaleen, but I never thought to ask her if she had lost a child.

Angela said she told people to look into her family history because there were other children who had died on her father's side. She didn't specify who she told, and I didn't get a chance to clarify during our brief conversation. But she did say that no one would listen. It made her feel powerless.

I told her that I believed what she and Anthony had said all along—that there must be an underlying medical condition that explained Athena's death—was credible, especially considering all the other infant deaths in the same branch of her family. "If a pathologist can narrow down the potential causes, maybe we can get you tested, find out if you're a carrier."

Angela said she and Anthony would think it over and get back to me.

I called Rosaleen Smith again. Angela was right. Her aunt did lose a baby. She was delivered at home. "I heard her cry, but they wouldn't show her to me," Rosaleen said. "They took her right to the hospital and that was it." Rosaleen said it was a normal pregnancy, and no one ever told her why or how the child died. "I couldn't find out nothing. They took her to the hospital and said she died and that's all I could find out. Same as with my little boy that died in the hospital."

"You lost a son as well?" I asked.

"Yeah." Rosaleen hadn't lost one child. She had lost two. "You never forget it. I took him to the Halifax hospital, and he wouldn't live. I don't know." Her son was a healthy baby until he was about nine months old, she said. "He was throwing up and had diarrhea. I took him down to the hospital one day and he died the next. You never forget it." Again, no one would tell her anything about why her child had died. "You don't get no answers when you ask."

Rosaleen couldn't remember exactly when the children were born or died. Maybe the late 1950s or early '60s. She didn't receive death certificates for either of them. She did have birth certificates, and she told me she would see if she could dig them out. If I knew their birth dates, I might be able to get their death certificates from the province. But I was never able to get any more information from Rosaleen or her family.

Six infants on the same branch of the family tree, all dead before their first birthday.

By now I was in near-daily contact with Heather Kirkwood. She threw a barrage of possibilities at me to consider. Maybe it went all the way back to the birth. Athena's white blood cell count was elevated when she was delivered, which meant she was fighting an infection. Kirkwood wondered if the Group B Streptococcus infection was truly gone; maybe it had just gone dormant after two days of antibiotics. "One problem with incomplete antibiotics is that bugs can lurk," she told me in one email. Or maybe Athena had some other, undetected viral infection. It was frustrating. There were so many possibilities, but Kirkwood had in mind a pathologist and radiologist who could review the case for me, and hopefully narrow them down.

Marta Cohen, a histopathologist at the Sheffield Children's NHS Foundation Trust, a children's hospital in Sheffield, England, specializes in the microscopic examination of tissues to understand the manifestations of disease. She has a special interest in the genetic causes of sudden infant death and vitamin D deficiency, and has additional certification in pediatric histopathology and forensic pathology. She has co-authored more than 120 papers, research studies and book chapters, and co-edited *The Pediatric and Perinatal Autopsy Manual*, published in 2014. She sits on a variety of professional bodies. In 2013, that included the Paediatric Pathology Society, the European Society of Pathology and the International Paediatric and Perinatal Association.

Kirkwood also connected me with Julie Mack, a radiologist at the Milton S. Hershey Medical Center, in Hershey, Pennsylvania, who agreed to review Athena's X-rays to correlate them with Cohen's pathological review.

Dr. Cohen was intrigued. "The case is fascinating," she wrote in one of her first emails. "However, it is very difficult to give an opinion on somebody else's description. If this is wrong, then my diagnosis will also be wrong as it is based on incorrect (histological) information."

When I told her it was a Charles Smith case, she was even more wary of building her opinion of the case off his autopsy findings. "30+ rib fractures: you would need to batter the child heavily, leaving bruises, etc.," she wrote. She immediately ruled out shaken baby syndrome. "Based on the liver issue, I would not believe anything from this report." She suggested I compile a full family history, including non-fatal medical conditions, to help narrow down the possibilities.

Shortly after that correspondence, we spoke on the phone. I hadn't yet managed to get any of the autopsy materials, and I hadn't sent her Smith's autopsy report so as not to contaminate any review she would eventually do. But as best I could I walked her through the clinical history of the case: the head injury—which she said didn't sound severe—and the acute liver laceration that the defence had been ready to argue was caused during CPR.

She zeroed in on the rib fractures. "The interesting thing is that you said thirty-odd fractures. A person with thirty-odd rib fractures would have a very unstable thorax, and that would be perceived," she said, especially if some of the fractures were caused at the same time. The child would have a hard time breathing. "The ribs help to keep the lungs in place, and it allows for the necessary expansion and collapse of the lungs to allow for the breathing and exchange of oxygen. So a person with thirty-plus fractures would have a non-stable thorax and it would have been evident to the GP or the parents or relatives that this child was having difficulty breathing and was in need of urgent medical treatment."

As well, I told her about the frequent visits to the doctor—five in the last month of Athena's life, including one within days of her death.

"The thing is, I am doubting things here. Just to play devil's advocate, I don't believe the child could have thirty-odd rib fractures and them not be evident to the GP or other relatives. So I wonder if there were rib fractures at all. There was something else, like vitamin D deficiency, which can cause many features [that look like fractures] but they can confuse those who are not trained to identify these features. What this case is screaming to me is a metabolic condition."

I'd been looking for a genetic or metabolic condition that explained how so many of Athena's ribs could break naturally. The possibility that she didn't actually have any traumatic fractures hadn't occurred to me.

In Angela's initial interview with police, she described Athena as a demanding, fussy child, but she sounded like a normal demanding, fussy child. Angela said she liked to be held; that she would cry when left alone in her crib or car seat. The only way she or Anthony could calm her was to pick her up and hold her. That didn't sound to me like a child who had thirty-two rib fractures, according to Smith. Of course, Angela could have been lying. But that would require a level of deception that police didn't suspect. Matt Crone said he considered Angela more of a witness than a suspect. What Marta Cohen was suggesting provided a viable explanation: maybe Athena didn't have rib fractures at all.

"I have done studies that three per cent of sudden deaths in childhood are actually due to a metabolic condition, and now more and more in science, protein and genes are discovered that can cause metabolic conditions that we are not currently able to test," she told me. "For instance, there are one thousand mitochondrial enzymes, and each of these can cause a metabolic condition. So we still don't know them all. We only know the tip of the iceberg."

She cautioned that without examining autopsy photos and slides, all this was conjecture and speculation, but something else suggested a metabolic condition: a history of sudden deaths on the maternal side of the family. "It's very interesting, because all the mitochondrial genes are transmitted through the mother," Cohen said.

She told me to look for a notation in Smith's autopsy report that a metabolic test was done on the child's fibroblast culture. But she doubted

I would find one. The test is more common today, but it would have been highly unusual in 1998, when Athena died.

She also told me to focus on doing a full breakdown of the family history: sudden infant or childhood deaths, stillbirths, even sudden adult deaths, deafness or hearing problems, heart abnormalities or arrhythmia, epilepsy, neurological impairment or deterioration, early aging. As well, she wanted a fuller clinical presentation of Athena's birth and illness: Was she born prematurely? When and how exactly did her neurological deterioration begin? When did her diarrhea and vomiting first appear? Did she have a subdural hemorrhage?

It was a long list of complicated questions. A lot of them, I hoped, would be answered in the autopsy report.

"What I should do," I suggested, "is send you the autopsy report and all the reviews that were done. Then, we could go through exactly what the findings are and what fits and what doesn't fit."

What Cohen really wanted to see were the slides and specimen blocks and any tissue that was preserved. She was going against her own advice— "Please don't show me his autopsy report. It could contaminate my opinions"—but in this context, it was the logical place to start.

Lastly, Cohen suggested I contact a clinical geneticist to see about genetic testing. If I couldn't persuade Angela to participate, Cohen said I should ask a female relative with the closest blood links to Athena, preferably one with her own history of child deaths.

I wanted to let Angela know where things stood. I hadn't heard from her since our first conversation weeks before, and I hoped that once she heard about the review team Kirkwood and I had put together, she and Anthony would get involved. I couldn't get her on the phone, so I left a couple of messages. In the end, we never spoke again.

What you take away from Angela's silence depends a lot on what you think about the case. If you think one or both of them is guilty of beating their daughter to death, then their reluctance to talk to me is a sign of their guilt. They didn't want me writing about their case because they were guilty.

But if you have doubts about the medical evidence against them, then their silence could point to something else. Angela told me they'd finally moved on from the darkest, most painful period of their lives, and they simply didn't want to go back. That sounded reasonable. She told me she and Anthony weren't sure about my motives, or whether they could trust me. That sounded reasonable too.

Smith's mistakes directly or indirectly sabotaged what everyone, even the defence, believed was a legitimate prosecution. That's why the Goudge Inquiry, though created in response to wrongful convictions, was interested in their aborted case—to find ways to stop a similar travesty from ever happening again.

But what if Angela and Anthony *weren't* guilty? What if the inquiry—specifically set up to find mistakes and fix a system that had failed before—failed again? The reviewers never considered Athena's family history. What if her true cause of death was hidden in there? What if it could be discovered by genetic or metabolic testing that was never done? If Angela and Anthony had nothing to do with Athena's death, then they had been burned by the very inquiry set up to root out the mistakes that Dr. Smith made.

The result of the Charter challenge guaranteed that Anthony and Angela would never be prosecuted for Athena's death, but it freed them on a technicality. An important technicality—unreasonable delay—but the result said nothing about their innocence or guilt. It also denied them a chance to defend themselves. Angela herself called the Charter challenge a double-edged sword. There can be no legal remedy for Angela and Anthony. There was no verdict, so there is no verdict to correct. They were left in a weird limbo, unable to challenge the validity of a prosecution that never happened. In that light, maybe Angela Veno and Anthony Kporwodu are Dr. Smith's biggest victims of all.

THREE

I CONTINUED TRACING the family tree. I didn't find any more child deaths, or any noteworthy medical conditions, in the maternal branches.

Without Angela's or Anthony's co-operation, I wouldn't be able to access any original autopsy materials. But I thought Smith's report might contain some obscure references that hinted at what the most likely genetic condition could be. I was hoping Angela's aunt Rosaleen might agree to genetic testing. It wouldn't be as definitive as testing Angela, but she was a close relative who had lost children herself. Finding out if she was carrying an undiagnosed genetic condition would provide more evidence of what Angela might be carrying and what might have killed Athena. The challenge was figuring out what to test her for. Genetic testing is not a catch-all; you need to know what you are looking for.

In the meantime I called Cohen to discuss her progress, and what she told me took the case in yet another unexpected direction.

We started with the liver laceration. Smith had noted the presence in the liver laceration of neutrophils, a type of white blood cell. Neutrophils take some time to appear after trauma, and the body has to be alive to produce them. So if the laceration was caused during CPR, neutrophils shouldn't be present, since Athena was presumably already dead at that point. (Emergency personnel and paramedics were unable to revive her at any point.)

"To me, it's not possible that it happened during CPR," Cohen told me. "This happened a few hours before she died. It's proof that she survived this liver laceration for a few hours.

"The other question I was asking myself," Cohen continued, "was what happened with the ribs? Why were there so many rib fractures? Were they really rib fractures? And actually, they're reported in the radiology report. That means they are healing fractures, because usually fresh fractures are not seen by the radiologist." It's not until fractures begin healing that they start to show up on X-rays. "So I believe that the fractures were most possibly real."

"You think they were real?" I repeated.

"Yes, and actually now, reading his report, I think that this child was abused."

"You do?"

"To be fair, this looks to be a very thorough report." Smith's autopsy report for Athena is fifteen pages long. It is very detailed. The breakdown of his microscopic findings for the ribs takes up more than three pages on its own.

The one area of concern Cohen saw was the lack of bruising. "Where are the bruises to explain this laceration?" she asked. In this type of injury, she said, she would expect to see a corresponding bruise on the child's abdomen, but there wasn't one (although there was one on the child's left side, leading Cohen to believe Athena was hit from the side rather than through the abdomen). She had similar questions about the ribs. "It's very difficult to interpret why there are so many fractures with no bruises that explain the rib fractures. This is something that makes you wonder."

But these lingering questions didn't lead her back to an undiagnosed but benign cause. An underlying metabolic condition couldn't explain the liver laceration. The presence of neutrophils made her believe the laceration wasn't caused during resuscitation efforts. And if Athena had a metabolic condition that explained bone fractures, why were only her ribs fractured? Conditions like osteogenesis imperfecta and rickets don't concentrate in one area; they affect all the bones in the body.

Based on Smith's report, Marta Cohen believed that Athena Kporwodu was beaten to death. She didn't think it was a case of shaken baby syndrome. This was straightforward abuse.

But how could she explain the lack of bruising?

"I don't know if she was dropped or something," Cohen said, "but I think that whoever did this, they maybe were cautious to use some pillow or some soft surface to not cause more marks."

"They would have done this multiple times?" I asked.

"I think so. This is what I perceive from reading this report. It struck me as a battered child."

Whoever killed Athena was not a parent who lost it on their newborn in a moment of exhaustion or frustration, as the police suspected. According to Cohen, this was a person who purposefully beat a defence-less child and took concrete steps to conceal the abuse.

Cohen was assuming that Smith was being truthful when he said neu-trophils were present in the liver laceration; without them, the laceration could have been caused during CPR. (She said it was highly unlikely that trained paramedics would cause such a laceration, though. An untrained parent such as Anthony theoretically might, but she had never seen a similar case of that happening.)

Cohen was doing exactly what she had said she would not do: she was basing her opinions on an autopsy report done by Charles Smith, a pathol-ogist whose work she had said she refused to trust.

"Did he make it up? I can't contradict that, because I am not making a firsthand assessment on the autopsy material. I am just following his descriptions," she said. "Maybe he copied this from a book. I don't know. Maybe he made it up. I don't know. There is nothing I can say without looking at the tissue. But reading this report, it looks thorough. It makes sense. And it looks like abuse to me."

There was still no evidence that any metabolic testing had been done at autopsy, but having taken a closer look at Athena's injuries, that was no longer an issue for Cohen. An underlying metabolic condition could still be a factor with the fractures, although she said it was unlikely given that they were all concentrated in the ribs. But a metabolic condition was definitely not responsible for the liver laceration.

Cohen said she would be happy to do a more thorough review if I could get the original autopsy material. I told her I was still going through all the court records on the off chance autopsy records had been filed on appeal (the court records filled more than six large boxes) and I would try one more time with Angela.

My appeals to Athena's parents went unanswered. But I did find thirteen of the more than eighty original autopsy photos in the court record. So I gathered them up, along with all the supplementary reports, and sent them to Cohen for one final look.

It was worth it. This time Cohen found what she believed were substantive errors in Smith's opinions. To begin with, she wasn't sure about his assessment of Athena's brain injury. Smith said he found evidence of multiple instances of subdural hemorrhage, or bleeding on the brain, caused by trauma. Cohen agreed there was evidence of old and new bleeding on the brain, but she thought it was more likely related to Athena's forceps delivery. There were no outward signs of trauma on her head, no scratching or bruising. (In 2004, six years after Athena died, a study of 111 healthy, full-term infants found that 8 per cent had subdural hemorrhage caused during birth. The findings were present in all types of births, but they went up dramatically, to 28 per cent, in those involving forceps. In all cases, the bleeding eventually resolved itself.)

Smith had found more recent signs of cerebral hypoxia, or reduced oxygen supply to the brain. Trying to resuscitate a child with hypoxia can cause subdural hemorrhage. Pathologists, though, often link that bleeding to trauma—as Smith had done. Hypoxia can be caused by natural and unnatural causes: a viral infection or blunt force trauma. Because of that, Cohen said hypoxia should be considered non-specific on its own—there need to be other signs of trauma to the head for hypoxia to be linked to a non-accidental injury. And Athena didn't have any such signs. The photos and the reports, Cohen told me, "don't describe any impact point. They don't describe any head injury as such. There is no scar bruising, there is no fracture to the skull. If you have trauma with a fracture and scalp laceration and then you have hypoxia, you know [the hypoxia] is because of the trauma. But if you don't have trauma . . . [the hypoxia] is not specific."

Hypoxia shouldn't be attributed specifically to trauma, which is what Smith had done. Cohen attributed the acute brain injury to hypoxic-ischemic encephalopathy, a brain injury caused by oxygen deprivation. She said in this case, its cause was unknown.

Cohen told me that if Athena's acute brain injury was her only injury, she would attribute her death to SIDS, or sudden infant death syndrome. And, she added, there is a link between SIDS and undiagnosed metabolic conditions. One study found that 3 per cent of SIDS deaths diagnosed at autopsy turned out to involve an underlying metabolic condition that contributed to the death. And that number may be even higher when you consider that metabolic conditions are still being discovered.

But Athena's brain injury was not her only injury. Cohen still believed the liver laceration was not accidental.

If Athena was punched in the abdomen, Cohen said, the force of the blow could push her liver upward, into the lower edge of the rib cage, lacerating it. CPR wouldn't move the liver in the same way, she said. "We do ninety post-mortem [examinations] a year, and all the babies come with CPR. I have never seen a laceration due to CPR. I have seen a laceration due to trauma, but not CPR."

The laceration itself is not visible in any of the photographs I have, but the liver is—and it's extremely bloody.

In several of the autopsy photographs, bruises can be seen on her chest and back, buttocks and left side. Most are not heavily pronounced, and it is hard to determine whether they are injury-related bruises or post-mortem artifacts caused during the autopsy or by natural changes to the body after death.

But three of the most distinct marks are round discolorations on the upper chest, positioned triangularly. To my eyes, they look like fingertips. Like someone pushing down on her chest with three fingers administering CPR.

Cohen agreed, but she still wasn't buying that CPR efforts were a factor.

"Maybe fingers left marks at some point, and then they punched her," she suggested. "I think she was punched from left to right. That's why there's bleeding from the left side of the rib cage, and from above, from the thorax to the abdomen and from the left to the right." She said it was hard to be definitive because she couldn't see the laceration itself. But the presence of neutrophils in the liver led her to believe the injury was eight to twelve hours old.

Cohen said there are other possible non-traumatic explanations for Athena's injuries. A vitamin D deficiency could lead the bones to fracture more easily. A blood-clotting disorder could lead to excessive bleeding and bruising. It was impossible to say for sure whether these were a factor in Athena's injuries because testing wasn't done for either, but Cohen thought the injuries were too localized for either to be likely. If she had a vitamin D deficiency, the fractures would be spread throughout her body, not concentrated only in her ribs. If she had a bleeding disorder, the bruising would similarly be found throughout her body, not concentrated in her abdomen and chest, where there are signs of other injuries.

"I'm sorry," Cohen told me, "I know you are writing a book about the possible innocence of these parents. And I do think there are some issues with the report that were not right. I don't think there was a head injury as such. But I do think that the bruising in the thorax and the laceration in the liver are possibly due to injury. If I were going to court, I would say it is due to injury."

This wasn't where I thought I would end up with this case. But the fact remains that every pathologist who reviewed Athena's case, including some who are world leaders in the field, had come to the same conclusion: Athena's fatal injuries were non-accidental. Marta Cohen specifically reviews cases with an eye to catching the mistakes of others, and she still ended up with the same basic finding: someone had beaten the child to death.

Nevertheless, there are aspects of this case that still don't sit well with me. Angela's family history of infant death is strange: six deaths in three generations, all on the maternal side, screams for more investigation. I went as far as I could, but I still don't know what those deaths point to, if anything. All I can say is what I started with: they're curious.

As well, Angela and Anthony's frequent visits to Athena's doctor suggest they were caring parents. If one or both of them was beating her enough to cause thirty-odd rib fractures, why would they risk taking her to the doctor five times in a month?

There is a rare mental disorder—Munchausen by proxy syndrome—in which a parent or caregiver repeatedly seeks medical attention for a child to get attention from and feel superior over medical professionals. But this disorder usually involves exaggerating or fabricating illness in relatively healthy children. Athena was not healthy. In rare cases, a parent will actually cause symptoms in the child in an effort to legitimize their concerns. Did Angela or Anthony beat Athena to the brink of death to get attention from their family doctor? I suppose that's possible. But they had another child who was healthy and showed no signs of abuse. I could find nothing to suggest Julius was being constantly dragged to the doctor.

And I keep coming back to Matt Crone's read of the case: he said he viewed Angela more as a witness than a suspect, and he viewed Anthony as a stressed-out, emasculated caregiver who—based on Athena's injuries—must have lost it on the child in a fit of exhaustion and frustration. Yet even that theory doesn't fit with the severity of the child's injuries.

If Athena had these severe injuries when she was taken to her doctor, why didn't the doctor notice them? It's possible it was an oversight. It's possible the doctor didn't examine her properly. But could he really miss, by Smith's count, thirty-two rib fractures? Marta Cohen had said the child's whole chest cavity would be so compromised that she would barely be breathing. It's highly unlikely a doctor would miss those kinds of symptoms during multiple visits.

Christopher Milroy did not recall investigating or considering the child's family history in his review for the Goudge Inquiry. In an email to me, he agreed there are non-traumatic explanations for each of her injuries. In his view, resuscitation efforts can cause a liver laceration, and rib fractures can be associated with metabolic bone disease. But he said the presence of three separate injury patterns—each needing its own distinct, unrelated cause—makes "a natural disease improbable." I understand that. What are the chances the child would have a lingering brain injury from her birth, a rare metabolic condition associated with rib fractures and also sustain a liver laceration during CPR? Each on its own is possible. All three together is improbable.

But is that any more improbable than a child having five relatives die in infancy, then die herself from another unrelated cause? I don't know. Without knowing more about what killed Athena's infant relatives, it's impossible to say.

Whatever happened to Athena Kporwodu, Charles Smith failed the system once again. Either his shortcomings allowed a child's intentional death to go unpunished, or he and all the others who failed to properly investigate the case cast a shadow of suspicion that Angela Veno and Anthony Kporwodu can never escape.

ONE

FORENSIC PATHOLOGIST CHRISTOPHER Milroy was tasked with reviewing Jenna Mellor's case for the Chief Coroner's Office. He found several problems with Smith's work on the case. The first was the most basic: "Dr. Smith showed a lack of appropriate knowledge of tissue responses to injury and clinico-pathological correlation." Smith could have answered the crucial question of when Jenna received her fatal injuries—crucial to determining the most likely suspect—during her autopsy if he'd understood the healing reactions of the fatal injuries to her pancreas and small intestine. Opinions from clinicians were eventually sought—not by Smith—but they shouldn't have been necessary.

Documentation in the case was also lacking, Milroy found. Smith gave no opinions in his final autopsy report, in which he should have outlined his reasoning on the crucial issue of timing and detailed the causes of Jenna's multitude of injuries. He should have discussed the discrepancy in the timing of her liver injury in relation to her fatal injuries. No exhibits were recorded in the reports. The hair found in the child's pubic area should have been properly photographed where it was found, then seized and given to police. Appropriate swabs should have been taken, as there was evidence of a possible sexual assault. Opinions were sought (specifically Dirk Huyer's consultation on a possible sexual assault) but not documented in the final autopsy report.

And Milroy believed Smith may have missed crucial evidence. Working from Smith's description of Jenna's injuries, Milroy agreed with earlier assessments by Dr. Michael Pollanen and Dr. Robert Wood that there were signs of a bite mark on the child's knee. Milroy said Smith should have investigated the mark more thoroughly in consultation with a forensic odontologist. If the bruising was in fact caused by a bite mark, it may have been possible to determine who inflicted the injury, since the two main suspects were a teenage boy and an adult woman. Furthermore, Milroy said that if Smith believed the child's behaviour throughout the day before her death would be a key consideration, he should have suggested an appropriate clinician with whom police could consult.

Lastly, Milroy pointed out that there did not appear to be any peer review or audit completed at the time of the final autopsy. When the various reviews were eventually completed, Smith appears to have had minimal involvement. "This case may well have had a different course if an early review of the case had been conducted with the appropriate experts," Milroy concluded.

At the Goudge Inquiry, Smith said he still believed his findings from Jenna Mellor's autopsy were correct. He testified that he did not agree with reviewers who believed the child suffered her fatal injuries within six hours of her death, while she was in JD's care. He pointed to an injury to Jenna's liver, arguing that it was older.

He claimed that he did an exam to rule out sexual assault. He said Dirk Huyer from SickKids' SCAN team assisted. He admitted he had found a hair in Jenna's vaginal area, but dismissed its relevance, believing it to be a contaminant. He kept the hair because, he said, the police didn't want it. He took it with him to Brenda's preliminary hearing but never mentioned it, even when asked about it. Smith said he never made the connection because he was questioned about a pubic hair and he believed the hair in his pocket was a contaminant.

It was more of the same incomprehensible rationalizations Brenda Waudby had been hearing for years. And then Smith apologized.

"I realize in Jenna's case the evidence that I gave concerning timing of the injury was not clear and concise, and I realize that it had the potential to be misunderstood. And I also realize that my handling of the hair was not what it should have been and gives reason for others to question not only that, but also thereupon my entire report. I'm sorry for that.

"I realize that those actions were not helpful. I realize that they served only to perhaps confuse the investigation. It was not helpful in Court. And so I would apologize to the investigators and the judicial system, but most importantly, I would apologize to Jenna's mom for what I did."

Smith's eyes stayed down when he spoke those words. He would not look at Brenda. And when he did look up, his eyes went past her to the back of the room, where a line of television cameras dutifully recorded his mea culpa.

Brenda Waudby did not accept his apology—could not accept it.

It didn't matter. She didn't need one. What she needed were answers.

Unfortunately, for her, the Goudge Inquiry did not provide them.

Brenda welcomed Christopher Milroy's report as further vindication of the criticisms that for years she had voiced about Smith's conduct in the case. Her calls for a public inquiry started shortly after the charges against her were dropped. She filed a complaint to the Peterborough Police Services Board. It was dismissed, but she continued her calls for a public inquiry, and she did after her complaint to the College of Physicians and Surgeons of Ontario was considered. Brenda wanted Smith's licence revoked. The College stopped short of that, although it did find that aspects of his conduct in the case were deficient. At each step along the way, Brenda was able to glean a little more insight. But each new bit of information just left her with more questions. The inquiry was supposed to answer them all, but in the end it didn't.

Milroy's review of Jenna's case was gratifying, yet the way it was handled only added to Brenda's frustration. JD had pleaded guilty to manslaughter on December 14, 2005, the same day the sexual assault charges against him were withdrawn. The very next day, Milroy completed his report pointing to signs of a possible sexual assault. While it did not say definitively that Jenna was sexually assaulted—stating that more testing should have been done—the report raised the possibility. And it came one day after JD's sex assault charges were withdrawn.

"It's heartbreaking to think that he got away with what he got away with because of one day, the lack of one phone call," Brenda said years later. "It's all it would have taken."

There was also the issue of Jenna's older rib injuries. They were the entire basis of Brenda's plea bargain and conviction, yet Milroy's report didn't even address them. Brenda wanted to know if those injuries were in fact older. But her own lawyer did not direct those questions to Milroy at the Goudge Inquiry. Jim Hauraney said the rib injuries simply weren't an issue at the time. He said Brenda never asked him to question Milroy about them—a claim Brenda angrily denies.

Brenda believes there is a reason Hauraney didn't ask about the timing of Jenna's rib fractures: he didn't want to introduce testimony that might suggest there was in fact no medical basis for Brenda's child abuse plea—a plea he had helped arrange.

Brenda's conflicted feelings about Jim Hauraney reflect the complexity of her case. On the one hand, she might have been tried and convicted of her daughter's murder had he not found medical experts to challenge Smith on the timing of Jenna's fatal injuries. However, Brenda believed he had saved her from one wrongful conviction only to play a crucial role in landing her another one.

Granted, the charges are not equal. Murder carries a potential life sentence; her child abuse conviction earned her probation. Even if the plea deal was a necessary evil, it was a small price to pay to correct a much larger wrong. I spoke with one lawyer familiar with the case and he all but laughed at the insignificance of the conviction. It wasn't even a Criminal Code charge. To go from a second-degree murder charge to a minor child abuse conviction was a ridiculously good swap, he said. Brenda Waudby should be grateful.

Except Brenda never abused Jenna. Still, to family, to friends, to people she'd never met, to the world, she would always be an admitted, convicted child abuser.

And she couldn't live with that.

After the Goudge Inquiry, Brenda decided to appeal her conviction. There were enough discrepancies between Jenna's injuries, Brenda's retracted confession and the agreed-upon facts in her plea deal that Brenda hoped the courts would see the value of a thorough review of the conviction.

She talked to her lawyer, Julie Kirkpatrick. To both the defence and the new Crown counsel, Alison Wheeler, Christopher Milroy seemed an obvious choice to do the review. In 2008 he had moved from England to take up a position at the Eastern Ontario Regional Forensic Pathology Unit at the Ottawa Hospital as well as a teaching post in pathology and laboratory medicine at the University of Ottawa. Everyone had been impressed with the work he had done for the inquiry. Perhaps he could finally answer the lingering questions about the older injuries to Jenna's ribs: Were they actually older? Or could JD have caused them on the night of her death? If the pathologist believed JD was responsible, Brenda would have grounds to get her child abuse conviction overturned.

Brenda remembers when Julie Kirkpatrick called her with the news. Her lawyer asked her to join her for a walk in the picturesque village of Millbrook, outside Peterborough, where her office was located. Brenda was worried; a walk with her lawyer never brought good news.

Kirkpatrick told her that officials with the Hospital for Sick Children had gone through Smith's office and catalogued everything they found. It was a long, and troubling, list. Jenna's rib cage was on it.

At first Brenda was horrified. But then she realized there might be an opportunity in the gruesome discovery. It was 2009, or maybe 2010. (Neither woman can remember exactly.) The Goudge Inquiry was over. Brenda was gearing up to challenge her child abuse conviction, which hinged on the timing of Jenna's rib injuries. Now they had the rib cage for forensic testing.

Milroy completed four reviews specifically related to Brenda's child abuse conviction. He found the damage to Jenna's ribs was extensive: twenty-three injuries, including twelve fractures, to thirteen ribs. He did not find any evidence of an underlying medical condition, such as a metabolic bone disorder or genetic disorder, to account for the injuries. While some of the damage could have been caused during the paramedics' resuscitation efforts, the extent and positioning of the injuries strongly suggested they were caused by trauma. "Fractures of a young child's rib cage require considerable force as the ribs are elastic and pliable," Milroy wrote in his report. "This force is beyond normal handling or simple falls or bumps against an object."

He also found that nothing Brenda had done, or allegedly had done, could account for the damage to the ribs. Brenda's accidentally dropping Jenna on the crib rail wouldn't have caused them. Even her recanted confession, in which she told police she swung her arms and may have hit the child once or twice, could not account for the injuries.

And then there was their timing. Milroy reasoned that, based on the microscopic findings in the case, all of Jenna's rib injuries occurred within twelve hours of her death, and they correlated with the other injuries that caused her death. In other words, they weren't older. Jenna's ribs were damaged during the same assault or assaults that killed her.

In his last two reports, Milroy dealt with the final lingering question surrounding Jenna's injuries: a laceration to her liver. It hadn't been used as evidence, and wasn't even mentioned, in Brenda's conviction, but it was the one injury that still didn't quite fit with the assaults that killed her.

Brenda and Julie Kirkpatrick were eager to clear the air; they didn't want to leave any doubt over whether Brenda was responsible for any of Jenna's injuries. But more than that, Brenda just wanted to know. More than fifteen years had passed since the murder, a long, painful journey for a mother just trying to understand what had happened to her daughter.

Milroy wrote, "The features suggest a time frame of more than six hours, and likely 24 hours. It is not days old, however." He added that the liver injury would have been caused by an impact to the child's abdomen, such as a punch or kick, leaving open the possibility that Brenda might have been responsible. If the injury occurred six to eight hours before Jenna's death, she was with JD. Any earlier put her in her mother's care.

For his final report, Milroy was asked to clarify if this wider window of opportunity for the timing of the liver injury was evidence that Jenna had been a victim of chronic abuse by her mother.

His answer: "I can confirm that there was no evidence of chronic abuse of Jenna and that the timing and causation of the injury to the liver are compatible with the statement given by the babysitter."

It was done. Brenda Waudby finally had all her answers. Now all she needed to do was clear her name.

COURTROOMS ARE SUPPOSED to be places of justice. For Brenda Waudby they hadn't been. But her lawyer promised her this day would be different. It was June 27, 2012. Two lawyers—Julie Kirkpatrick for Brenda, Alison Wheeler for the Crown—gave prepared speeches to the judge. They detailed Brenda's suffering, and for the first time, there were no caveats. Jenna's death was not her fault.

"The bottom line is that the rib injuries were not old and they were not caused by Ms. Waudby, and there is no forensic evidence that Jenna was chronically abused," Wheeler said. "There is a liver injury that has been described as older but, given the amount of time that the babysitter had the child—some seven and a half hours—and, given the extent of his confession, the most reasonable explanation is that it, too, was caused by the babysitter. The conviction should be set aside as a miscarriage of justice and the only appropriate order would be for this court to enter an acquittal."

Wheeler would not budge, however, on one of Brenda's key claims: that the Crown required she plead to child abuse in exchange for dropping the murder charge. "The Crown adamantly denies that it was a precondition." Brenda bristled when she heard those words. She had even launched a Charter application, in part, over the issue: that the Crown's demand violated her right to life, liberty and security of the person under Section 7 of the Charter. (The application's primary focus was the Crown's non-disclosure of JD's confession after his plea, even during the Goudge Inquiry.)

She knew the Crown's position. She and her lawyer Julie Kirkpatrick had discussed it at length. They could continue to fight it, but the Charter challenge would be a long, fraught court battle that they might not win. Or Brenda could get on with her life, which is what she had been trying to do from the very beginning. So she had dropped the Charter application. Brenda Waudby took a deep breath and let it go.

"Apart from the concession on this appeal and the request that an acquittal be entered," Wheeler continued, "the most important aspect today is that the Crown apologizes to Brenda Waudby. The Crown is deeply sorry for how Ms. Waudby has suffered as a result of being wrongfully convicted of abusing Jenna. Her daughter was murdered. I should correct that," Wheeler clarified, catching herself. "Her daughter was the victim of a homicide; the young person pleaded guilty to manslaughter.

"Ms. Waudby should have been treated like a grieving parent. She was not. Due to flawed forensic pathology, she had to deal with being the focus of a police investigation, being charged with murder and being stigmatized as an abusive mother.

"Although the Children's Aid Society had legitimately been involved with the family because of other issues—which I note did not have to do with abuse—when all things are considered it would seem that she was wrongfully deprived of her two other children for periods of time largely because of Dr. Smith's opinions.

"She was wrongly placed in the position of having to rebuild a parental relationship with her older daughter who, at one point, came to believe that her mother might have been responsible for Jenna's death.

"She was wrongly stigmatized in a small community over a long period of time, and it has taken a very long time for all of this to be set straight.

"For all of this, the Crown is deeply sorry."

Brenda struggled to keep her emotions in check. When Wheeler was finished, Kirkpatrick asked the judge if Brenda could address the court. It was an unusual request—appellants are not usually given the chance to speak—but these were unusual circumstances and everyone in the courtroom knew it. Madam Justice Michelle Fuerst allowed it. Brenda unfolded the piece of paper on which she had prepared some words. It was dog-eared and worn from where she had held it tightly throughout the morning.

"Good morning, Your Honour. My name is Brenda Waudby. I am Jenna Mellor's mother." She cleared her throat, trying to calm herself. "I almost can't believe that this day has arrived and that I have just heard the Crown state that my plea of guilty was a miscarriage of justice. I can't describe the feeling that I have now as I stand before this court in the presence of my daughter, Justine, and the rest of my family. Not only has the Crown offered an apology, but it has been committed to righting the wrongs in my case, and that has meant everything to me and my children . . .

"On the first of March, 2007, when Jenna's killer was sentenced, I read a victim impact statement to the court. I would like to read a short part of that today."

Brenda turned the page. She had read these words five years earlier in a courtroom just down the road. She remembered the day, remembered the satisfaction of seeing JD in that courtroom, finally being held accountable for his crimes. But that satisfaction was short-lived and had led to only more frustration: the pittance of a sentence he received, and the blank stares she faced when she gave her speech. There was empathy in that courtroom, but it was clipped, contained, as if it was her who was still being judged.

This time, as she glanced around the room, it felt different. People were listening. The court was finally ready to hear her speak.

"'Jenna was gone forever. I could never say goodbye to her. My baby had barely started to live her life. She was just learning to talk. Her first word was "Mom." I believed Jenna had great potential, but I will never know. She had a smile that would light a room. Her eyes sparkled with love. She loved me and I loved her. I was to be her safety and security. I let her down. I failed her. Do you have any idea the guilt a mother feels for failing a child?'" Brenda read, tremors of sorrow shaking her hands.

"'I was charged with murder. I pled guilty to a Child and Family Services Act charge in June of 1999. I was innocent of this charge. I understood from my lawyer that my choice was I plead guilty or fight the murder charge, while the CAS puts Justine up for adoption. I was terrified at the prospect of losing another child forever.'

"That decision to plead guilty to save my family is the reason why I am before this court today. It worked. I did save my family."

Brenda looked over at her two children, who stared back. Justine was so young when all this started; now she was a fully grown woman.

Alex had never known Jenna. This nightmare was the only reality he had ever known.

After describing her efforts to find the truth about Jenna's death, Brenda said, "I knew that I didn't harm Jenna, and I knew the only reason I pled guilty to the charge of child abuse was because I believed at the time I had no choice.

"The consequences, however, were enormous—not only legally, but privately. Because of that conviction, I was unable to have my young son in my care until he was almost a year old. The Children's Aid Society entered Jenna's autopsy photographs into evidence before the family court, and I was repeatedly accused of causing the injuries that were evident on her body . . . It didn't matter how often I said that I hadn't and couldn't have done that to her, very few people would believe me . . .

"We are all human, and we all make mistakes. I have made many mistakes, and I have had to learn to live with the biggest mistake of my life—leaving Jenna with my neighbours to babysit, and returning home to find sirens in my driveway and my baby dead in the hospital morgue. Somehow, the fourteen-year-old boy was able to sexually assault and beat my baby to death while his mother was upstairs, and nobody at the time believed that was possible. They thought it must have been me. I live my life wishing I could turn back the clock, that I had stayed home that night. But I didn't, and I have to learn to live with that.

"Because I have had to learn to live with the horror of what happened to Jenna, I know that I have become far stronger than I ever knew I could be, more determined to seek the truth, more committed to seeing that justice is done and, I hope, more understanding of others, less judgmental and more determined to be kind and to choose to forgive whenever possible . . .

"I knew that if I didn't give up this day would come . . . My beautiful children have made it worth the fight, and because of me they know that anything is possible if you believe deeply in finding the truth.

"Your Honour, thank you for giving me the time today to say the things that I've needed to say for a long time. I very much appreciate that. Thank you."

384 - JOHN CHIPMAN

Justice Fuerst adjourned court for the morning break. Brenda's appeal was a joint submission, so ordinarily a simple endorsement from the judge would be enough to resolve the case. But given the extraordinary circumstances, the judge had more to say and needed a moment to prepare herself.

When court returned at noon, Justice Fuerst reviewed the facts of the case, slowly coming to the most contentious issue: the circumstances surrounding Brenda's guilty plea.

"She decided to enter the guilty plea, even though she had not, in fact, harmed Jenna at any time, because she was terrified that if she continued to fight the murder charge her older daughter would be put up for adoption by the Children's Aid Society, and she would lose her forever."

Since Brenda had withdrawn her Charter challenge, it was no longer necessary for the court to rule on whether her plea had been voluntary, but the judge still felt compelled to address it. "The Crown who appeared on the guilty plea and on the subsequent withdrawal of the murder charge denies that the plea of guilty to the child abuse charge was a precondition of withdrawal of the murder charge. I note, however, that the transcript of the guilty plea proceedings reveals that, at their outset, Crown counsel advised the presiding judge that the Crown would be withdrawing the murder charge. Crown counsel did so, a few days after Ms. Waudby entered her guilty plea to the child abuse charge, stating that because of a shift in medical opinion there was no reasonable prospect of conviction.

"It is not my role today to make a finding on this disputed issue. I will simply say that it is understandable that Ms. Waudby would believe that withdrawal of the murder charge was conditioned upon her plea of guilty to the child abuse charge."

Julie Kirkpatrick slipped her hand in Brenda's and gently squeezed. After much thought, they had decided that the fight wasn't worth it, that trying to prove Brenda had been coerced into accepting the plea would be too long and arduous. And now the judge said she accepted her explanation anyway.

Justice Fuerst continued reading the corrected facts of the case into the record, and then she said the words Brenda had been waiting thirteen years to hear: "Ms. Waudby did not inflict the fatal injuries to her daughter. She did not inflict the rib injuries to her daughter. She did not inflict the injury to her daughter's liver. There was no factual basis for the charge of child abuse, or for Ms. Waudby's guilty plea to it. Her guilty plea along with the ensuing conviction for child abuse was a miscarriage of justice. Accordingly, the appeal is allowed. The guilty plea and conviction are set aside, and an acquittal is entered."

A long, level breath escaped Brenda's throat. It felt as if she had just expelled thirteen years of anguish and frustration.

Madam Fuerst then ordered her name be removed from the Child Abuse Register.

"This has been a long and time-consuming process," the judge continued. "It is my hope that today's proceedings will, once and for all, put to rest any lingering doubts or concerns that Ms. Waudby was in any way responsible for her daughter's horrific death. She has been wrongly accused and stigmatized; first as a murderer and then as a child abuser. She should have been treated over these many years as the person she is—a victim, not a perpetrator; a loving parent who suffered the excruciating loss of her daughter's life at the hands of someone else."

After eleven years, Brenda was finally free from her child abuse conviction. There was only one thing left to do: make Jenna whole.

Funeral director Patrick Benson, along with government officials, oversaw the exhumation at Little Lake Cemetery in Peterborough. They had erected a canopy over the site for privacy. The media wasn't informed and didn't find out. Brenda was there, together with Justine, Julie Kirkpatrick, and Brenda's brother and his wife. They stood away from the gravesite, but Benson kept Brenda apprised as the exhumation began.

It was difficult for the workers to bring Jenna up. The casket had crumbled. Jenna had been buried more than fifteen years earlier. Brenda was expecting to find a skeleton, but Jenna's body was still decomposing. In the casket, her remains were contained within a plastic bag. Patrick Benson took the remains back to his mortuary.

At Jenna's funeral in 1997, her casket was closed. The funeral home wouldn't let Brenda see her body. The director told her it was for her own good, since the autopsy had been very intrusive. What Brenda didn't know was that the funeral home had not taken any steps to prepare the body for burial. Jenna Mellor was buried in a plastic bag, her body still stuffed with rags from SickKids after the autopsy.

Benson told Brenda what had happened. He told her she could view the body, but advised against it. He would be taking pictures, he explained, if she needed to see. He and his wife washed and trimmed Jenna's hair. He put some in a keepsake box and some more in lockets for Brenda and Justine. In turn, Brenda and Justine also cut their hair, and the funeral director placed strands inside the casket.

A memorial was held three days later. Brenda invited her immediate family and a small cadre or friends who had stuck with her over the years. About thirty people attended.

Justine spoke at the memorial, along with a minister. Brenda tried. Her emotions blotted out the words, but she struggled through. She's not sure anyone understood her. It didn't matter. Everyone understood the pain.

The burial was held the next day, at the same plot. A violinist stood at the top of the hill, playing as the same small group gathered. Julie Kirkpatrick brought a hawk's wing, bundled in sage. She and Brenda and Justine used it to cleanse the grave.

Benson had brought carnations for everyone, and one by one, they dropped their flower into the grave. Justine placed a stuffed dog at the foot of the casket. Brenda took a handful of dirt and dropped it in. Then Justine did the same.

People slowly started leaving, until it was just Brenda, Justine, Julie Kirkpatrick and the cemetery worker, filling the grave. Justine picked up a shovel and helped for a while. And then it was done. The violinist stopped.

Brenda slipped her hand in Justine's, and mother and daughter walked away.

KENNETH

ONE

SO WHO IS the man at the centre of so much pain suffered by so many people?

Despite a week of public testimony at the Goudge Inquiry, Charles Smith said almost nothing under oath about his personal history. Snippets of his story have been reported in the media, though, and much of it appears to have come directly from him.

Kirsty Duncan, Canada's minister of science under Prime Minister Justin Trudeau, came to know Dr. Smith in the early 1990s while researching for a project about the 1918 Spanish flu outbreak in Norway. Smith agreed to act as a consultant on her project. He told her he was of Norwegian descent and that his grandfather had immigrated from Norway and founded Mandel, a Norwegian town, in Saskatchewan. In her book *Hunting the 1918 Flu: One Scientist's Search for a Killer Virus*, Duncan described Smith as "what the Irish call a *seannachie*, a storyteller." She wrote, "The *seannachie* looked into the distance, 'Norwegian culture gave me so much. This will give me an opportunity to give something back to Norway.'" He told a newspaper reporter that he was born at the Salvation Army's Grace Hospital in downtown Toronto and that he was given up for adoption at three months. His adoptive father was in the Canadian Armed Forces, so Smith had a nomadic childhood, living all over Canada and in Germany. He went to high school in Ottawa and summered in Saskatchewan.

Finding his biological mother became a lifelong obsession. Smith told the reporter he spent years searching for her. He finally tracked her down, on her sixty-fifth birthday, only to have her reject him. "She hung up the phone," he said. The search for his biological mother did lead to the discovery of a half-brother in Toronto—who, he told the reporter, also happened to work at the Hospital for Sick Children.

Smith went to medical school at the University of Saskatchewan and completed residencies in surgery and pathology from 1975 to 1978, before moving to the University of Toronto for two more years of residency in pathology. He started out at the Hospital for Sick Children as a research fellow in 1980, before being hired as an anatomic pathologist the next year. Smith received certification in anatomic pathology in 1980 from the American Board of Pathology, but it would be another nineteen years before he received a diploma in pediatric pathology. He never received one in forensic pathology. Nevertheless, he started doing child autopsies for the Ontario Chief Coroner's Office in 1980.

Smith rose quickly in prominence at both SickKids and the Coroner's Office. He sharpened his style of testimony over years of practice. While his testimony wasn't always aesthetically pleasing—he was sometimes described as bland, even plodding in the witness box—it was highly effective. He was always confident in his findings, forceful and in control. His oratorical style would often come across as lecturing; he would chide lawyers on both sides for interrupting him. Defence lawyers feared facing him in court. They often had to search out of the province for pathologists who would challenge his findings on the stand.

By the mid-1980s, Smith was teaching law students how best to examine expert witnesses like himself. His curriculum vitae would eventually run to twenty-two pages. He openly boasted about one day writing "the definitive textbook on pediatric pathology."

He had many influential supporters. "He's a friend," Jim Cairns told Jane O'Hara, a reporter with *Maclean's* magazine. "I admire his work and he is greatly admired at the Hospital for Sick Children. He's done a tremendous amount of good over the years. His sincerity is beyond reproach."

Even some defence lawyers came to admire him. In 1988, Charles Ryall defended a man convicted of manslaughter in the death of his nine-week-old son. Smith did the autopsy and testified for the Crown. Ryall told O'Hara, "I told him that he'd done an excellent job as a witness and that it was a pleasure to have been in court with him."

Smith was heavily involved in his Protestant evangelical church, the Christian and Missionary Alliance. It boasts some two million members in forty countries, with more than four hundred churches in Canada alone. In 1999, Smith and his then wife, Karen, left their old parish to help start a satellite church in Richmond Hill, north of Toronto.

An important event in the early years of Dr. Smith's burgeoning career might shed some light on what was to follow. In 1980, when he began as a research assistant at SickKids, the hospital was going through a volatile time. In June of that year, babies in the hospital's cardiac ward had started to die in disturbing numbers. Sudden deaths of newborns were not uncommon or unexpected—it was a hospital for sick children, after all— but the rate of deaths that summer and fall jumped so dramatically that nurses on the ward were alarmed. The first death to trigger concern was on June 30, followed by five more in July. In the next nine months, there had been thirty-two deaths in the hospital's two adjoining cardiac wards.

Nurses began raising the alarm about the mortality spike almost immediately, but they were assured by their supervisors and doctors that the children were dying because of their medical conditions. That view started to change in January 1981, when eighteen-week-old Janice Estrella died. The child was the first to receive a test for digoxin levels at autopsy. (Digoxin slows down the heart rate, but it is so effective that patients must be monitored closely to make sure the heart does not stop completely. Policy at SickKids at the time required two nurses to monitor the patient's heartbeat while the drug was administered.) Estrella's result came back for digoxin nearly thirty times higher than therapeutic levels—so high that the number was dismissed as a laboratory error or due to contamination.

No one thought much of this anomalous result until a twenty-five-day-old named Kevin Pacsai died two months later. His digoxin levels were six times higher than normal. Less than two weeks later, three-and-a-half-month-old Justin Cook died. He had not been prescribed digoxin at all, yet elevated levels were found at autopsy.

Three days after Cook's death, police had a suspect in custody: a pediatric nurse named Susan Nelles. Shift charts showed she had been working when most of the children died. When the arresting officers arrived at her apartment, she asked for legal counsel, which police and the Crown took to be a sign of her guilt. Nelles was charged with four murders, but the case fell apart at her preliminary hearing, when the judge ruled that the evidence against her was circumstantial, the Crown had never established a motive and there was insufficient evidence for the case to proceed to trial.

The judge believed someone was murdering children at the hospital; it just wasn't Susan Nelles. Three reviews did little to appease the mounting public furor. In 1983, a royal commission of inquiry was called to re-examine the baby deaths and the case against Nelles. The inquiry, led by Mr. Justice Samuel Grange, examined thirty-six deaths on the cardiac ward. It concluded that eight children had died from digoxin overdoses and poisoning could be suspected in another fifteen. Justice Grange agreed that there was insufficient evidence connecting Susan Nelles to the murders.

The police continued to investigate. Suspicion fell on another nurse at the hospital, but no further charges were ever laid.

Charles Smith would have seen these baby deaths and the police investigation up close. He would have witnessed the moral panic that gripped the hospital and then the public. He would have watched as murder charges were laid but didn't stick. And he would have known that whoever was responsible for poisoning those children got away with it.

For Charles Smith, one of the driving forces of his career was to find justice for children the system had failed. The poisoning epidemic at SickKids would have given him more fuel for that quest.

Was Tammy Marquardt's son Kenneth one of the children for whom Dr. Smith was attempting to find justice?

Tammy survived her suicide attempt in the summer of 1998. A prison guard found her unresponsive in her cell, and she spent three days in hospital. When she was discharged, she was transferred back to the Prison for Women. Correctional Services must have decided there were too many triggers at Grand Valley. Or the warden there didn't want to deal with a suicidal inmate.

For Tammy, one prison or the other prison, it didn't matter. But she couldn't muster the strength to try killing herself again. It was harder to get pills in P4W, and she was on suicide watch. It wasn't that she wanted to live. It's just that her suicide attempt had terrified her. She had even failed at that.

A year and a half later, just before P4W was shuttered for good, she was transferred back to Grand Valley. The verbal abuse resumed. Inmates taunted her relentlessly. "She nuked her kid!" they screamed. "She put him in a roasting pan and ate him for Thanksgiving dinner!" The threat of physical violence was ever-present. Tammy continued to profess her innocence, to inmates, prison guards, psychiatrists—to anyone who asked and many who didn't. Tammy had been seeing psychiatrists since the start of her sentence. She always refused to admit she had killed her son, and the psychiatrists always insisted that acceptance was essential for her to move on.

"Acceptance!" she would yell in frustration. "I. Didn't. Do. It. *You* need to accept that I am not supposed to be here."

"Tammy, you were found guilty," was always the response. "You're here for a reason. You killed your son. You're only hurting yourself by not admitting the truth."

Dr. Gjylena Nexhipi had assessed Tammy in 2000. In her report, she suggested Tammy review Smith's autopsy report. "[It] offers a very clear and comprehensive account reflected in the conclusion of non-accidental asphyxiation in the form of suffocation as the likely cause of death."

Nexhipi didn't think Tammy was actively trying to deceive herself or anyone else. She accepted that Tammy believed she had not killed her son. The psychiatrist concluded that she had developed amnesia to deal with the trauma and guilt.

Two years later, another psychiatric assessment noted Tammy's contin-ued reluctance to admit what she had done. "Tammy did become weepy when discussing her feelings of injustice that she was found guilty of a crime that she states she did not commit . . . [She] is unable to take responsibility for the offence that she was convicted of. When confronted with the obvious discrepancies between her version of events and that of pathological findings, Ms. Marquardt could offer no explanation."

Tammy continued to struggle with depression; she struggled to keep the suicidal thoughts at bay. And the guilt. It was hard to shake the feeling that a life lost to prison is what she deserved—not because of what she purportedly did, but because of what she hadn't done. If she had only remembered how to do CPR, she could have saved Kenneth, she could have saved Keith and Eric, she could have saved herself. But she hadn't, so here she was.

Tammy rarely had visitors, but she did find solace and support from an unexpected source: the Native Sisterhood, a First Nations inmate group at Grand Valley. Tammy's father, Donald, was a member of the Oji-Cree First Nation, yet she'd never explored that part of her heritage. She did in prison, first out of necessity, then out of honest curiosity. The Native Sisterhood not only gave her a sense of belonging; most important, it introduced her to people on the inside who looked out for her well-being.

The Native Sisterhood helped immensely. She joined the inmate committee. She signed up for computer training and other professional development courses. She asked about volunteering outside the prison. And she connected with Epilepsy Waterloo-Wellington, in Kitchener. She wanted to help out in person.

Kenneth had had epilepsy. Tammy was convinced it must have played some role in his death. If she could help another parent avoid the trauma and loss that she had suffered, then some good could come from Kenneth's death. The parole board agreed. It took note of the progress she was making at Grand Valley and her increased involvement at the institution. It granted Tammy escorted temporary passes to the epilepsy agency.

She had one friend on the outside, Melinda Harbinson. Tammy had met her when she was awaiting trial. Melinda believed Tammy when she said she was innocent, and continued to believe her even after she was convicted. She brought her son for visits and let Tammy change his diapers and feed him his bottle. It meant the world to Tammy that Melinda trusted her with the baby. In light of the success of her off-site volunteering, the parole board granted her escorted visits to Melinda's home as well.

In 2002, her security clearance was lowered from medium to minimum. The next year, she started regularly attending meetings of Alcoholics Anonymous at a branch outside the prison. In 2004, she was granted supervised visits to the Elizabeth Fry Society offices in Toronto. She became a facilitator in the Alternatives to Violence program inside the prison.

In 2004, she contacted a lawyer to help her prepare for her parole application. The conversation, naturally, turned to her crime. Tammy told the lawyer she didn't kill her son, just as she had told anyone who would listen for more than a decade. But for the first time, someone heard her. The lawyer suggested she get in touch with a group called the Association in Defence of the Wrongly Convicted.

In late 2005, Tammy applied for an unescorted temporary absence permit so she could go to the Elizabeth Fry Society on her own. This would mark the first time she had stepped outside the prison without an escort in almost a decade. Elizabeth Fry was on board, and so was Grand Valley. Her case management team supported her application, noting Tammy's excellent work ethic as well as the work she was doing addressing her "contributing factors." It felt she was at low risk to reoffend. The permit was granted.

It was a surreal feeling to step outside prison on her own—untethered, unsupervised and free—equal parts exhilarating and terrifying. Tammy had not made a decision on her own in almost a decade. In prison, guards tell you when to eat, when to sleep, when to work, when to shower. Her autonomy had increased as her security clearance dropped, but it was largely an illusion. She was still in prison.

Her sentence had been life in prison with parole ineligibility for ten years. By October 2005 she had survived a decade on the inside. She had worked diligently on her parole application for more than a year, ticking off all the steps she needed to take, all the milestones she needed to reach. It felt like the end was in sight.

On December 13, 2005, Tammy was granted day parole and released to a halfway house in Toronto. She would be on parole for the rest of her life, but she was free again.

JAMES LOCKYER FOUND his life's calling in the summer of 1992. He had immigrated from England in 1971 and taught law at McGill and the University of Windsor before joining a law firm in 1977, where he took on criminal and immigration cases with a civil rights component. In 1980, he teamed up with legendary defence lawyer Jack Pinkofsky. He had his first encounter with Charles Smith in 1990, as part of the defence team for Julie Bowers. Smith's conduct in the case didn't make much of an impression on Lockyer, perhaps because Bowers was acquitted.

For Lockyer, everything changed in August 1992, when he took on the appeal of Guy Paul Morin—the first time Lockyer had challenged a wrongful conviction. Morin had just been convicted of first-degree murder in the 1984 death of his nine-year-old neighbour Christine Jessop. (He'd been found not guilty at his first trial, in 1986, and the Crown had appealed.) And the lawyer wasn't the only one in Guy Paul's corner. A grassroots group sprang up, calling itself the Justice for Guy Paul Morin Committee. Its members were motivated by what they saw as a miscarriage of justice, and they became determined and ferocious allies for Lockyer.

Lockyer was set to argue the unreliability of Morin's purported jailhouse confession and the hair and fibre analysis that tied him to Christine's body, but he never got the chance. DNA test results on semen stains found on Christine's underwear came back negative for a match to Guy Paul. The Crown conceded that this new evidence was "indisputable scientific fact that Mr. Morin is not guilty of the first-degree murder of Christine Jessop, and should be acquitted."

The case gave Lockyer—and several members of the Justice for Guy Paul Morin Committee—a new-found legal focus: wrongful convictions of any Canadian. With Morin's exoneration, the group was reconstituted as the Association in Defence of the Wrongly Convicted, or AIDWYC. A team of volunteer lawyers would review cases to look for possible miscarriages of justice. James Lockyer was a founding member.

Tammy's 2004 letter to AIDWYC initially went to lawyer David Bayliss, one of that team of volunteers, and Smith's involvement in her case immediately piqued his interest. He went to visit Tammy at Grand Valley in the fall of 2005, just before she was released on bail. Several months later, when Chief Coroner Barry McLellan ordered the review of all Smith's suspicious child death cases, Lockyer was appointed to the committee established to oversee the reviews. Tammy's case was on that list. When Lockyer found out she had also reached out to AIDWYC requesting assistance, he approached Bayliss to find out more about the case and offer his assistance. Her case was being reviewed by an independent pathologist. If he found problems with Smith's opinions or conduct, AIDWYC would take the case.

Dr. Pekka Saukko was assigned to review Kenneth's death. His résumé is impressive. Unlike Smith, he was a certified specialist in forensic medicine, but his qualifications went far beyond that. Saukko led the Department of Forensic Medicine at the University of Turku, in Finland, and served as visiting professor in forensics at universities in Japan, China and Hungary. He was a founding member and president of the European Council of Legal Medicine and held similar positions or fellowships at societies of forensic medicine in Hungary, Belgium, Germany and Great Britain. He published widely on issues of forensic pathology and was the editor-in-chief of *Forensic Science International*, one of the leading international peer-reviewed forensic journals.

After reviewing Smith's autopsy report and his testimony at both the preliminary hearing and the trial, Saukko was very concerned. To begin with, several of Kenneth's organs had been removed for donation *before* the autopsy—something Smith had brushed off at the time as "a minor inconvenience." "It is impossible," Saukko wrote in his 2007 review, "to know in advance with certainty to which extent organ harvesting may or may not hamper the subsequent autopsy." The problem is that organs that were harvested could contain clues to how and why the person died. Without examining them, pathologists can never know if they missed something important. But that's only one of the problems. "Surgical intervention may destroy or obscure evidence or cause artefacts that make the interpretation of the findings more difficult, if not impossible," Saukko wrote. The surgery required to remove organs often damages the body, further complicating the autopsy and making it even more difficult to determine the cause of death. Smith had compromised his post-mortem exam before it even began.

And then there was the autopsy itself. Saukko thought Smith had wildly overstepped the evidence to reach his conclusion of asphyxia caused by suffocation or smothering. Smith had diagnosed asphyxia based solely on the presence of petechiae—tiny blood spots—on the thymus and on the outer linings of the lungs and the heart. But Saukko said the presence of petechiae alone is "generally known to be non-specific." In other words, the tiny spots don't mean anything on their own.

Overall, Saukko found Smith's testimony unscientific, confusing and contradictory. Smith testified, for example, that the presence of petechiae was significant "and sufficient to make a diagnosis of asphyxia." But later he said he didn't "have concrete evidence of asphyxia." When asked if Kenneth could have suffered some form of epileptic seizure, Smith replied, "That would be the other major explanation or the other possibility . . . I cannot assure you that he did not die from a seizure." Yet later he contradicted himself again, stating his findings were consistent with manual or ligature strangulation and with suffocation.

At one point, Smith testified that the harvesting of Kenneth's organs could have caused the petechiae on Kenneth's epicardium. Later, he contradicted himself, stating that "petechiae don't make the diagnosis . . . other causes of petechiae have to be considered."

Saukko wrote, "It is illogical and completely against scientific evidence-based reasoning to give any cause of death if there is one or several causes that cannot be reasonable ruled out. In such a case, the death has to be classified accordingly as unascertained."

Adjusting to life on the outside was difficult. After more than ten years, Tammy had earned her freedom, but she had not won it. Her murder conviction was still an albatross around her neck; she would have to comply with her parole conditions for the rest of her life. In some ways, she felt she had missed her chance to prove her innocence. Now that her incarceration was behind her, was it even worth holding on to the injustice? Although AIDWYC had taken on her case, she found it hard to invest much hope in it. If no one believed her when she was inside, why should anyone believe her now?

And there were the simpler challenges of adjusting to life on the outside. She needed to find a job, needed to find a way to support herself. She found odd jobs at a restaurant, at a bookstore, at a factory. She spent a short stint working at Canada's Wonderland. But she couldn't hold on to any of the work. And the spectre of October was looming.

October was the anniversary of both Kenneth's death and her conviction. She stopped taking her antidepressant medication. She started drinking again, and getting high. What little money she earned went into dangerous self-medication. Illicit drug use was strictly prohibited under the terms of her parole, and she was subject to regular drug testing. She tested positive for cocaine use in the fall of 2006, which landed her back in Grand Valley for a few weeks.

Being sent back to jail was a stark warning that the authorities could lock her up again at any time. Tammy needed to stay clean—but she couldn't. In the spring of 2007, she again tested positive for cocaine. This time it cost her a month back in Grand Valley.

By the time she got out, the Goudge Inquiry was building up steam. She met with Commissioner Stephen Goudge that June. He told her that international experts were reviewing Kenneth's death. If mistakes had been made, they would find them.

It was surreal to hear: everything Tammy had prayed for was finally starting to unfold. It was wonderful news, but it was overwhelming. It's one thing to know you are innocent; it's another thing to watch the world slowly come to that realization. Tammy turned back to drugs and alcohol to cope and quickly spiralled out of control.

In July, staff at the halfway house where she was living found a crack pipe in her room. Later that month, she signed herself into a detox and treatment centre in Toronto for its intensive three-week residential program. But sobriety didn't take, and Tammy quickly relapsed. In August, her parole was revoked once again and she was returned to Grand Valley. Tammy had used up all her second chances. In November 2007, her parole was revoked for good.

James Lockyer now had Pekka Saukko's damning review of Smith's opinions on Kenneth's death. That review, which became a key part of the Goudge Inquiry, was powerful and compelling. Smith argued at the inquiry that listing asphyxia as the cause of death—without explaining what caused the asphyxia—was reasonable in 1994, when he had completed the report. "I believe that it was in line with the practice standards at the time," he testified. "[It] may have been inadequate, but that was a normal or accepted practice and so I think I was in the mainstream of my work pattern when I did that."

Saukko's findings, however, were unequivocal: Smith had overstepped his own findings by suggesting there was pathological evidence of foul play in Kenneth's death.

James Lockyer believed he had the makings of an appeal of Tammy's conviction based on fresh evidence. But he wasn't taking any chances. He needed corroborating opinions, another pathologist, or even two, who could review the medical evidence.

Lockyer approached Simon Avis, the chief forensic pathologist and chief medical examiner for Newfoundland and Labrador. He was certified in general and anatomical pathology by the Royal College of Physicians and Surgeons of Canada in 1989 and received further training in forensic pathology in the United States.

Avis's review of Kenneth's death eviscerated Smith's medical opinions and testimony. He, too, pointed out that the findings of petechial hemorrhages have no diagnostic significance and are of no assistance in determining Kenneth's cause of death. The finding of a hypoxic brain injury, or an oxygen deficiency in the brain, was likewise a non-specific injury, and one that was to be expected, given that Kenneth suffered a heart attack that cut off blood flow. Avis wrote, "Based on the autopsy, the cause of death should have been listed as undetermined. The manner or death likewise was undetermined."

Like previous reviewers, Avis pointed out that the organs removed before the autopsy could have been relevant to determining the cause and manner of death. "Some inborn errors of metabolism, capable of causing sudden death, may only become apparent on examining individual organs such as the liver," he wrote. He noted that when Smith was asked about the organ harvesting at trial, he testified that it "was a minor inconvenience in terms of [his] examination, but it doesn't affect the conclusions at all." Avis, his disbelief almost jumping off the page, wrote, "No forensic pathologist would support this statement."

He found Smith's testimony in general either unsupported by his findings or incomprehensible to medical experts, let alone a jury. And often both.

At one point, Smith had testified that he found evidence suggesting that Kenneth had been suffocated with a soft object. "There were no findings made at autopsy to justify this answer," Avis said. "The unspoken inference that Kenneth may have been suffocated with something like a pillow is not available as a conclusion from the autopsy findings."

Likewise, Smith had suggested that microscopic hemorrhages in the neck were consistent with a neck injury. His testimony on the issue was confusing and imprecise—Avis wrote that Smith himself admitted during his testimony that he was "rambling"—but the pathologist left the impression that Kenneth may have suffered a neck injury. Avis wrote, "There was no evidence of neck injury or neck compression found at autopsy. The microscopic hemorrhage in the neck structures has no pathological significance."

So if there was no anatomical evidence indicating Kenneth's cause of death, how did he die? While Avis believed the cause and manner of death ultimately should have been declared "undetermined," there were other issues that needed to be considered. The most obvious was Kenneth's history of seizures. "Sudden unexpected death in epilepsy (SUDEP) is a well- recognized cause of unexpected death in infants and adults," Avis said in his report. "Deaths due to disorders of the central nervous system (CNS) are second only to cardiovascular disease as the cause of sudden unexpected deaths, and seizure disorder is the most common disorder of this type."

Kenneth had experienced at least seven seizures. Most were diagnosed as febrile, benign seizures often seen in infants and young children during a fever. But Avis said Kenneth's seizures were likely misdiagnosed. "None of Kenneth's seizures were associated with a documented increase in body temperature," he wrote. When Avis reviewed Kenneth's medical records, he found that when his temperature was taken on the four days he suffered one or more seizures, it was in fact lower than normal. "Despite this, Kenneth's medical record indicates that six of his seven seizures were associated with a fever. The available medical documentation does not support this conclusion."

Avis said that Kenneth's EEG was normal, but he argued that that didn't exclude the possibility of a seizure disorder. He said that epilepsy is intermittent, and because EEG testing is often done in between seizures, evidence of the condition may not show up in the results. "An abnormal EEG finding can be diagnostic, but a normal EEG does not exclude the occurrence of a seizure disorder."

According to Avis, Kenneth's seizures were serious enough that his doctors had prescribed medication to help manage them, first phenobarbital and then Dilantin. When Kenneth was admitted to hospital, the levels of Dilantin in his system were below therapeutic, increasing his predisposition to seizures. "Death from a seizure disorder can occur as a result of respiratory arrest or cardiac arrest. Many seizure deaths occur in individuals with sub-therapeutic levels of anti-seizure medication," he wrote, adding that Tammy herself had once been treated with seizure medication and another relative was diagnosed with a seizure disorder. And Avis argued that a person can die from a partial seizure but be conscious in the moments before death, which would explain how Kenneth was able to call out to Tammy before he died.

Avis pointed to two other possible medical explanations for Kenneth's death. "Errors in fatty acid metabolism are becoming increasingly recognized as a cause of sudden death in infants and young children," he wrote. He said seizures may be seen in people with a genetic condition called medium-chain acyl-coenzyme A dehydrogenase, or MCAD, deficiency. "[It] may only be apparent when examining the liver under the microscope . . . Unfortunately, due to harvesting, Kenneth's liver was never examined."

The other possibility was a cardiac conduction defect, but these would have been hard to detect in the early 1990s, when Kenneth died. "Today these can sometimes be diagnosed post-mortem as a result of improved molecular genetic technology," Avis wrote. "At the time of Kenneth's death they would have simply presented as a sudden unexplained death."

James Lockyer believed his appeal was on solid ground with Avis's report and Saukko's work on the case for the Goudge Inquiry. It was time to see if he could get Tammy out of jail.

It had been sixteen months since Tammy's parole was revoked for the last time. But prison was different this time. When she was sent back in the fall of 2007, the Goudge Inquiry was front-page news. Revelations about Charles Smith rippled through Canada's judicial and penal systems. For the first time, Tammy's psychiatrists stopped dismissing her claims of innocence. Prison administrators began treating her with a new-found respect. Prisoners she once worried were plotting to kill her now nodded at her wordlessly as someone railroaded by a broken system.

Her bail hearing was held on March 12, 2009. Tammy made the hour-long drive from Grand Valley to Ontario's Court of Appeal in downtown Toronto. Madam Justice Kathryn Feldman presided. The bailiff led Tammy into the prisoner's box, her hands still shackled in front of her. The hearing was a formality; Lockyer had already told her that Crown counsel Gillian Roberts would be consenting to her bail request. Tammy would be leaving court as a free woman. She smiled as she surveyed the crowd of people who had come to witness her release. An old high school teacher was in the gallery. Bill Mullins-Johnson was there too. And Rick

Marquardt. Tammy couldn't believe it. What was her ex-husband—the man who'd deserted and divorced her after her arrest, who testified against her at trial—doing there? There was warmth in his eyes, and something else. She couldn't place it at first, and then it hit her.

Remorse. Tammy looked away.

Lockyer made his submissions to the court, specifically citing the findings of Dr. Saukko and Dr. Avis. Tammy was granted bail.

"Do up your coat," Lockyer said to her as she stepped into the glaring sunshine of a late-winter day. "It's cold outside."

THREE

TAMMY'S LEGAL FIGHT was far from over. Lockyer had convinced the Supreme Court of Canada to consider reopening her case. If it agreed, the case would be sent back to the Ontario Court of Appeal, which would decide what to do with her conviction. The best-case scenario would be that the appeal court would set aside the conviction and enter an acquittal in its place. That's what it had done in Bill Mullins-Johnson's case. But it was a very high bar. It meant the court would have to decide that no reliable evidence, medical or otherwise, implicated Tammy. The more likely outcome would be a decision to send the case back for a retrial that would incorporate the medical opinions of Saukko and Avis.

The Crown then would have to decide if it wanted to mount a new trial, considering the thirteen years Tammy had already spent in prison. Setting aside the conviction wouldn't be as satisfying as an outright acquittal, but if the Crown declined to retry her it would have the same practical outcome and it was more easily attainable.

The Crown was doing its own due diligence. Gillian Roberts commissioned yet another pathologist to review Avis's report. Chris Milroy agreed that the pathological findings in the case did not point to a definitive cause of death. He, too, believed Smith should have classified it as "unascertained" or "undetermined." And he agreed that a seizure disorder could not be excluded as a potential factor. But he said an expert in pediatric neurology should be able to determine whether Kenneth's earlier seizures were febrile or epileptic convulsions. And a pediatrician with expertise in childhood epilepsy might be able to say whether Kenneth could have called out to Tammy in the midst of a seizure.

Milroy considered Avis's other explanations to be on shaky ground. He argued that although MCAD deficiency should have been considered, signs of it would not have been in Kenneth's liver. "Changes in MCAD may be found in the heart, but were not present in this case. The decision to harvest the liver for transplantation in this case was not unreasonable," Milroy argued. He added that Kenneth had not had other clinical signs and symptoms of MCAD, such as vomiting and lethargy. Lab findings typically show low blood glucose levels, but Kenneth's blood glucose levels were elevated when he was admitted to ICU.

Milroy thought MCAD deficiency was likely not a factor in Kenneth's death. Likewise, he thought Tammy's description of Kenneth's behaviour before his collapse precluded a cardiac conduction disorder, since those usually present as a sudden loss of consciousness or heart stoppage.

But Milroy's most pointed criticism of Avis's review was not for something *in* his report but rather for something he left out. "Dr. Avis is correct when he states that there is no evidence in the pathology to support a finding of 'asphyxia,'" Milroy wrote. "However, what Dr. Avis does not state in his report is that in smothering deaths there are characteristically no positive pathological findings. Thus, the pathological findings do not exclude smothering. Dr. Avis should have listed smothering as a possible cause of death."

Milroy's report was a setback for Tammy. An esteemed pathologist thought smothering could have been a cause of death. Nothing pointed directly to it, but nothing excluded it, either.

"The full determination of the cause of death," Milroy concluded, "requires an examination of not only the pathological evidence, but other evidence including the clinical evidence and the evidence of other non-medical witnesses. Whether this evidence is accepted is a matter for the tribunal of fact."

Milroy was practically crying out for a new trial, the outcome Lockyer was most trying to avoid. Tammy had already lost more than a decade of her life behind bars; her lawyer didn't want to put her through the stress and trauma of a new trial. Although more jail time seemed unlikely, given the sentence she had already served, Lockyer felt another conviction would be another miscarriage of justice.

The lawyer was determined to stop it before it got that far.

—

Simon Avis wrote a rebuttal to Milroy's report, defending his findings. He agreed that smothering could occur in the complete absence of any anatomical findings. (He noted that Lockyer had asked him to look for new potential medical explanations for Kenneth's death, which was why he had left aside smothering, since that was one of the existing theories that underpinned Tammy's conviction.) And he added that, given Tammy's description of Kenneth's struggles in the bedsheet, he could not exclude accidental suffocation as a cause and manner of death.

The trio of reports had left smothering as a possible cause of death. Lockyer needed another heavy hitter. He also needed to keep his eye on the target. Milroy was an esteemed pathologist who had contributed to uncovering Smith's shoddy work in other cases for the Goudge Inquiry. Trying to discredit him would be counterproductive. Discrediting Smith was still the key.

Both Avis and Milroy agreed that a pediatric neurologist might be able to figure out what type of seizures Kenneth had suffered in his short life: benign fever-related seizures or potentially fatal epileptic seizures.

Elizabeth Donner is a pediatric neurologist at Toronto's Hospital for Sick Children and a leading expert in sudden unexplained death in epilepsy. Donner was the lead author on the largest-ever research study into cases of SUDEP in children, which was published in the peer-reviewed journal *Neurology* in 2001. (Interestingly, one of her co-authors was Charles Smith.)

Lockyer knew most medical experts wouldn't have a problem challenging Smith's findings. He'd been thoroughly discredited during the Goudge Inquiry. But Smith wouldn't be the only target. At Tammy's trial, several medical experts had testified for the Crown, including William Logan, another pediatric neurologist at SickKids. In 2010, when Lockyer approached Donner, Logan was the senior staff neurologist at the hospital.

Lockyer was up front about the possibility that Donner might end up challenging the work of an esteemed colleague from her own hospital, one with more seniority and standing than she had. She told him she was certain she would be able to remain objective. She wouldn't hold back her own opinion of the case.

And she didn't. Her report was even more damning than Dr. Avis's.

Donner listed five criteria a person must have at the time of death for it to be classified SUDEP. First, and most important, the person must have epilepsy, defined as a history of two or more unprovoked seizures. Donner agreed with earlier assessments that Kenneth's first seizures were febrile, but she said his medical records clearly show that, starting just before his second birthday, he had five seizures that, did not involve a fever. Moving from febrile to afebrile convulsions is a common progression for patients with epilepsy.

"His epilepsy was significant enough, in the opinion of his treating physicians, to warrant treatment with an anticonvulsant medication," Donner wrote, adding, "It is not standard practice, nor was it in 1993, to treat febrile seizures with these anticonvulsant medications."

Second, SUDEP involves a person dying unexpectedly while in a reasonable state of health. "From review of the medical records and court testimony, it seems that Kenneth was in good general health at the time he died," Donner wrote, noting that while he did have asthma, neither his pediatrician nor his family doctor believed that affected his general health.

Third, in cases of SUDEP, deaths either happen suddenly or occur later from complications of cardiac or respiratory arrest. Donner noted that while Kenneth's death wasn't sudden, he did suffer a sudden heart attack, from which he later died.

Fourth, SUDEP deaths happen during normal activities in benign circumstances. Tammy said Kenneth was calling her name and kicking his legs when she found him entangled in his sheets. "Seizures may take many forms; a seizure may involve kicking or jerking both legs. A seizure may also include a child being able to call out. A combination of these symptoms, however, is unlikely," Donner acknowledged. But she added that a seizure does not always precede death in SUDEP. "Most reported cases of SUDEP are not witnessed, making it difficult to ascertain whether a seizure preceded death. There is evidence of a seizure before death in up to 67% of

SUDEP cases." However, the presence of seizures preceding death is even less common in child SUDEP cases. Donner cited two of her own reviews in which only half of witnessed child SUDEP deaths followed a seizure.

The final criterion for a SUDEP finding is that the autopsy must demonstrate no toxicological or anatomic cause of death. Smith's initial autopsy report identified an anatomic cause of death—asphyxia—but the subsequent reviews by Saukko, Avis and Milroy all found his opinion to be unfounded. All three thought Kenneth's cause of death should have been classified as "undetermined" or "unascertained."

"In my opinion," Donner concluded, "the death of Kenneth Wynne meets the criteria for SUDEP." But she added that a SUDEP finding could not have been made at trial because of Smith's incorrect finding of asphyxia. That finding, which went unchallenged by Tammy's defence team, effectively removed SUDEP as an alternative cause.

Donner's report was everything Lockyer needed. Not only did it criticize Smith's work on the case (which Saukko, Avis and Milroy had also done), but it also provided a feasible explanation for Kenneth's death. Still, Lockyer was taking no chances. He wanted a second opinion on SUDEP, so he approached Carter Snead, another pediatric neurologist at SickKids and Donner's other co-author on her landmark 2001 study. Snead also found that SUDEP could not be ruled out as the cause of Kenneth's death.

James Lockyer now had five experts—three pathologists and two pediatric neurologists—all of whom believed Smith's findings at autopsy and his testimony at trial were not supported by the medical evidence. Several pointed to other possible natural causes of death, including sudden unexplained death in epilepsy.

It would take two trips. Lockyer and the rest of Tammy's legal team had already argued before the Supreme Court, back in 2009, that in light of the questions being raised about the legitimacy of Smith's medical opinions in the case, Tammy needed a new hearing to consider the fresh evidence. The top court had ruled in her favour, sending the case back to the Ontario Court of Appeal for consideration.

The first appeal hearing was held on February 10, 2011. More than fifteen years after Tammy's conviction. More than seventeen years after Kenneth's death. The hearing was, once again, a formality, Lockyer assured her. The Crown was on board. It agreed that the fresh evidence should be admitted, the appeal allowed, the conviction quashed and a new trial ordered.

It was that last detail—a new trial—that was so difficult for Tammy to stomach. Hadn't she suffered enough already? Lockyer told her not to focus on that. They'd won. The court was going to set aside her conviction. She would no longer be a convicted child killer. The question of a new trial was for another day. Lockyer thought it was unlikely the Crown would push the case that far, and assured her he would do everything he could to make sure it never happened.

She looked around the courtroom at the Ontario Court of Appeal. Newfound supporters—people she barely knew—had come out en masse.

Lockyer made his submissions to the three judges on the bench. Gillian Roberts made submissions for the Crown. And then one of the judges addressed Tammy directly.

"We recognize this has been a terrible ordeal for you, and it's tragic it has taken so long to uncover the flawed pathology that led to your conviction in 1995," Mr. Justice Marc Rosenberg said. "We agree . . . There was a miscarriage of justice."

As expected, the court quashed her murder conviction and ordered a new trial.

"Finally, the nightmare is coming to an end and I'm waking up," Tammy told reporters afterwards.

But the prospect of another trial—however remote—made real celebrations feel premature.

Four months later, she was back in court again—and Lockyer was right. Crown counsel Greg Driscoll notified the judge that the Crown was withdrawing the murder charge and would not be proceeding with a new trial.

"I appreciate that my words today may seem inadequate," Mr. Justice Michael Brown told Tammy, "but I offer to you, Ms. Marquardt, my

410 - JOHN CHIPMAN

deepest expression of regret for all you have endured as a result of the miscarriage of justice in this case. Nothing I can say to you today will repair the damage that has been caused to you. Nothing I can say can bring back your son Kenneth for whom you still grieve. This has been a terrible ordeal."

And then the hearing ended.

"You are free to go, ma'am," the judge said. Tammy was greeted by applause from supporters and reporters in the hallway outside the courtroom.

"The one thing that never should have happened has ended," she told them. "Honestly, I never thought I would see this day. I. Am. Free. Now Kenneth can rest in peace."

FOUR

KEITH STARED AT his parents blankly.

Brian and Eileen had just told their oldest son everything they knew about Tammy. About his older brother, Kenneth, a brother he hadn't known existed until only hours before. About Kenneth's death and Tammy's conviction for murdering him. About her life sentence, and the adoption. About the medical experts who had got it wrong. Keith's birth mother was wrongfully convicted. And now she was out.

Keith wanted to believe his birth mother wasn't a murderer.

He asked his parents if they knew how to reach Tammy. They were sitting in his mother's hospital room. Brian and Eileen suggested he contact Children's Aid. But they warned him he might have to wait until he was eighteen before they could do anything. Brian took Keith home, and Keith immediately began searching online news sites. He found story after story about his birth mother. She was almost famous.

Keith called *W5*, the investigative program that had done an episode on Tammy, but he couldn't find anyone there who could help him. He called CP24, the twenty-four-hour news channel. He called the *Toronto Star*, which just kept hanging up on him, and the *Toronto Sun*. The person at the *Sun* was sympathetic, but didn't know how to find Tammy.

Brian suggested he try Facebook. Keith wasn't on Facebook himself, so he used his mother's account. He found Tammy almost immediately. At least he thought it was her. Her profile photograph was of a wolf. He sent her a friend request. Then he found a Rick Marquardt and skimmed through his pictures, thinking he saw a resemblance to himself. He sent Rick a friend request too. Then he went back to Tammy's page and started going through her list of friends. Maybe one of these people would know her phone number. He started sending out friend requests and quickly got a response. He explained to the woman who he was and why he was looking for Tammy.

"Can you help?" he asked.

The woman said she would get in touch with Tammy.

At last, a friend request came from Tammy, then a flurry of Facebook messages. He got her phone number, then thought better of it. He wanted their first conversation to be in person.

"Can we meet?" he messaged.

Tammy gave him her address.

Keith rode the GO train into Toronto. It was a long walk to the train station from their suburban home—forty minutes, at least—but Keith welcomed the time to gather his thoughts.

The train car was empty. Keith sat in a window seat and watched the scenery race by. The train pulled into the Danforth GO station in Toronto's east end. He double-checked her address, then braced himself against the bitter winter wind. It felt surreal, walking unfamiliar streets to an unfamiliar house to meet his mother for the first time.

Keith Hutton knocked on the door.

The tiny woman who answered introduced herself as Tammy. And Keith introduced himself as her son.

EPILOGUE

CHARLES SMITH—DR. SMITH's medical licence in Ontario expired on August 9, 2008, when he failed to renew it with the College of Physicians and Surgeons of Ontario.

On February 1, 2011, the College's Discipline Committee found that Smith had committed acts of professional misconduct in his practice of forensic pediatric pathology and in his work providing expert-opinion evidence. The committee found Smith was incompetent. He failed to maintain the standard of practice of the medical profession, and engaged in conduct or acts or omissions that could reasonably be regarded as disgraceful, dishonourable or unprofessional. In particular, and in multiple cases, the discipline committee found that:

— Dr. Smith failed to gather relevant information, undertake appropriate investigations and properly detail relevant information;
— Dr. Smith expressed opinions about the cause of injuries or death that were either contrary to or not supported by the pathology evidence at the time the opinion was first expressed or were no longer supported after receipt of additional information;
— Dr. Smith formed erroneous opinions about the cause of death based on non-specific findings, and he misinterpreted autopsy findings;
— Dr. Smith referenced aspects of the social history of the parents or caregivers of the deceased child that were irrelevant to the pathology;
— Dr. Smith opined on the manner of death rather than exclusively on the pathological cause of death;

— Dr. Smith failed to respond to communications from coroners, Crown attorneys, police officers and other pathologists in an appropriate and timely manner. Furthermore, Dr. Smith attempted to unfairly shift responsibility for these failures to others. These failures compromised the administration of justice;

— Dr. Smith failed to create, maintain and preserve pathology materials relevant to criminal investigations in the manner expected of a pathologist acting pursuant to the Coroners Act. These failures compromised the administration of justice;

— Dr. Smith exaggerated his experience, or conversely, failed to disclose his lack of experience in the area of forensic pathology. Dr. Smith offered opinions outside of his area of expertise. Dr. Smith gave evidence that was unbalanced, overly dogmatic or failed to acknowledge uncertainty or controversy, and which was speculative, unsubstantiated and not based on pathology findings;

— Dr. Smith failed to provide his opinions to coroners, the police, Crown attorneys and/or the Court in a manner that met the standard expected of a forensic pathologist in Ontario at the time. He gave his evidence in a manner that was misleading, overly casual, unfairly critical of other experts or unscientific. In other cases he acted as an advocate rather than expressing an unbiased opinion. Dr. Smith failed to adequately prepare for court; and

— Dr. Smith failed to respond to inquiries from regulating bodies, including the CPSO, with the candour expected of a member regarding his involvement in certain cases under investigation. This lack of candour prevented the regulating bodies from exercising the degree of oversight that might otherwise have been exercised.

The Discipline Committee ordered that Smith's certificate to practise medicine in Ontario be revoked. He was ordered to appear before the panel to be formally reprimanded, and to pay costs of $3,650 to the College.

Charles Smith was licensed to practise medicine in Saskatchewan through parts of 2005 to 2007. On July 16, 2006, the Saskatchewan College of

Physicians and Surgeons charged Smith with unbecoming, improper, unprofessional or discreditable conduct. On February 2, 2007, Smith pleaded guilty to providing false and misleading information to the Saskatchewan College. On his licence application, he answered negatively to the question of whether he had ever been the subject of an inquiry or investigation by a medical licensing authority or hospital. Smith received a formal reprimand and was ordered to pay costs of $2,407.82. After his plea, restrictions were added to his his licence but it was active in the province until January 1, 2008, when it went inactive for non-payment of licensing fees.

As of August, 2016, Charles Smith is not licensed to practise medicine in any jurisdiction in Canada. He has never been charged, prosecuted or convicted of a criminal offence for anything related to his work as a pediatric forensic pathologist.

JIM CAIRNS—Dr. Cairns's licence to practise medicine in Ontario expired on June 1, 2009, when he resigned his membership with the College.

The former deputy coroner of Ontario signed an undertaking with the College in 2010 in which he agreed never to apply or re-apply for a licence to practise medicine in Ontario or any other jurisdiction. In exchange, the College dropped its investigation of him under the Health Professions Procedural Code. As of August, 2016, Jim Cairns is not licensed to practise medicine in any jurisdiction in Canada. He was never charged, prosecuted or convicted of any crime related to his work with Charles Smith or with the Office of the Chief Coroner of Ontario.

JAMES YOUNG—Dr. Young's registration as a licensed medical practitioner also expired on June 1, 2009, when he too resigned his membership with the College.

On Jan. 19, 2010, the former chief coroner of Ontario agreed to an undertaking with the College. In it, Young acknowledged that he has no intention of applying again for a medical licence in Ontario, and agreed to notify the College if he changes his mind. In exchange, CPSO agreed not to proceed with an investigation of him. But if he decided to re-apply, Young acknowledged that the College could re-open its investigation. As of August 2016, he is not licensed to practise medicine in any jurisdiction in Canada.

James Young has never been charged, prosecuted or convicted of any crime in relation to his time working with Charles Smith or in his duties as Chief Coroner of Ontario.

DR. DIRK HUYER—The former SCAN team member at the Hospital for Sick Children worked with Charles Smith on several cases, most notably the death investigation of Jenna Mellor. During the autopsy, the two doctors decided there was no evidence of sexual abuse. Huyer did not put his opinion in writing. He did not file a report. He later told me that he viewed his involvement in Jenna's autopsy as an opportunity for professional development more than a formal consultation.

After consulting Dr. Huyer, Smith decided not to complete a full sexual assault evidence kit for Jenna, a decision that had a profound impact on the direction of the police investigation.

No disciplinary action was taken against Dr. Huyer for his role in the Jenna Mellor case, or any others. In March 2014, he was appointed Chief Coroner of Ontario.

DR. BARRY MCLELLAN—As Chief Coroner of Ontario, Dr. McLellan ordered the review of Dr. Smith's cases in 2005, which eventually led to the Goudge Inquiry. In 2007, Dr. McLellan left OCCO to become the President and CEO of Sunnybrook Health Sciences Centre in Toronto.

NOTES AND SOURCES

THE STARTING POINT for my source and reference material was the *Inquiry into Pediatric Forensic Pathology in Ontario*, by the Honourable Stephen T. Goudge, released in 2008. Dozens of witnesses testified at the Goudge Inquiry in late 2007 and early 2008, including Charles Smith. Smith did not respond to numerous requests to speak to me for this book, so I relied heavily on his testimony at the inquiry, along with his notes and reports that relate to the cases that I examined. Dr. Jim Cairns declined my requests for an interview, and I could not locate Dr. James Young, despite concerted efforts, so I also relied heavily on their testimony and files.

Lawyers for the Goudge Inquiry prepared overview reports examining the twenty cases that were the focus of the inquiry. They also released thousands of documents to assist testimony before the inquiry and support these overview reports. I reviewed and referenced hundreds of these documents in researching this book. I haven't listed them all here, but they are referenced in each of the reports I used for Jenna, Nicholas and Kenneth. There was no overview report for Athena. And there are extensive court records from the criminal prosecutions surrounding Kenneth, Jenna and Athena, which I also used.

Below is a breakdown of the testimony and other material I reviewed and/or used in each of these cases.

TESTIMONY
Transcripts for the following testimony is available online at http://www.attorneygeneral.jus.gov.on.ca/inquiries/goudge/index.html and was accessed between March 1, 2013, and May 1, 2016. All titles listed were current at the time of testimony.

Dr. Barry McLellan, former 1 Coroner of Ontario, November 12–16, 2007.

Dr. Michael Pollanen, Chief Forensic Pathologist for Ontario, November 12–16 and December 5–6, 2007.

Dr. Jack Crane, State Pathologist for Northern Ireland, November 19–23, 2007.

Dr. Christopher Milroy, Chief Forensic Pathologist (Forensic Science Service), Professor of Forensic Pathology (University of Sheffield) and Consultant Pathologist to the U.K. Home Office, November 19–23, 2007.

Dr. John Butt, Forensic Pathologist and former Chief Medical Examiner (Alberta and Nova Scotia), November 19–23, 2007.

Dr. Jim Cairns, Deputy Chief Coroner of Ontario, November 26–29, 2007.

Dr. James Young, former Chief Coroner of Ontario, November 29–30 and December 3–4, 2007, and February 8, 2008.

Dr. David Chiasson, Director of the Pediatric Forensic Pathology Unit (Hospital for Sick Children [HSC]) and former Chief Forensic Pathologist for Ontario, December 7 and 10–11, 2007.

Dr. Helen Whitwell, Forensic Pathologist (U.K.), December 12–14, 2007.

Dr. Pekka Saukko, Professor of Forensic Medicine (University of Turku, Finland), December 12–14, 2007.

Maxine Johnson, Administrative Coordinator (Pathology Division, HSC), December 17, 2007.

Dr. Glenn Taylor, Head of the Division of Pathology (HSC), December 18–19, 2007.

Dr. Ernest Cutz, Pathologist (HSC), December 18–19, 2007.

Dr. Bill Lucas and James Edwards, Regional Supervising Coroners, January 7–8, 2008.

Dr. Dirk Huyer and Dr. Katy Driver, HSC Suspected Child Abuse and Neglect (SCAN) team, January 9–10, 2008.

Insp. Robert Keetch, Sudbury Police, January 14, 2008.

Sgt. Larry Charmley and Const. Scott Kirkland, Peterborough Police, January 15, 2008.

Michele Mann and Elizabeth Doris, College of Physicians and Surgeons of Ontario, January 16, 1998.

Dr. Chitra Rao, Regional Pathology Unit, January 17–18, 2008.

Brian Gilkinson, Crown Counsel, January 21–22, 2008.

Dr. Robert Wood, Odontologist, January 23, 2008.

Dr. Charles Smith, January 28–February 1, 2008.

CHARLES SMITH

The story of Smith's birth mother rejecting him appears to have originated from an interview Smith gave *Toronto Star* reporter Dale Brazao in 2005. When I asked Smith's former wife, Dr. Karen Smith, about it she dismissed the story as a media fabrication. The details, however, appear to have originated from Smith himself.

Documents

Report titled "Evidence of Dr. Smith," prepared for the Goudge Inquiry, undated.

Books/articles cited

Kirsty Duncan, *Hunting the 1918 Flu: One Scientist's Search for a Killer Virus* (Toronto: University of Toronto Press, 2003).

Elaine Buckley Day, "The 20th Century Witch Hunt: A Feminist Critique of the Grange Royal Commission into Deaths at the Hospital for Sick Children," *Studies in Political Economy* 24 (Autumn 1987).

KENNETH

Interviews

Brian Hutton, October 28 and November 12, 2013; Keith Hutton, November 20, 2013; James Lockyer, May 30, 2013, and September 29, 2015; Rick Marquardt, May 24, 2013, and September 2015; Tammy (Marquardt) Wynne, May 13, 14, 28 and June 14, 2013, and September 2015; Margaret Wynne, October 14, 2016.

1   In one instance Brian and Keith Hutton had different versions of an event. Keith's
     version is recalled on pp 3–4. Brian recalls Keith's discovery of his adoption papers a
     little differently. He said it didn't happen all on the same day. Brian said he went to the
     bank in the summer to get the boys' adoption papers. Keith was with him and when the
     teenager asked him what the documents were, Brian said he told him the truth. He said
     he would share them with Keith when he was older. Brian brought the entire file home
     and put it in a lockbox. He had meant to bring it back to the bank, but never did. In
     December, one of the boys needed some personal information for a school project so he
     got the adoption papers out, but didn't lock them up again. Brian had an argument with
     the boys on the day he was going to see his wife in the hospital. One of them demanded
     more information about their adoption and birth mother. Brian refused. When he went
     to the hospital that night, Keith searched the house and found the adoption papers.

Court decisions
R. v. Marquardt, 1998 CanLII 3527 (ON CA).
R. v. Marquardt, 2011 ONCA 281 (CanLII).
Tammy Marie Marquardt v. Her Majesty the Queen, 2009 CanLII 21729 (SCC).

Transcripts
Tammy's 911 call, October 9, 1993.
Preliminary inquiry on September 27 and 29–30, 1994, three volumes.
Trial on October 2–6, 11–13, 16–20 and 23–24, 1995, ten volumes.
Appeal in the Superior Court of Justice, June 7, 2011.

Documents
Kenneth Wynne Overview Report, prepared by Commission Counsel for the Goudge
     Inquiry, including all available supporting documentation.
Tammy's statement to Det. S. Naccarato, October 9, 1993.
Admission forms from the Hospital for Sick Children for Kenneth Wynne, November 23,
     1991, November 8, 1992, and June 4 and 5, 1993.
Letter from Dr. D. Filek to Dr. S. Caspin, December 9, 1991.
Letter from Dr. M. Mian to Dr. S. Caspin, May 31, 1993.
Ambulance Call report, June 4, 1993.
HSC Emergency Nursing Record, June 15, 1993.
Oshawa General Hospital records, July 6, 7 and September 6, 1993.
Final Autopsy Report by Dr. Smith, undated.
Report of Post-Mortem Examination by Dr. Smith, April 15, 1994.
HSC Social Work report, October 9, 1993.
Report of Dr. Simon Avis examining the death of Kenneth Wynne, October 30, 2008.
Supplementary report of Dr. Avis, September 4, 2009.
Report of Dr. Christopher Milroy, July 30, 2009.
Comments of Dr. Milroy, August 2, 2010.
Supplementary report of Dr. Milroy, November 13, 2010.
Report of Dr. Elizabeth Donner, April 5, 2010.
Report of Dr. O. Carter Snead, June 30, 2010.
Supplementary report of Dr. Snead, August 9, 2010.

Tammy's Impact Statement to CPSO, February 1, 2011.

Tammy's Victim Impact Statement, October 2011.

Tammy's Affidavit filed with the Court of Appeal for Ontario, January 4, 2011.

Original indictment against Tammy alleging second degree murder, December 12, 1994.

Bail recognizance pending trial, February 11, 1994.

Order of Justice J.A. Feldman granting bail pending appeal, March 12, 2009.

Order of Justice J.A. Rosenberg ordering release pending re-trial, February 10, 2011.

Medico-legal report in respect of the death of Kenneth Wynne, conducted by Dr. Pekka Saukko for the Goudge Inquiry, undated.

NICHOLAS
Interviews
Miguel Bonin, June 20, 2013; T.C. Chen, June 19, 2013; Angie Gagnon, June 18, 2013; Maurice Gagnon, June 17–18, 2013; Berk Keaney, June 18 and September 24–25, 2013; Lynne Monk, June 20, 2013; Carolle Thibeault, June 19, 2013; Lianne (Gagnon) Thibeault, June 17–19, 2013; Pete Thibeault, June 19, 2013.

Transcripts
Lianne's interview with Sudbury Police, undated.

Reasons for Decision by Honourable Justice Louise L. Gauthier on July 28, 1998.

Submissions before Justice Gauthier by Roy Sullivan on August 10, 1998.

Reasons for Judgement by Justice Gauthier on September 22, 1998.

Order of Justice Gauthier on March 26, 1999.

Arbitration decision of Justice Gauthier on January 17, 2000.

Documents
Nicholas Overview Report, version 2, prepared by the Commission Counsel for the Goudge Inquiry, including all available supporting documentation, October 29, 2007.

Autopsy Final Report for Nicholas Gagnon, by Dr. T.C. Chen, August 14, 1996.

Autopsy Final Report for Nicholas by Dr. Charles Smith, August 6, 1997.

Statement by Dr. James Deacon, Coroner, May 27, 1997.

Letter from Dr. E. Uzans to Dr. James Cairns, November 25, 1996.

Consultation Report by Dr. Charles Smith, January 24, 1997.

Letter from Dr. Paul Babyn to Dr. James Cairns, January 13, 1997.

William Halliday report on the death of Nicholas Gagnon, February 27, 1999.

Police investigation notes and reports by Sgt. R. Keetch, February 14, 1997, and November 30, 2005.

Statement of Lynn Monk, June 20, 1997.

Statements of ambulance attendants André Groulx and Barry Ross Stenabaugh, November 30, 1995.

Statement of Dr. Miriam Mann, December 1, 1995.

Letter from Dr. Smith to Dr. Cairns, May 6, 1997.

Review by Dr. Mary Case, March 6, 1999.

Correspondence between Berk Keaney, Réjean Parisé and CAS of the Districts of Sudbury and Manitoulin, May 20, June 18 and December 30, 1998, and February 19, 22, 27 and March 24, 1999.

Berk Keaney letter to Réjean Parisé, October 27, 1998.

Memos and correspondence between Berk Keaney and Dr. Smith, December 10 and 16, 1998, and January 9, 21, 25 and 27, 1999.

Roy Sullivan handwritten note, June 22, 1998.

Court appearances log, file C-368-98.

Letter from Colette Kent to Lianne regarding Child Abuse Register, July 30, 1998.

Offer to Settle Agreement, July 3, 1998.

Letter from Maurice Gagnon, June 22, 1998, to Janet Ecker, Minister of Community and Social Services.

Correspondence between Maurice Gagnon and Dr. James Young, Chief Coroner, May 6, 1999; October 16, November 6, 9, 19, December 4 and 5, 2001; January 23, March 11, May 23, 30, June 3, 7, November 29, December 5 and 16, 2002; and January 8, 2003.

OCCO Memorandum #99-02: Forensic Pathology Pitfalls.

Consultation report by Dr. Mark Montgomery, January 9, 2002, and related correspondence, February 1, 2002.

Correspondence between Maurice Gagnon and Dr. Barry McLellan, Deputy Chief Coroner, February 17 and March 4, 2002.

Correspondence between Maurice Gagnon, College of Physicians and Surgeons of Ontario, and Dr. Young, October 5 and 27, 1998, and March 9, 1999.

Report by CPSO titled "Complaints Committee Decision and Reasons," November 15, 2002, and related correspondence between October 5, 1998, and September 6, 2002.

Partially redacted letter to CPSO from OCCO, March 4, 1998.

Review by Dr. Derek J. de Sa, Children's and Women's Health Centre of BC, of the Nicholas Gagnon death investigation.

Correspondence between Maurice Gagnon and Dr. Jim Cairns, March 26 and April 27, 1999.

Revised Coroner's Investigation Statement into the Death of Nicholas Gagnon.

Document titled "Chronology in the Matter of the Death of Nicholas Gagnon (Infant) and the Persecution of Lianne Gagnon (Mother)," prepared by Maurice Gagnon, undated.

Statement of Sgt. L. Thibeault, Sudbury Regional Police Service, regarding the first autopsy of Nicholas Gagnon, undated.

Complaint to the Coroner's Council by Maurice Gagnon against Dr. Smith, February 17, 1999.

Correspondence between Maurice Gagnon and Ian Davidson, Chief of Police, Sudbury Police Services, January 16, 27, November 30 and December 7, 2004, and January 15, 2005.

Letter to Mr. Gagnon from S.D. (Dave) Crane, Detective Chief Superintendant, Commander, Investigation Bureau, OPP, November 25, 2003.

Correspondence between Maurice Gagnon and Robert A. Keetch, Sudbury Police, October 24, November 15 and 21, 2001, and November 29, 2002.

Correspondence between Maurice Gagnon and Virginia M. West, Ontario Deputy Minister of Public Safety and Security, April 22, July 8 and November 25, 2002.

Correspondence between Maurice Gagnon and John Luczak, Crown Attorney, Sudbury District, January 20 and 21, 2005.

Report by Clare Lewis, Ombudsman Ontario, dated September 24, 2001, and related correspondence, June 26, November 10 and 30, 2000.

Maurice Gagnon's complaint against Dr. James T. Cairns, submitted to David Tsubouchi, Solicitor General of Ontario, March 6, 2000, and related correspondence, April 13, 2000.

Affidavit of Julie Boivin, worker with CAS of the Districts of Sudbury and Manitoulin, October 4, 1999, including handwritten notes.

Affidavit of Gisèle Haines, worker with CAS of the Districts of Sudbury and Manitoulin, October 19, 1999.

Affidavit of Louise Huneault, lawyer with CAS of the Districts of Sudbury and Manitoulin, October 21, 1999.

Home Study & Safety Assessment, CAS of the Districts of Sudbury and Manitoulin, prepared by Gisèle Haines, June 29, 1998, along with related endorsements and correspondence.

Affidavits of Dr. William Halliday, June 16 and July 10, 1998.

Affidavit of Dr. James Cairns, June 19, 1998.

Affidavits of Dr. Charles Smith, June 29 and July 20, 1998.

Affidavit of Dr. T.C. Chen, June 23, 1998.

Minutes of Settlement between CAS of the Districts of Sudbury and Manitoulin, and Lianne Gagnon, Pierre Thibeault, Angela Gagnon and Maurice Gagnon, June 26, 1998.

Protection Application by CAS of the Districts of Sudbury and Manitoulin, regarding Nicole Melanie Thibeault, June 29, 1998.

Complaint against the CAS of the Districts of Sudbury and Manitoulin, submitted to the Minister of Community Services by Maurice Gagnon, March 23, 2000, and related correspondence, April 26, 2000.

Reasons for Judgement by Judge P.W. Dunn in the matter of Her Majesty the Queen v. S.M., May 24, 1991.

Complaint against CAS of the Districts of Sudbury and Manitoulin, submitted to the Child and Family Services Review Board by Maurice Gagnon, August 7, 2000.

JENNA
Interviews
Jim Hauraney, March 1, 2016; Julie Kirkpatrick, March 6, 2016; Maja Schlegel, December 5, 2014; Justine Traynor, April 20 and June 27, 2013; Brenda Waudby, April 20 and June 27, 2013, and March 6, 2016.

Court decisions
Waudby v. The Queen, 2012 ONSC 4005.

Court filings
Notices of Application, filed in Superior Court of Justice, October 7 and 19, 2011.
Amended Notice of Application, May 24, 2012.
Respondent's Factum, filed by Crown Alison Wheeler, June 20, 2012.
Indictment for second degree murder, November 2, 1998.
Information regarding guilty plea to child abuse charge, filed June 11, 1999.
Probation order, June 11, 1999.
Affidavits of Brenda Waudby, May 4, 7, July 5 and 30, 1999, October 7, 2010, and May 29, 2012.
Affidavit of Linda Mitchelson, August 20, 1997.

Affidavit of Ken Munks, July 29, 1999.
Affidavit of Jennifer Brown, May 6, 1999.

Transcripts
Witness video statements of Brenda Waudby on January 22 and 23, 1997, and March 19, 1997.
Project Jenna Incident reports, surveillance intercept, September 5 and 8, 1997.
Brenda's two statements to police on September 18, 1997.
Police undercover operation targeting JD, December 16, 2005.
Proceedings on Adjournment before the Honourable Justice C. Marchand, April 29, 1999.
Proceedings at an Examination for Discovery of Sylvia Sullivan, May 31, 1999.
Proceedings at Sentencing and Plea before the Honourable Justice T.C. Whetung, June 11, 1999.
Proceedings before Justice H.R. McLean, June 15, 1999.
Proceedings on Appeal before the Honourable Justice M. Fuerst, June 27, 2012.
Reasons for Judgment by Judge A.P. Ingram, July 30, 1997.
Reasons for Judgment by Madam Justice K.E. Johnston, May 27, 1999.
Proceedings at plea before the Honourable Justice J.A. Payne in the matter of R. v. JD, December 14, 2006 (corrected transcript).
Proceedings in the matter of R. v. JD, February 27, 2007.
Proceedings on Sentencing before the Honourable Justice J.A. Payne in the matter of R. v. JD, March 1, 2007.

Documents
Jenna Overview Report, prepared by Commission Counsel for the Goudge Inquiry, including all available supporting documentation, dated November 12, 2007.
Report of Post-Mortem Examination of Jenna Clare Ann Mellor, by Dr. Smith, September 8, 1997.
HSC Internal Tracking Document for Jenna Ann Mellor, by Dr. Smith, undated.
Report of The Centre of Forensic Sciences, April 2, 1997.
Autopsy Report Review Form, by Dr. Milroy, December 14, 2006.
Medico-legal report reviewing the death investigation of Jenna Mellor, conducted by Dr. Christopher Milroy for the Goudge Inquiry, undated.
Warrant for Post-Mortem Examination, January 22, 1997.
Hospital records, January 22, 1997.
Witness Statement by Sally Kater, dated October 4, 2010.
Diagnostic Imaging Consultation Reports for Jenna C. Mellor, by Dr. Paul S. Babyn, dated January 29 and February 9, 1997.
Handwritten notes of Dr. Smith, undated.
Handwritten notes of Dr. Sigmund Ein, November 3 and 26, 1998, and April 23, 1999.
Letter from Dr. Ein to Jim Hauraney, January 25, 1999.
Review by Dr. P. Fitzgerald, May 14, 1999.
Review by Dr. B.M.B. Porter, May 26, 1999.
Review by Dr. K.C. Finkel, June 28, 1999.
Review by Dr. Ken Feldman, April 22, 2002.
Review by Dr. Michael Pollanen, June 16, 2004.

Review by Dr. J. Mark Walton, January 15, 2005.

Reviews by Dr. Christopher Milroy, September 30 and October 6, 2011, and April 4 and 21, 2012.

Letter by Julie Kirkpatrick to Dr. Milroy, April 18, 2012.

Letter by Alison Wheeler to Dr. Milroy, July 13, 2011.

Handwritten notes by Alison Wheeler regarding interview with Brian Gilkinson, November 29, 2010.

Notes by Helena Gluzman of Alison Wheeler's interview of Jim Hauraney, March 2, 2011.

Toronto Police Service press release, "Police officer of the Year - 1998 - awarded to Police Constable Maja Schlegel."

Peterborough Police General Occurrence Report, prepared by Det. Const. Lemay, covering March 4–10, April 30–May 1, May 24, 26 and July 9–August 18, 1997.

Police notes of Det. Const. Lemay, April 23–June 7, 1999, various others, undated.

Supplementary police report of Det. Const. Lemay, April 19 and April 28, 1997.

Supplementary Occurrence Report of Det. Const. Lemay, September 18, 1997.

Police notes of Sgt. Gord McNevan, undated.

Police notes of Const. Schlegel, April 8, 21, 29 and September 18, 1997, various others, undated.

Police notes of Const. Scott Kirkland, January 22, 1997.

Police supplementary report by Const. J. Chartier, January 23, 1997.

Jenna Mellor Homicide Review by Det. Const. Larry Charmley, undated.

Notes of CAS worker Melissa Graham, January 22, 1997.

Notes of CAS worker Sylvia Elgaly, January 24, 1997.

Notes of CAS worker Sylvia Sullivan, March 9, April 6, 9, 26 and 28, 1999.

Notes of CAS worker Jennifer Brown, May 6 and 7, 1999.

Notes of Dr. Smith's interview with CPSO, June 18, 2002.

Letter from Laird Meneley to Brenda, August 22, 1997.

Phone message memos by Mr. Meneley, September 8 and 9, 1997.

Fax message from Mr. Meneley to Robert Lightbody, September 5, 1997

Fax messages from Mr. Meneley to Mr. Hauraney, May 18 and June 2, 1999.

Memo by Alvin Schiek, September 18, 1997.

Handwritten letter by Brenda to Jim Hauraney, September 18, 1997.

Letter by Brenda to Jim Hauraney, undated.

Letter by Colleen Ward, September 23, 1999.

Letters by Dr. J.G. van Dorsser, October 9, 1996, and May 5, 1999.

Notes by Dr. van Dorsser, January 10, 1997.

Email from Brian Gilkinson to Rita Zaied, November 26, 2002.

Memo by Elizabeth Doris, CPSO investigator, September 12, 2001.

Letter from Mr. Meneley to Premier Michael Harris et al., December 15, 1999.

Studies cited

Saul M. Kassin and Katherine Neumann, "On the Power of Confession Evidence: An Experimental Test of the Fundamental Difference Hypothesis," *Law and Human Behaviour* 21, no. 5 (1997).

Steven A. Drizin and Richard A. Leo, "The Problem of False Confessions in the Post-DNA World," *North Carolina Law Review* 82 (2004).

Richard A. Leo and Richard J. Ofshe, "Consequences of False Confessions: Deprivations of Liberty and Miscarriages of Justice in the Age of Psychological Interrogation," *Journal of Criminal Law and Criminology* 88, no. 2 (1998).

Saul M. Kassin and Holly Sukel, "Coerced Confessions and the Jury: An Experimental Test of the 'Harmless Error' Rule," *Law and Human Behavior* 21, no. 1, (1997).

Saul M. Kassin and Lawrence S. Wrightman, "Prior Confessions and Mock Juror Verdicts," *Journal of Applied Social Psychology* 10, no. 2, (1980): 133–146.

Aldert Vrij, Par Anders Granhag and Stephen Porter, "Pitfalls and Opportunities in Nonverbal and Verbal Lie Detection," *Psychological Science in the Public Interest* 11, no. 3 (2010): 89–121.

Saul M. Kassin and Katherine L. Kiechel, "The Social Psychology of False Confessions: Compliance, Internalization, and Confabulation," *Psychological Science* 7, no. 3 (May 1996).

Melissa B. Russano, Christian A. Meissner, Fadia M Narchet and Saul M. Kassin, "Investigating True and False Confessions Within a Novel Experimental Paradigm," *Psychological Science* 16, no. 6 (June 2005).

Brent Snook, Joseph Eastwood, Michael Stinson and John Tedeschini, "Reforming Investigative Interviewing in Canada," *Canadian Journal of Criminology and Criminal Justice* 52, no. 2 (2010).

The Honourable Rene J. Marin, *Admissibility of Statements* (Aurora: Canada Law Book, 2004).

Gisli H. Gudjonsson, *The Psychology of Interrogations and Confessions: A Handbook* (Wiley, 2003).

ATHENA

Everything I wrote about Athena's case was drawn from public court records filed in her parents' case and at the Goudge Inquiry, as well as the interviews listed below. I did not speak to Anthony Kporwodu, and I had one brief phone conversation with Angela Veno, which is detailed in the book.

Interviews

Wade Carver, undated; Shir Churchill, undated; Dr. Marta Cohen, February 5, 2014, January 21 and May 31, 2015, and various dates via email; Matt Crone, October 9, 2014, and January 28, 2015; Breese Davies, undated; Del Doucette, April 15, 2013; James Grosberg, April 11, 2013; Heather Kirkwood, December 10, 2014, May 13, 2015, and various dates via email; Dr. Chris Milroy, April 7, 2015, via email; John Rosen, September 30, 2014, and various dates via email; Rosaleen Smith, October 7, 2014, and undated; Angela Veno, undated; Betty Veno, October 17, 2014, and March 15, 2015; Dan and Sonia Veno, October 7, 2014; Cindy Wasser, April 17, 2013, and December 16, 2014; Rita Zaied, April 15, 2013.

2   When I first spoke to each member of Angela's and Anthony's defence teams, I had not uncovered Athena's family history. I emailed each later to ask if they were aware of it, and what impact it might have had on their defence strategy had the Charter challenge failed and the case proceeded. Delmar Doucette and Cindy Wasser deferred to John Rosen for a response. Breese Davies did not respond.

Court decisions

R. v. A.K.1, 2003 CanLII 46118 (ON SC).

R. v. Kporwodu, 2003 CanLII 30947 (ON SC).

R. v. Kporwodu, 2005 CanLII 11389 (ON CA).

Judgment on Voir Dire by Justice P. Harris, November 27, 2001.

Final Order of the Honourable Judge Katatynych regarding custody of Julius Kporowdu, January 7, 2000.

Court Filings

Notice of Application for a Stay of Proceedings pursuant to ss. 7, 11(b) and 24(1) of the Charter, filed in the Ontario Superior Court of Justice, September 19, 2002.

Notice of Application to adduce further evidence on the application for a Stay of Proceedings, Charter, s. 11(b), April 4, 2003.

Amended Factum of the Applicants, dated May 26, 2003.

Supplementary Factum of the Respondent, Unreasonable Delay, May 27, 2003.

Written Submissions on behalf of the Office of the Chief Coroner of Ontario and Denise Dwyer, May 29, 2003.

Respondent's Factum, Unreasonable Delay.

Affidavit of Angela Veno, September 17, 2002.

Affidavit of Anthony Kporwodu, September 19, 2002.

Affidavit of Det. Matt Crone, October 7, 2002.

Affidavit of Cindy Wasser, April 4, 1993.

Affidavit of Jennifer Jenkins, September 19, 2002.

Affidavit of James J. Grosberg, October 27, 2002.

Affidavit of Dr. Jim Cairns, October 23, 2002.

Supplementary Affidavit of Dr. Jim Cairns, November 20, 2002.

Transcripts

Anthony's interviews with Toronto Police on March 6 and 7, 1998.

Angela's interviews with Toronto Police on March 6 and 7, 1998.

Det. Matt Crone's testimony at trial, voir dire, undated.

Preliminary Inquiry before Honourable Justice P. Harris on February 5, November 5, 6, 7, 8, 13, 19, 20 and December 17, 2001.

Judgment on Preliminary Inquiry before Justice P. Harris on January 17, 2002.

Hearing before Honourable Justice Brian Trafford ruling on The Production of Third Party Records to the Court, November 27, 2002.

Trial before Justice Trafford on November 28, 2002, and May 22, 2003.

Documents

Report of Post-Mortem Examination by Dr. A.J.A. Hunt, March 12, 1998.

Report of Post-Mortem Examination by Dr. Smith, October 26, 1998.

Letter from Dr. Smith to Det. Sgt. Crone containing his addendum to his post-mortem report, April 3, 2000.

HSC Internal Tracking Document by Dr. Smith, undated.

Two Ambulance Call Reports, both dated March 6, 1998.

Diagram form and handwritten hospital notes, March 6, 1998.

13 autopsy photographs, undated.

Central Nervous System Report by Dr. Laurence Becker, April 29, 1998.

Diagnostic Imaging Consultation Report, by Dr. David E. Manson, March 13, 1998.

Diagnostic Imaging Consultation Report by Dr. Paul S. Babyn, July 20, 1998.

Criminal Subpoena for Angela Veno, October 28, 2002.

Review by Dr. Robin P. Humphreys, May 30, 2002.

Review by Dr. Graeme Dowling, April 10, 2001.

Insurance documents for Athena Kporwodu, February 26, 1998.

Letter from Det. Crone to Dr. Smith, February 1, 2000.

Graph of 17 pediatric/child cases being considered for review, undated.

Letter from John B. McMahon, Director of Crown Operations, Ministry of the Attorney General, to Assistant Crown Rita Zaied, including graph of 19 pediatric/child deaths to consider for review.

Supplementary affidavits of Jennifer Jenkins, April 4 and May 16, 2003.

Memo from Cabbagetown Women's Clinic, November 6, 2002.

Chronology of Important Dates, January 17, 2004.

Report of six-case review by Dr. Blair Carpenter, June 1, 2001.

Chronology of Pre-trial Motions, undated.

Det. Crone's police notes, November 21, 29, 30 and December 14, 1999.

Letter from Denise Dwyer regarding Third Party Records, November 6, 2002.

Personal Medical History of Anthony Kporwodu, November 1, 2002.

Letter from Dr. William Sy to John Rosen, August 20, 2002.

Note from Dr. William Lucas, October 27, 1998.

Document titled "Preliminary Observations on Smith Cases for External Review," undated.

Memo by Dr. Pollanen to Dr. McLellan, January 8, 2007, regarding Smith review process.

Minutes: Review of Dr. Charles R. Smith (Reconciliation Meeting Week Two), December 15, 2006.

Notes from briefing of Minister re Charles Smith, April 21, 2005.

Letter to Michael Bryant, Attorney General of Ontario from Melvyn Green, president of AIDWYC, April 21, 2005.

Letter to Dr. McLellan from Melvyn Green, April 4, 2005.

Report by Dr. Pollanen titled "Preliminary Observations on Smith Review," November 20, 2006.

Letter from Crown Shawn Porter to Dr. McLellan, concerning Cindy Wasser, January 20, 2006.

Report titled "Coroner's Review" of Smith cases, undated.

Letter from Crown Rita Zaied to Dr. Smith, March 13, 2000.

Letter from Cindy Wasser to Dr. Chiasson, November 9, 2001.

Letter from Cindy Wasser to Dr. Cairns, November 9, 2001.

Notes of Det. Larry Linton, March 6, 1998, to July 10, 2002.

Summary of Memo Book notes by Det. Sgt. Matt Crone, March 6, 1998, to November 11, 2002.

Memo from Dr. Chiasson to Dr. Lucas regarding Forensic Pathology Case Review for Athena Kporwodu, October 27, 1998.

Coroner's investigation summary for Athena Kporwodu, by Dr. William Lucas, dated December 18, 1998.

Memo to Dr. Lucas, February 23, 1999.

Letter from CAS worker Colin So to Coroner Dr. William Lucas, August 17, 1998.

Report titled "Dr. Charles Smith Review: The Coroner's Death Investigation for
   Athena Kporwodu," February 27, 2007.
Report by Dr. Dirk Huyer on death investigation of Athena Kporwodu, February 9, 2002.
Review by Dr. Patricia McFeeley, September 7, 2001.
Letter from Det. Sgt. Crone to Dr. Smith, February 1, 2000.
Autopsy Report Review Form for Athena Kporwodu, completed by Dr. Milroy,
   December 13, 2006.
Email from Cindy Wasser to Robert Clark regarding Smith review, November 21, 2002.
Correspondence between John Rosen and John McMahon regarding Smith review,
   November 21, 25 and 26, 2002.
Correspondence between John Rosen and Rita Zaied, December 4, 11, 16 and 17, 2002.
Correspondence between Julie Battersby and John McMahon, April 25 and 29, 2003.
Memos from Rita Zaied to John McMahon, May 11, 2003, regarding the chart of Smith
   cases under consideration for review, and the disclosure of Crown material.

Studies cited

E.H. Whitby, P.D. Griffiths, S. Rutter, M.F. Smith, A. Sprigg, P. Ohadike, N.P. Davies,
   A.S. Rigby and M.N. Paley, "Frequency and Natural History of Subdural
   Haemorrhages in Babies and Obstetric Factors," *The Lancet* 363, no. 9412 (March 13,
   2004): 846–51.
M. Arnestad, L. Crotti, T.O. Rognum, R. Insolia, M. Pedrazzini, C. Ferrandi, A. Vege,
   D.W. Wang, T.E. Rhodes, A.L. George Jr. and P.J. Schwartz, "Prevalence of
   Long-QT Syndrome Gene Variants in Sudden Infant Death Syndrome," *Circulation*
   115, no. 3 (January 23, 2007; ePub January 8, 2007): 61–7.

Additional interviews

Mary Ballantyne, April 22, 2013; Todd Barron, April 15, 2014; John House, April 16,
2014; Tim Moore, November 25, 2013; Brent Snook, April 10 and 11, 2014; Jim Trainum,
January 7, 2014; Mike Trodd, April 18, 2013.

INDEX

Agatha (P4W inmate), 85
Alcaire, Antonio, 110–12
American Academy of Forensic Sciences, 324
Arbour, Justice Louise, 82–83
Armstrong, Derek, 114, 116
Armstrong, Frank, 322
Association in Defence of the Wrongly Convicted (AIDWYC), 351–52, 393, 395–96
autopsies
  categories for cause of death, 38, 195
  identification of contaminants, 154
  pace of completion, 300–302
  variability of outcomes, 110–12
Avis, Simon, 399–402, 406

Babyn, Paul, 114, 116, 118–19, 124, 138, 168
Baden, Michael, 324
Ballantine, Det. Const. Mark, 153
Barker, Geoffrey, 203
Battersby, Julie, 335
Baumer, Julie, 351–52
Baxter, Alex, 246–52, 383
Baxter, Steven, 244, 245
Bayliss, David, 396
Becker, Laurence, 301
Ben-Aron, Mark, 36, 258
Bennett, Ross, 210, 283, 286, 299–300, 336, 339
Benson, Patrick, 385–86
Bernardo, Paul, 109–10

Black, Karen, 286, 297, 306–7, 321–22
Blenkinsop, Barry, 123
Boivin, Julie, 196, 197
Bonin, Miguel, 220
Bowers, Dustin, 317–21
Bowers, Julie, 317–21, 395
Boynton, Ted, 187
Bradley, Ed, 325
breath-holding spells, 281
Brody, Judy, 25
Brown, Clayton, 82
Brown, Jennifer, 249, 250
Brown, Justice Michael, 409–10
Bryant, Michael, 343

Cairns, Jim, 104–5, 133, 274, 327, 388, 415
  and Athena Kporwodu case, 301, 332
  complaint against, 346
  and Halliday affidavit, 218–19
  and Nicholas Gagnon case, 108, 113–17, 118, 130–31, 134–35, 195–96, 228–30
  qualifications, 194–95, 229–30
  and Sharon Reynolds case, 324–25
  testimony at Goudge Inquiry, 109–10
Cameron, Lisa, 43, 44, 49, 57–58, 59, 74–78
Canadian Charter of Rights and Freedoms, 329, 333–34, 335, 380
Carpenter, Blair, 330–32
Carroll, Det. Sgt. Paul, 24–25, 31–34, 39
Case, Mary, 231
Caspin, Shirley, 14, 53

Centre of Forensic Sciences, 135, 260, 301

Charmley, Det. Sgt. Larry, 258–68, 274

Chen, Teh-Chien, 99–100, 107, 108, 113, 115, 116, 195, 218, 219, 223, 225

Chiasson, David, 301, 309, 324, 326, 327, 330, 332

child abuse
  coroners' heightened suspicion of, 108–14
  "duty to report," 193–94
  false indications of, 352–54, 361–62

Child and Family Services Act, 193–94, 198

Children's Aid Society of Sudbury-Manitoulin, 136–37, 193–98, 218–20, 223, 226–28, 230–32, 346

Children's Aid Society of Toronto, 51, 294–95, 303

Clark, Peter, 157

Clark, Steven, 37, 45, 47–48, 51–56, 60, 64, 69–74, 78–79

Cohen, Marta, 360–70

College of Physicians and Surgeons, 210–12, 261–62, 375, 413–15

confessions
  false, 188–91
  impact on trials of, 182
  and Reid Technique, 183–92

Cook, Justin, 390

coroners
  heightened suspicion of child abuse, 108–14
  vs. forensic pathologists, 38

Coroner's Council, 345–46

Craig, Stacey, 28, 43, 47

Creal, Margaret, 309

Cressman, Sheila, 41–43, 47, 52, 54–56, 60, 62, 63

Crone, Det. Sgt. Matt, 285–97, 305–16, 333, 336, 350, 362, 371

Cunningham, Deputy Chief Jim, 132, 138

Deacon, James, 99–100, 107–8, 113, 115, 132

death
  categories of, 38, 195
  manner vs. cause, 61

"Diagnosis: Murder," 314, 346

DNA evidence, and wrongful convictions, 183

Donner, Elizabeth, 406–8

Dorion, Robert, 324–25

Doucette, Delmar, 321–22

Driscoll, Greg, 409

Driver, Katy, 203

Duhaime, Ann-Christine, 204, 205

Duncan, Kirsty, 387

Dunn, Justice Patrick, 205–10, 216, 346–47

Durham Children's Aid Society
  and custody of Eric Hutton, 88–90
  and custody of Keith Hutton, 37, 79–80
  and Kenneth Wynne, 8, 10, 11–12, 24, 52

Dwyer, Denise, 334–39, 340

Edwards, Maureen, 8, 46, 50, 69

Ein, Sigmund, 240–44, 248

Elgaly, Sylvia, 146

Elizabeth Fry Society, 393

Elliott, Mark, 187

epilepsy, 9, 14, 54, 63, 65–66. See also sudden unexplained death in epilepsy (SUDEP)

Epilepsy Waterloo-Wellington, 392

Estrella, Janice, 389

febrile seizures, 9

Federal Bureau of Investigation (FBI), 261

Feldman, Justice Kathryn, 402

Feldman, Ken, 261

Ferris, Rex, 324–25

the fifth estate, 314, 346

Finkel, K.C., 240

Fitzgerald, Peter, 240

Friesen, Dale, 148, 153, 154, 239, 259

Fuerst, Justice Michelle, 381, 384–85

Gagnon, Angie, 91, 94, 98, 100, 102–3, 124, 134, 136, 220–21

Gagnon, Lianne, 91–108, 344, 345
  custody of Nicole, 217–22, 226–28, 231–32
  and disinterment of Nicholas, 119–22
  exoneration, 137–40

placement on Ontario Child Abuse Register, 228

police interrogation, 100, 102–6

pregnancy with Nicole, 140

and reinterment of Nicholas, 124–25

and reopening of police investigation, 125–30, 132–35

Gagnon, Maurice, 91–94, 97, 100, 124, 139–40, 220–22

   complaint against Charles Smith, 120–22, 345–46

   efforts to exonerate Lianne, 193–97, 206–9, 217

   and Nicholas's death investigation, 133–35, 136

   reaction to Nicholas's death, 101

   suspicions about Steve Tolin, 126–27, 129–30

Gagnon, Nicholas, 92–108

   autopsies, 99–100, 108, 113–15, 116, 123–24, 134–39, 194–95

   death, 95–99

   disinterment of remains, 117–22

   missing heart, 224–25

   reinterment of remains, 124–25

   reopening of death investigation, 115–22, 125–30

Garrett, Brandon, 183

Gauthier, Justice Louise, 226–28

Gilkinson, Brian, 243–44, 247, 249, 254–55, 265, 267, 274–76

Gilles, Floyd, 207

Goudge, Justice Stephen, 203, 204, 332, 343, 398

Goudge Inquiry, 109–10, 155, 203, 323–24, 343–49, 374, 376, 398

Grange, Justice Samuel, 390

Grosberg, James J., 299, 313, 314

Groulx, André, 97–98

Group B Streptococcus, 279, 283, 360

Habgood, Marc, 187

Haines, Gisele, 196

Haley, Kathy, 21

Halliday, William, 217–19, 223–26, 229

Harbinson, Melinda, 392–93

Harding, Sheila, 20–22, 25, 56

Hauraney, Jim, 172, 182, 234, 236–45, 252–55, 259, 376

Higald, Ray, 135

Hogan, Chris, 146–47

Holmes, Frances, 51, 52

Homolka, Karla, 86, 109–10

Homolka, Tammy, 109–10

Hospital for Sick Children

   baby deaths in 1980s, 389–90

   Ontario Pediatric Forensic Pathology Unit, 60–61, 301

   Suspected Child Abuse and Neglect (SCAN) program, 14, 26, 32–33, 67, 155, 203, 210

Humphreys, Robin, 322, 333

Hunt, Allan, 283–84, 286

Hutton, Brian, 3–5, 81–82, 90, 411

Hutton, Eileen, 3–5, 81–82, 90, 215, 411

Hutton, Eric, 3, 88–90, 213–15

Hutton, Keith, 3–5, 37, 44, 48, 49, 79–82, 213–15, 411–12

Huyer, Dirk, 26, 32–33, 67, 155, 265–67, 274, 275, 333, 373, 374, 416

Inbau, Fred, 183

Ingram, Justice Alan, 248, 256

Innocence Canada. *See* Association in Defence of the Wrongly Convicted (AIDWYC)

Innocence Project, 183, 352

Inquiry into Pediatric Forensic Pathology in Ontario. *See* Goudge Inquiry

Jaffe, Fred, 67–68

Jay, Venita, 223

JD (babysitter of Jenna Mellor), 143–49, 152, 159–61, 166–67, 234, 238, 240–41, 257, 258, 262–64

   confession, 268–75

   plea bargain, 275–76

Jessop, Christine, 395

Johnson, Valin, 330

Kassin, Saul, 189–90
Kawartha Haliburton Children's Aid
    Society, 142, 146–47, 255
    custody of Alex Baxter, 167–68, 169,
        246–52
    custody of Justine Traynor, 151, 157–58,
        164
Keaney, Berk, 196–98, 223, 228–30, 346
Keeley, Fred, 203
Keetch, Robert, 99–100, 102–3, 108, 195,
    312
    reopening of Nicholas Gagnon
        investigation, 115–20, 122, 127–29, 130,
        132–39
    and second Nicholas Gagnon autopsy,
        123–24
Kelly, Edward, 37, 45, 53–54, 58–59,
    64–67
Kirkland, Scott, 153–56, 236, 260
Kirkpatrick, Julie, 377, 378, 380–81, 385,
    386
Kirkwood, Heather, 351–53, 355–56, 360
Kleum, Det. Const. Rolf, 22
Kporwodu, Anthony, 277–83, 285–86,
    290, 303
    author's contact with, 355, 358–59
    bugging of residence, 305–8
    custody of Julius, 294–95, 317
    manslaughter charge, 310
    murder charge, 311–13, 317, 333
    police interrogation, 291–95
    polygraph test, 300
    preliminary hearing, 317, 322, 325, 329,
        332
    suicide threat, 306–7
    trial, 333–38, 349–50
Kporwodu, Athena, 277–89, 353–57
    autopsy, 283–88, 300–304, 310–11, 331,
        365–67, 368–70
    cremation, 299
    family history, 356–60
    insurance policy on, 309–10, 333
Kporwodu, Julius, 278, 286, 294–97, 358,
    371

Laframboise, Sophie, 93, 135
Laidley, Maureen, 322
Langford, Jane, 344–45, 349
Leestma, Jan, 207
Lemay, Det. Const. Dan, 150–52, 156–57,
    162–68, 171–78, 182–87, 234, 243, 247,
    249, 257
Levine, Lowell, 324
Lewis, Dale, 25
Lightbody, Robert, 251
Linton, Larry, 285–87, 294, 297–98, 300,
    304–9, 336
Little Lake Cemetery (Peterborough), 164,
    385
Lo, Tak, 280, 281, 293, 297, 354
Lockyer, James, 318, 330, 395–96, 399,
    402–3, 404, 406, 408, 409
Logan, William, 26, 57–59, 406
London Life Insurance, 309–10
Loparco, Anthony, 309
Loukras, Lucinda, 153
Lucas, William, 110, 301, 303, 309

MacDonald, Colleen, 262
Mack, Julie, 361
Macklin, Richard, 334
Maclellan, Silvana, 26–27, 52
Maggie (neighbour of Brenda Waudby),
    143–49, 152, 159–62, 166–67, 234, 260,
    263
Mann, Michelle, 216–17
Mann, Miriam, 98–100
Marquardt, Eric. See Hutton, Eric
Marquardt, Keith. See Hutton, Keith
Marquardt, Rick, 7, 11–14, 20–23, 26–31,
    36, 44, 64–65, 70–71, 74–76, 402–3
Marquardt, Tammy, 5–38
    appeal of conviction, 404–10
    bail conditions, 36
    bail hearing, 402–3
    contact with sons, 213–15
    conviction, 79
    defence testimony, 69–78
    drug and alcohol abuse, 5–7, 9, 72–73,
        398–99

granted parole, 393–94
incarceration, 82–88, 390–93
murder charge, 33–34
murder trial, 45–79
police interrogation, 22, 31–34
pregnancy with Keith, 35
preliminary hearing, 38–44
psychologists' reports, 391–92
relationship with Rick, 7, 11, 44, 70–71, 74–76
reunion with Keith Hutton, 411–12
suicide attempt, 215, 390–91
Marshall, Jillian, 136–37
Massey Centre for Women, 9–11
McAuliffe, Noel, 111–12
McCauley, Chief Alex, 115, 132, 138–39
McFeeley, Patricia, 329, 331
McGinnis, Barry, 83
McIntosh, Dave, 209–12, 216
McIntosh, Paulina, 201–2
McIntosh, Samantha, 200–206
McIsaac, Justice John, 45–46, 60
McLellan, Barry, 265, 274, 332, 343, 396, 416
McMahon, John, 310, 314, 327, 328, 337
McMullan, Cory, 171–72
McNamara, Jody, 9–10
McNevan, Gord, 163, 171, 173, 176, 182–83, 184, 243
medium-chain acyl-coenzyme A (MCAD) deficiency, 402, 404–5
Mehta, Sunil, 54–56
Mellor, Jenna, 142, 143, 144–49
    autopsy, 153–57, 241, 259–60, 265
    death investigation, 150–52, 156–57, 159–68
    hair in pubic area, 153, 154, 155, 239, 259–60, 374
    reinterment and memorial, 385–86
    reopening of death investigation, 258–68
    review of case by Milroy, 373–79
    sexual assault assessment, 266–67
Mellor, Randy, 141–42, 144, 147, 168, 169
Meneley, Laird, 151, 170, 244–47, 250–53
meningitis, 283, 284

Mian, Marcellina, 14
Milroy, Christopher, 355, 371–79, 404–6
Mr. Big stings, 268–74
Mitchelson, Linda, 169–70, 250
Monk, Lynne, 94, 95–99
Monk, Ron, 95, 96
Montans, Graciela, 110–12
Morin, Guy Paul, 301, 395
Mullins-Johnson, William, 330, 402
Munchausen by proxy syndrome, 371
Munks, Ken, 255–56

Naccarato, Det. Sgt. Sal, 22, 24–25, 31–34, 39
Narcotics Anonymous, 163–64, 179–80
National Registry of Exonerations, 183
Native Sisterhood, 392
Nelles, Susan, 389–90
Nelson, Robert, 7, 8, 39
Nevin, Alex, 26
Newport, Duncan, 211–12, 216
Nexhipi, Gjylena, 391

Oakley, Christine, 296–97
Ommaya, Ayub, 205
Ontario Child Abuse Register, 228, 232, 303, 385
Ontario Court of Appeal, 338–40
Ontario Homicide Investigators Association, 312
Ontario Pediatric Forensic Pathology Unit, 60–61, 210, 301
Ontario Provincial Police (OPP), 109, 127–29, 133
Ophoven, Janice, 318–21
Ort, Miroslav, 53–54
osteogenesis imperfecta (OI), 354–56, 366

Pacsai, Kevin, 389
Parisé, Réjean, 218, 230–31, 232
PEACE interviews, 191–92
Pediatric Death Review Committee (PDRC), 113–15, 249
pediatric forensic pathology, 60–61
Peterborough Police Services Board, 375

Phillips, M. James, 210
Pinkofsky, Jack, 317, 320, 321, 395
Pollanen, Michael, 265–66, 298
polygraph tests, 184
  of Anthony Kporwodu, 300
  of JD, 161, 257, 264
  of Maggie, 166–67
  of Tammy Marquardt, 31
Porter, Bonita, 249, 250–51, 259
Powell, Stewart, 12, 28, 29–30, 43, 47
Prison for Women (P4W), 82–88, 214
Prousky, Brian, 294–95

Queen Street Mental Health Centre, 35

Rao, Chitra, 67–68, 240
Reid, John, 183–84
Reid Technique, 183–92
Renaud, Gilles, 208
Reynolds, Louise, 322–25, 328
Reynolds, Sharon, 322–25
rickets, 352, 354, 366
Roberts, Gillian, 402, 404, 409
Rodgers, Greg, 132, 137–39
Rorke, Lucy, 206–8
Rosalie Hall, 8, 36, 37
Rosen, John, 313, 314, 317, 321–22, 331
Rosenberg, Justice Marc, 409
Rubenstein, Arnold, 257
Rumball, Caswell, 54
Runciman, Bob, 193
Russano, Melissa, 190
Ryall, Charles, 388–89

St. Joseph's Health Centre, 195, 220
Salmon, Tyrell, 322
Sanders, Ann, 25
Sarmiento, Melissa, 286, 297, 321–22
Saukko, Pekka, 396–97, 399
Sayer, Det. Pat, 31
Schieck, Alvin, 172, 173
Schindelheim, Robert, 287, 310
Schlegel, Maja, 163–65, 169–70, 178–81
shaken baby syndrome, 203–5, 284, 351–52
Shemie, Sam, 25–27, 57

Sheridan, Amber, 200–208, 211
Sheridan, Faith, 200, 201
SickKids. See Hospital for Sick Children
Smith, Aaron, 120–22
Smith, Charles, 249, 309, 314
  and Amber Sheridan case, 204–8
  and Athena Kporwodu autopsy, 286–89,
    299, 303–4, 310–11, 331, 349–50
  biography, 387–89
  at Brenda Waudby hearing, 234–40
  closed-mindedness, 208, 219
  complaints filed against, 120–22, 210–12,
    261, 375
  conduct at Gagnon gravesite, 120–22
  criticism of work, 206–8, 217–19, 325,
    337, 373–74, 396–97
  disorganization, 130–31, 300–302,
    312–18, 336–37
  and Dustin Bowers case, 318–21
  flawed methodology, 117, 265–66
  at Goudge Inquiry, 344–45, 349, 374–75,
    399
  inconsistency, 224, 242–43, 248, 312, 321,
    350
  independent review of work, 326–28,
    343–49
  internal review of work, 330, 332, 337
  and Jenna Mellor autopsy, 153–57, 259–60
  lawsuits against, 258, 328
  misrepresentation of conversation with
    Justice Dunn, 346–47
  misrepresentation of findings, 114, 168
  and Nicholas Gagnon case, 104–6, 113–19,
    123–24, 130–39, 194–96, 197, 222–30
  permission to perform non-criminal
    autopsies, 330–31
  qualifications, 61
  revocation of licence, 413–15
  and Sharon Reynolds case, 322–25
  suspension from performing autopsies,
    326
  at Tammy Marquardt hearing, 38–42
  testimony in Tammy Marquardt trial,
    60–67
  and Tyrell Salmon case, 322

Smith, Rosaleen, 357, 359–60
Snead, Carter, 408
Sorichetti, Cathy, 8, 50, 69–70, 76
Spiegel, Ramona. *See* Schlegel, Maja
Spinks, Philip, 147
Stenabough, Barry, 98
Struthers, John, 322
Sudden Unexplained Death (SUDS), 107–8
sudden unexplained death in epilepsy
    (SUDEP), 58–59, 401, 407–8
Sullivan, Roy, 198, 250–51
Sullivan, Sylvia, 247
Suspected Child Abuse and Neglect
    (SCAN) program, 14, 26, 32–33, 67,
    155, 203, 210
Symes, Steven, 325

Terry, Scott, 56–57
Thibeault, Carolle, 221, 222
Thibeault, Leo, 99, 115, 119, 120, 222
Thibeault, Lianne. *See* Gagnon, Lianne
Thibeault, Louie, 222
Thibeault, Nicole, 220–22
Thibeault, Pete, 102–4, 119, 124, 125, 132,
    139, 196–97, 221, 228
Thompson, David, 234, 236, 238
Thompson, Donald, 145, 148–49, 153,
    156–57
Titus, Dave, 147–49
Tolin, Steve, 91, 93, 125–27, 129–30, 132
Trafford, Justice Brian, 302, 330, 331,
    334–40
Traynor, Joe, 145
Traynor, Justine, 141–48, 151, 157–58, 159,
    168, 171–72, 192, 382, 385
    placed under hypnosis, 262–63

Uzans, Elmer, 108, 115, 117, 118–19, 122

Van Allen, Det. Sgt. Jim, 127–29, 133
Vandervelde, Insp. Ray, 153
Van Dorsser, John, 246
Veno, Albert, 356
Veno, Angela, 277–86, 291–92
    abortion, 303

author's contact with, 355, 358–59, 363–64
    bugging of residence, 305–8
    custody of Julius Kporwodu, 294–95, 317
    insurance policy on Athena Kporwodu,
        309–10, 333
    murder charge, 310–13, 317, 333
    police interrogation, 289–91, 306–8
    preliminary hearing, 317, 322, 325, 329, 332
    trial, 333–38, 349–50
Veno, Betty, 357
Veno, Dan, 357
vitamin D deficiency, 354, 362

Wallace, Aaron, 10–11
Walton, Mark, 266–67
Ward, Colleen, 252–53
Wasser, Cindy, 317–22, 350–51
Waudby, Brenda, 141–52, 156–88, 192,
    375–79
    access to Justine, 233
    appeal of conviction, 377, 380–85
    attempt to recant confession, 182–83
    complaint against Smith, 261
    confession, 176–78
    custody of Alex Baxter, 246–52, 256
    custody of Justine Traynor, 168, 169,
        248, 255
    drug abuse, 141–43
    lawsuits against police and Smith, 258
    murder charge, 171–72
    at Narcotics Anonymous, 163–64, 179–80
    plea bargain, 252–55
    police interrogation, 150–52, 160–63,
        165–66, 172–78, 184–88, 190
    polygraph test, 161
    pregnancy with Alex, 244
    preliminary hearing, 234–40
    reaction to charges against JD, 275–76
    release on bail, 192
Waudby, Gladys, 151, 169, 252
Waudby, Robert, 252
Waudby, Tom (brother of Brenda), 151,
    157–58
Wesson, David, 266–67
West, Dave, 102–6

Wheeler, Alison, 377, 380–81
Whetung, Thomas C., 254
Wikaruk, Marlene, 52, 70
Wood, Robert, 265, 323–25
Wynne, Carol, 21, 23, 26, 28, 44, 46–47,
    75
Wynne, Kenneth, 7–28
  autopsy, 38–42
  death, 16–19, 20, 27
  death investigation, 22, 31–33
  donated organs, 27, 65, 66, 396
  funeral, 28
  review of autopsy, 396–402

seizures, 9, 12, 13–14, 53–59, 63–64,
    400–401, 407–8
Wynne, Margaret, 5–7, 23, 26, 28
Wynne, Tammy. *See* Marquardt, Tammy

Young, James, 112, 205, 210, 327–28, 332,
    415–16
  and Amber Sheridan case, 216–17
  and Nicholas Gagnon case, 122
  and Sharon Reynolds case, 324, 326
YWCA, 52, 70

Zaied, Rita, 310–15, 329–40, 350

ACKNOWLEDGEMENTS

I'd like to say a big thank you to all the people who spoke to me during the course of my research and writing, especially Tammy Marquardt, Brenda Waudby and Lianne Thibeault. Thank you for trusting me enough to share your stories.

A lot of people had a hand in helping me shape this book, but none more so than my editor Martha Kanya-Forstner. Thanks Martha, for your patience, compassion, insights and professionalism. You are a marvel.

Others who deserve a nod: Shaun Oakey, Brad Martin, Kristin Cochrane, William Adams, Ward Hawkes, Susan Burns, Kim Hesas, Carla Kean, Scott Sellers, Val Gow, Sean Ward, Helen Heller, Win Wahrer, Rebecca Valero, Gillian Findlay, Dr. Shaku Teas, AJ Strauss, Chris Harbord, Harold Levy, Brett Throop.

And a special thanks to my wife, Monica Matys, and our kids Hana and Cole, for their support along the way.